Canvassing COVID-19 Responses

Facts and Analysis:
Canvassing COVID-19 Responses

edited by

Linda Chelan Li

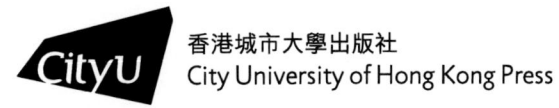

香港城市大學出版社
City University of Hong Kong Press

ISBN: 978-962-937-596-6

Published by
        City University of Hong Kong Press
        Tat Chee Avenue
        Kowloon, Hong Kong
        Website: www.cityu.edu.hk/upress
        E-mail: upress@cityu.edu.hk

Printed in Hong Kong

This book presents a timely and multi-disciplinary assessment of country responses to the first wave of the COVID-19 pandemic. It will be a rich resource for other scholars and commentators, encompassing as it does not only public health responses but also economic and social policy developments, and the popular and political reactions that followed. In the "post-truth" era, such careful documentation of the facts is especially welcome.

Dr Tania Burchardt
Associate Professor, Department of Social Policy
Associate Director, Centre for Analysis of Social Exclusion
London School of Economics and Political Science

There can be no doubt that the year 2020 will go down in world history because of the Covid-19 Pandemic. It will also almost certainly prove to be a major turning point in the social, economic, and political development of the world and individual countries, even if the precise direction in each case remains uncertain. This volume presents evidence of the impact of the Pandemic, and how governments and peoples have reacted. In the process it highlights the factors that make the crisis a truly global phenomenon while at the same time challenging in some ways the inherent globalization from which it has emerged. All of a sudden medical science is required to recognize national boundaries; governments dysfunctionally retreat into the local; outsiders are once again regarded with suspicion; and all of this made matters of intense domestic debate not least because of the existence of that most global of information sources, the Internet and all it brings. The end is not yet in sight for the Pandemic but in these pages the key factors in its development and some possible solutions for the future are laid out in ways that make it indispensable reading.

Prof David S. G. Goodman
Professor of China Studies and former Vice President, Academic
Xi'an Jiaotong-Liverpool University, Suzhou

Covid-19 is a public health issue with enormous social, economic, and political consequences, making public policy responses critical for outcomes. This book is a groundbreaking effort by social scientists to examine these critical policy responses globally and in Asia.

States have managed the Covid-19 health crisis. They will also be responsible for managing the enormous social, economic, and political costs and for driving post-pandemic recoveries. This book is an important and groundbreaking effort by social scientists to understand on how states have been managing the crisis. With cases on both rich and poor countries, the social, economic, and political outcomes provide valuable perspectives on crisis management.

Kevin Hewison
Weldon E. Thornton Distinguished Emeritus Professor, University of North Carolina at Chapel Hill
Adjunct Professor, Centre of Macau Studies, University of Macau
Editor-in-chief, *Journal of Contemporary Asia*

Although everyone on earth is deeply affected by Covid-19, the global pandemic has hit the world quite unevenly. Countries have undertaken different preventive strategies and containment policies in combating the virus. Some have successfully curbed the spread while many others remained in the limbo. It is thus imperative to know which approaches are successful under what conditions and which should be avoided. This volume offers informative comparative case studies that will shed light on this key question. Each country case is perceptively analyzed in the volume. Taken as a whole the collection offers invaluable comparative insights during this critical juncture. Beside the development of a vaccine, this is exactly the kind of research that will contribute to our fight against Covid-19.

Tak-Wing Ngo
University of Macau

A well-researched book on Covid-19 highlighting the value of the meticulous fact-based groundwork by an international team. It helps to enhance a practical and detailed understanding of complex issues of immense real life significance. It is most timely!

Carlson Tong, GBS, JP
Former Chairman, Securities and Futures Commission, Hong Kong
Chairman, University Grants Committee, Hong Kong

Table of Contents

About the Research Centre for Sustainable Hong Kong (CSHK)

The Research Centre for Sustainable Hong Kong (CSHK), established in June 2017, is an Applied Strategic Development Centre of City University of Hong Kong (CityU). Professor Linda Chelan Li, Professor of Political Science at Department of Public Policy, is its founding and current director. The mission of CSHK is to analyze and develop solutions to meet critical sustainability issues in Hong Kong from a multi-disciplinary perspective. Members come from a wide range of disciplines, including public policy, philosophy, international relations, applied social sciences, communication, law, economics and finance, accountancy, management science, civil engineering, biological engineering, electronic engineering and environmental science.

CSHK houses the Sustainable Hong Kong Research Hub (SusHK Hub) and supports all the research and collaborative activities with stakeholders from different sectors and regions. SusHK Hub is an open platform and network for facilitating synergies and collaborations of our members from the academia, industry, professional services and business sectors, as well as government. Currently, it has over 2,000 local and overseas hub members, and has been supporting our research work and events closely.

Website: www.cityu.edu.hk/cshk

Preface

This project is a product of Covid-19 lockdown. Tucked away in our respective neighborhoods, in different regions of the world, we shared our labor in making sense of the displacements caused by the new virus.

By now there is no doubt that the virus that is known as SARS-COV-2, and the global disease it caused, Covid-19 (literally meaning the Disease (D) of Corona- (CO) virus (VI) of 2019), has been a disruptor of our lives. Its impact has been unprecedented in modern human history, in terms of scale, depth or resilience, whether compared to other epidemics plaguing the world in recent decades, often much more "deadly", or to the advance of technologies which scientists have described as "revolutionary". From politics to economics, spanning families or across religions, Covid-19 has unsettled the accustomed norms. The global village is being atomized with "new normal" in routines. Cultures clash; politics is ever more polarized; regional tensions are on the rise. Global trade patterns and supply chains are increasingly being questioned and redrawn.

Old fault lines have resurfaced and deepened. Whilst the virus knows no boundaries, social equities remain a thorny issue. As the world focuses its effort in breaking new scientific grounds to find a cure, distribution may turn out to be our biggest challenge.

This struggle will continue for quite a while, we suspect. Not because a successful vaccine is still in its making – though it is certainly. But because the old problems won't go away with a vaccine, good and curing as it is. Human societies will need to mull over our clashes over beliefs, habits and ideas of knowledge – those of yours and mine and theirs – and hopefully out of some bubbles of reflections and struggles we emerge wiser and more resilient of the hard fact of co-existence. Amongst people of different colours, genders, religions and politics, and between humans and other lives, and non-lives, on earth.

Perhaps we should learn how to live with less hassles. We need to learn how to communicate better. As things become increasingly complex, perhaps it is time to go simple.

We seek simply, here, to lay out what we notice as the major events on Covid-19. Period. Some assessments are inevitable in the reports, and even in the selection of the "facts". There is nothing called "value free"; we are humans with minds. We have sought, nonetheless, grounded analysis and accounts to guide our making sense of the complexities. This is how, we hope, this work will be used and judged.

Conceived during my lockdown in London in March 2020, this project quickly took shape with the formation of a collaborative team with colleagues and friends from different regions of the world. We are often humbled by the weight of the developments, as we reflected upon the fruits of our labor. Sharing and communications have re-energized us and kept us on track, however, and here the product is.

We have leveraged on the excellent work of a huge number of people, including the many sources we cited. Peers and students with the Research Centre for Sustainable Hong Kong and Department of Public

Policy have provided essential assistance and suggestions. Professor Martin Painter, professor emeritus at City University of Hong Kong and long-time friend and colleague, read the drafts of a few reports, at the busy time of welcoming a new member to his family. The editors at City University of Hong Kong Press embraced the project idea and delivered efficiently the final product. Our sincere thanks to their efforts. The faults (and certainly there are) that remain are ours.

Linda Chelan Li
January 2021, Hong Kong

About the Contributors

(Arranged in alphabetical order by surname)

Lai-Ha CHAN

Lai-Ha Chan is a Senior Lecturer in the Social and Political Sciences Program, Faculty of Arts and Social Sciences, University of Technology Sydney, Australia. She was a Fung Global Fellow (2016-2017) at the Princeton Institute for International and Regional Studies, Princeton University, New Jersey. Her broad range of research interests cover global health governance, military intervention, development aid and international politics of the Indo-Pacific. Her current research centres on the impact on regional order of China's economic statecraft and infrastructure investment; and on Australia's hedging policy in the Indo-Pacific.

Andy CHIU

Andy Chiu is a PhD candidate in Sociology at University of Warwick. His research areas focus on the sociology of sports, social stratification, Hong Kong studies, race and ethnicity, and nationalism.

Jeffrey Shek Yan CHUNG

Jeffrey Chung is Research Assistant of the Research Centre for Sustainable Hong Kong (CSHK) and former Senior Research Associate of Department of Public Policy, City University of Hong Kong. He attained Master of Arts in International Political Economy from University of Warwick, UK in 2014.

Robert GREGORY

Robert Gregory is Emeritus Professor, School of Government, Victoria University of Wellington, New Zealand. He was a Visiting Professor at the then Department of Public and Social Administration, City University of Hong Kong, in 2010-11. He has published widely in public administration and management, and public policy, and in 1995 won the Sam Richardson Award for the most influential article in that year's volume of the Australian Journal of Public Administration. Much of his published work has focused on issues of public accountability and responsibility.

Lawrence Ka Ki HO

Lawrence Ka Ki Ho received his PhD in Sociology at the University of Hong Kong (HKU) and is currently Assistant Professor in the Department of Social Sciences at the Education University of Hong Kong (EdUHK). He is appointed as an Honorary Fellow of Centre for Criminology, The University of Hong Kong. His research interest includes history and sociology of policing, comparative policing practices, public order management; private policing, and policing youth and deviance.

Pak K. LEE

Pak K. Lee is a senior lecturer in Chinese politics and international relations in the School of Politics and International Relations at the University of Kent, United Kingdom. His current research interest is order contestation between China's Belt and Road Initiative (BRI) and the Free and Open Indo-Pacific (FOIP). His recent book examines the South China Sea disputes from the perspectives of order contestation and ontological security (https://www.palgrave.com/gp/book/9783030348069).

Linda Chelan LI

Linda Chelan Li is Professor of Political Science in the Department of Public Policy and the Director of the Research Centre for Sustainable Hong Kong (CSHK), City University of Hong Kong. Her research interests include good governance, central-local relations, government reform, public finance and sustainable development. She initiated "CSHK on Covid-19", a collaborative project to collate and analyze essential data on the case developments and policy response of different jurisdictions to Covid-19, with an international team spanning Europe, Asia, America and Australasia.

Lue LI

Lue Li is professor and the coordinator of public administration program, School of Humanities and Social Science in Macao Polytechnic Institute. He received his bachelor and Master degree of Law in Political Science and Public Administration from Peking University and his PhD from City University of Hong Kong. His research interests include public policy and public administration reform.

Yuqing LIANG

Yuqing Liang is Assistant Professor of College of Management at Shenzhen University. Her research interests are local government reform, institutional changes and One Belt One Road strategy.

Socheat OUM

Socheat Oum holds a Master Degree in Public Administration from Seoul National University in 2015 and obtained a Diploma of High Ranking Civil Servant in 2007. He has served in various posts in the Ministry of Foreign Affairs and International Cooperation of the Kingdom of Cambodia since 2007 and is currently a director of the Foreign Languages Department, National Institute of Diplomacy and International Relations. He is also a PhD candidate at the City University of Hong Kong.

Bennis Wai Yip SO

Bennis Wai Yip So is Head and Professor at the Department of Public Administration, National Chengchi University, Taiwan. His recent research interests are in civil service systems in East Asia, performance management of the public sector, and application of design thinking to public service.

H. Christoph STEINHARDT

H. Christoph Steinhardt is Assistant Professor in the Department of East Asian Studies, University of Vienna. His research focuses on state-society relations in China, examining popular protest, environmental politics, trust and political identities. His writings have appeared in journals such as *European Political Science Review*, *Journal of Contemporary China*, *Modern China* and *The China Journal*.

Fanny UNTERREINER

Fanny Unterreiner is former research intern of CSHK. She is currently studying political science at Amsterdam University.

Kin Man WAN

Kin Man Wan is a PhD candidate in the Department of Government and Public Administration at the Chinese University of Hong Kong. His research interest includes the political economy of regime type, inequality, politics of sport, and Hong Kong politics. His recent articles have been published in *World Development*, and *Social Indicators Research*.

Cleo Lok Hei WONG

Cleo Wong is former Research Assistant of CSHK and a member of the Sustainable Hong Kong Research Hub of CSHK. She currently works in the field of art administration.

Natalie W. M. WONG

Natalie Wong is a Visiting Fellow in the Department of Public Policy, City University of Hong Kong. She researches on environmental governance and activism in the Greater China region, and her publications have appeared in several international journals. Natalie had rich practical experience as researcher at a Hong Kong-based labor NGO working on the labor conditions in the Pearl River Delta and an international environmental NGO investigating into the air quality of Beijing in the context of Olympus 2008.

Lanlan XU

Lanlan Xu is Associate Professor at the Department of Public Administration, Law School, Shantou University. Her research addresses local governance, social gender and public policy.

Yamin XU

Yamin Xu is an independent researcher currently living in Washington, DC. She is trained in politics and information science and has participated in various research projects in China (Hong Kong and mainland) and US.

Layla Xin YAN

Layla Yan is Research Assistant of CSHK and a member of the Sustainable Hong Kong Research Hub of CSHK. She is interested in gender studies.

Bria Yifei YAN

Yifei Yan is an LSE Fellow at the Department of Social Policy, London School of Economics and Political Science, a Founders' Fellow with the American Society for Public Administration. Broadly interested in comparative public policy and administration, she is more specifically interested in the intersection of policy and governance, education and development, and China and India. She holds a PhD in Public Policy from the National University of Singapore.

Dingyi YOU

Dingyi You is PhD candidate at City University of Hong Kong and University of Chinese Academy of Sciences (joint degrees). Her major research interests are science and innovation policy and third sector development.

Guilan ZHU

Guilan Zhu is Assistant Professor of Taiwan Research Institute of Tsinghua University, China. Her research interests are in the areas of public policy, political anthropology and Taiwan Study. She has published in *Management World* and *Journal of Higher Education* and a monograph, *Rethinking the National Identity of Taiwan Region*, is forthcoming.

Canvassing COVID-19 Responses

The Development of the Global Pandemic[1]

Linda Chelan Li, assisted by Xin Yan and Fanny Unterreiner

The trend of global spread, from January to August 2020, is from East and South East Asia to Europe and North America, and onto Eurasia, South Asia and Latin America. Whilst China was the original epicentre, the U.S. has stayed the longest in the top-10 infected regions, followed by Brazil. Global cooperation has been put to the most severe stress test.

The COVID-19 outbreak had its first cases in Wuhan, China, in early December 2019.[2] The World Health Organization (WHO) declared the outbreak a pandemic on 11 March. This chapter outlines the development of the COVID-19 pandemic from its initial phase in December 2019 until 18 September, the date global cases of COVID-19 passed 30 million (30,232,252), reporting 946,778 deaths.[3] The overall death rate is about 0.031.[4] As shown in Figure 1.1, the highest point of the daily new cases reached 314,271 on 18 September, and the daily confirmed number goes up and down over time with an overall upward trend. Figure 1.2 shows the global deaths per day. The figures are of a relatively low level initially, with a daily average of 81 deaths from 23 January to 9 March. The number has been on the rise from March to April, however. It goes lower thereafter throughout May but bounces up again since middle of June. The highest record of daily deaths is 10,491 on 16 April, the only five-digit number since January.

Figure 1.3 depicts the pattern of the upward climb of cumulative cases, where the line steepens from the late March to exceed 20 million on 11 August, and 30 million on 18 September. The total confirmed cases globally first reached 100,000 on 7 March. Then quickly in just 27 days it reached 1 million on 3 April. Speeding up, the number surpassed 2 million on 16 April, only 13 days after. It reached 5 million on 22 May. On 29 June, the number reached 10 million. The leap from 10 million to 20 million on 11 August took 42 days. From 20 million to 30 million on 18 September, it took 38 days.

---

1 Data used in this report on the global development of the pandemic draws from the Global Timeline, unless otherwise specified. The case statistics are from Our World in Data (OWID): https://ourworldindata.org/coronavirus-data-explorer and Coronavirus Resource Center of Johns Hopkins University: https://coronavirus.jhu.edu/.

2 WHO, "Novel Coronavirus – China," January 12, 2020, www.who.int/csr/don/12-january-2020-novel-coronavirus-china/en/

3 Our World in Data (OWID), https://ourworldindata.org/coronavirus-data-explorer, accessed on 21 September, 2020.

4 This is arrived by a simple division of the reported deaths and the global total cases. But the death toll statistics and the calculation of the death rate due to the pandemic are complicated by definitional issues and varied scope of testing and reporting of cases amongst regions and countries, however. There have been abundant discussions on this theme. See for one at www.webmd.com/lung/news/20200901/what-changing-death-rates-tell-us-about-covid, accessed 20 September 2020.

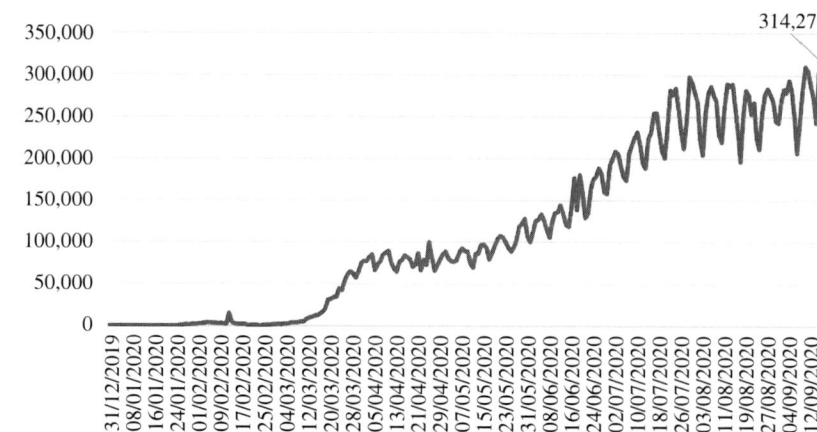

Figure 1.1
Global daily new cases, as of 18 September 2020

Source: OWID

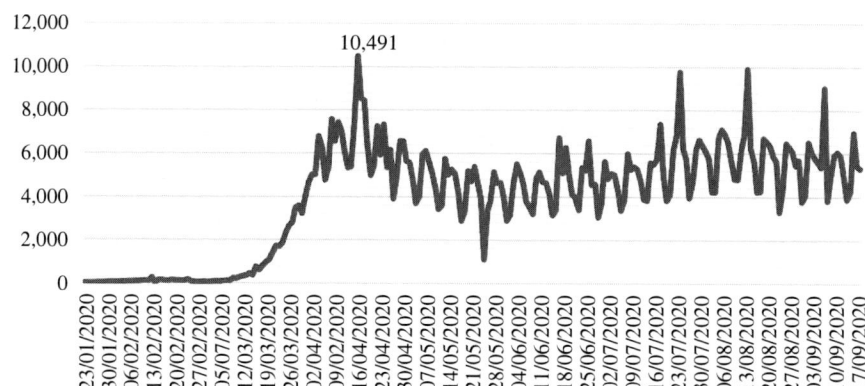

Figure 1.2
Global daily deaths, as of 18 September 2020

Source: OWID

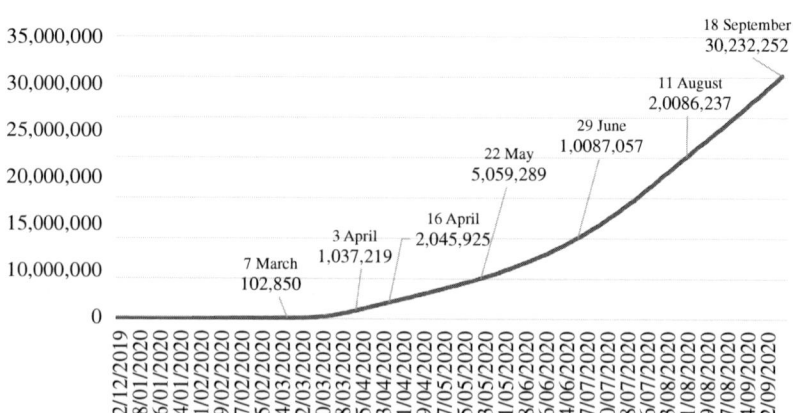

Figure 1.3
Global cumulative cases, as of 18 September 2020

Source: OWID

The Global Spread: Evolving Top-10 Countries

Starting with a few patients seeking help for pneumonia-like symptoms with unknown sources in Wuhan, China, during the first week of December 2019, and then dozens of patients with similar symptoms by 31 December, cases have spread to most provinces in China within January 2020.[5] Towards the end of January a few regions outside of mainland China saw their first cases, including Hong Kong, Thailand, Japan, South Korea and U.S., which almost invariably could trace to a prior travel history to the city of Wuhan. The South China Seafood Wholesale Market in Wuhan, where a portion of the early cases were closely connected, was closed for environmental disinfection on 1 January 2020, which some medical experts subsequently criticised as counter-productive to a scientific inquiry into the origins of the outbreak, as possible environmental evidences were eliminated prematurely.[6] After WHO's Strategic and Technical Advisory Group on Infectious Hazards held a first meeting, the WHO published its first batch of guidance documents on the new virus. The first-ever publication of the genome sequence of the new virus by Professor Zhang Yongzheng and his team at Shanghai Public Health Center on 11 January facilitated further research into it.[7] Zhang's laboratory was, however, shut down for "rectifications" one day after.

Figure 1.4 Countries of top-10 confirmed cases worldwide, January to August 2020

No.	JAN	FEB	MAR	APR	MAY	JUN	JUL	AUG
1	CHINA	CHINA	US	US	US	US	US	US
2	THAILAND	S.KOREA	ITALY	SPAIN	BRAZIL	BRAZIL	BRAZIL	BRAZIL
3	JAPAN	ITALY	SPAIN	ITALY	RUSSIA	RUSSIA	INDIA	INDIA
4	SINGAPORE	DIAMOND PRINCESS	CHINA	UK	UK	INDIA	RUSSIA	RUSSIA
5	S.KOREA	IRAN	GERMANY	GERMANY	SPAIN	UK	SOUTH AFRICA	PERU
6	TAIWAN	JAPAN	IRAN	FRANCE	ITALY	PERU	MEXICO	SOUTH AFRICA
7	AUSTRALIA	SINGAPORE	FRANCE	TURKEY	INDIA	CHILE	PERU	COLOMBIA
8	MALAYSIA	GERMANY	UK	RUSSIA	GERMANY	SPAIN	CHILE	MEXICO
9	US	FRANCE	SWITZERLAND	IRAN	PERU	ITALY	IRAN	SPAIN
10	FRANCE	KUWAIT	TURKEY	BRAZIL	TURKEY	IRAN	UK	ARGENTINA

Source: Constructed with data from John Hopkins University (https://coronavirus.jhu.edu/data)

Figure 1.4 shows the changing profile of the "top-10" countries, measured by cumulative confirmed cases at the end of each month since January 2020. The evolution sees considerable shifts in the pattern. China being the epicentre of the original outbreak ranked the first during January and February and was at the fourth place by end of March, overtaken by U.S., Italy and Spain, and since April fell outside the top-10 list. By end of August, mainland China registered cumulative cases of 85,058 which is 20% of Argentina's 417,735 total, the tenth place on the top-10 league.[8] Ten countries have occupied the top 3 places across

---

5   When the first case emerged in Wuhan is not exactly clear as current evidence gives two "first case" patients, one on 1 December in a report published in The Lancet and the other on 8 December according to the Wuhan official sources. See Mainland China Timeline.

6   *The Standard*, "Wuhan destroyed virus evidence early, Yuen Kwok-yung says", www.thestandard.com.hk/breaking-news/section/4/151892/Wuhan-destroyed-virus-evidence-early,-Yuen-Kwok-yung-says

7   The sequencing was shared at the Virologic.org and GenBank websites on 11 January. "Severe acute respiratory syndrome coronavirus 2 isolate Wuhan-Hu-1, complete genome (GenBank: MN908947.3)," National Center for Biotechnology Information, www.ncbi.nlm.nih.gov/nuccore/MN908947

8   National Health Commission of the PRC, "截至7月31日24时新型冠状病毒肺炎疫情最新情况," www.nhc.gov.cn/xcs/yqtb/202009/170661a5589542c497b5822270d8eb7c.shtml

the 8-month period. U.S. appears most frequently: 6 of the 24 slots and all at the top rank from March to August. This is followed by Brazil with 4 slots and then Italy with 3 slots. Italy is between the top second and third place during February to April and is the first European country in the top three position. Brazil is second place after U.S. during May to August. It is at the tenth place in April, suggesting a rapid sharp surge during May. China, Spain, Russia and India each have appeared twice in the top three slots, and Thailand, South Korea, and Japan have one appearance each. Thailand, South Korea and Japan are places of early outbreaks which have since been successfully contained, whilst India enters into the seventh place in May, rising quickly to the fourth in June and the third in July and August. India has been reporting the most cases in Asia and third worldwide, at the time of writing in September 2020. The trend of global spread is from East and South East Asia to Europe and North America, and to Eurasia, South Asia and Latin America. The main developments in each month within the top-10 are summarised below.

January 2020: Early Responses

The global total reached 9,824 cases on 31 January, when the outbreak was still predominantly within China. Countries/regions in Asia started to report a handful of cases, so had Australia, U.S. and France. China, with 9,802 cases, accounted for 99% among the top-10 countries, as well as the world total. The rest of the countries except China in the top-10 list had an average of 11 cases.

The first death in China due to the new virus was registered on 10 January 2020. The epicentre of the outbreak, Wuhan city, was locked down on 23 January with the city cut off from the rest of China and all movements away and into the city prohibited. During January, the virus spread to many parts of China. On 13 January, the first case outside China was reported in Thailand: an imported case from a traveller from Wuhan. On 16 January, Japan's Ministry of Health informed the WHO of its first case, from a person who had recent travel history to Wuhan. On the 20th, the U.S. and South Korea both reported their first cases, again, from travellers who came back from their trips to Wuhan. Despite cases rising in China, to set a Guinness world record, Wuhan's government on 18 January hosted a banquet attended by 40,000 families to celebrate the forthcoming Chinese New Year. Wuhan officials reportedly distributed 200,000 free tickets to attend festive activities to Wuhan residents.

WHO's Americas regional office issued the first epidemiological alert on 16 January. On 21 January, during its visit in China, WHO revised its previous claims on 14 and 19 January to acknowledge that it is "now very clear from the latest information that there was at least some human-to-human transmission, and that infections among health care workers strengthened the evidence for this".

Figure 1.5 Countries of top-10 confirmed cases, as of 31 January 2020

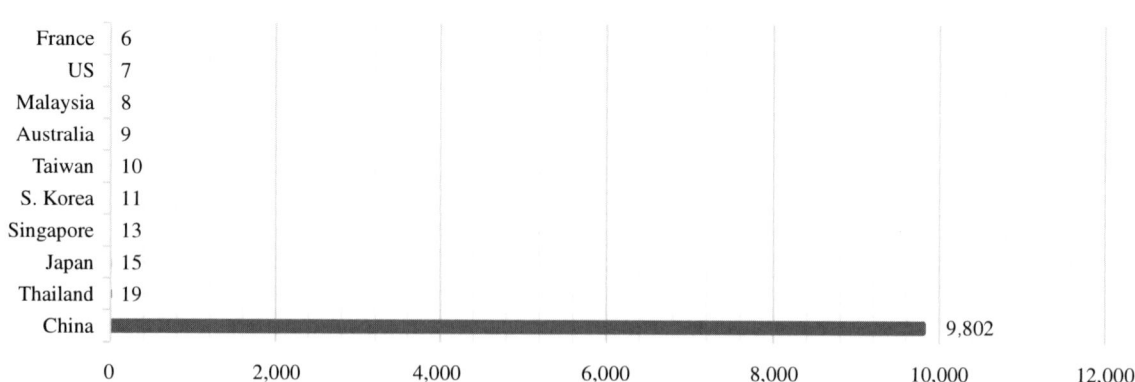

Source: Graph constructed based on data from Johns Hopkins University

February 2020: Asia Hit First

Global total reached 85,236 by 29 February from 9,824 as of 31 January, a huge increase of 768%. Global death was 2,921. The leap of cases was mainly due to the large-scale outbreak within China, especially in Wuhan after its shutdown on 23 January. The epidemic spread to a few countries of Asia and started to affect Europe and the Middle East. By end of February, the share of cases in China dropped to 93% of the top-10 total from 99% in January. South Korea accounted for 4% and the rest were all around 1%. The total top-10 countries still took up about 97% of global cases.

The major outbreak in China happened from late January to mid-February, after Zhong Nanshan, the Chinese respiratory expert, announced on 20 January that the COVID-19 had human-to-human transmission. Before Wuhan was totally locked down on 23 January, about 300,000 Wuhan citizens fled, en masse, mostly to the rest of the country and others overseas, during the several hours between announcement and execution of the lockdown measures.[9] In addition, an estimated 5 million migrant workers and residents had left the city for home in other provinces since early January for the celebration of Chinese New Year, which in 2020 fell on 25 January.[10] Soon, provinces in China reported new cases. On 25 January, the construction of an emergency hospital (Huoshenshan Hospital) started in Wuhan. A second hospital (Leishenshan Hospital), was soon added, following the experience of the SARS response in 2003, when the Xiaotangshan SARS hospital in Beijing was completed in 7 days to assist with treating patients. In addition, 16 "cabin" hospitals were set up in Wuhan for patients with mild symptoms. Medical teams from across China were sent to Wuhan to support the anti-epidemic work and the overloaded local medical system. During these weeks, the Wuhan local administration was strongly criticized by the public for the chaotic management of medical supplies, and its failure to protect its medical staff and treat patients of suspected cases efficiently.

Chinese researchers reported on 7 February their finding that the virus found in pangolins have a 99% match with the new coronavirus. The WHO deployed, on 8 February, an advance team for the WHO-China joint mission to examine the origin of the virus. China announced a permanent ban on wildlife consumption 20 days later, whilst exempting medical use and some other purposes.[11] WHO published home care guides for those suspected with the infection.

Outside mainland China, the outbreak in a leisure cruise, the Diamond Princess cruise, on 5 February off Japan saw 3,600 passengers quarantined on board. Passengers were given tests whilst on board, and only those tested negative were allowed to leave, excepting those who shared rooms with infected passengers. In total 705 people were found to be infected.

South Korea surpassed Diamond Princess to the second place on 24 February, with cumulative 3,150 cases by end of February. South Korea also reported their first death from the virus on 20 February. 200 cases were attributed to one cluster, arising from activities in Shincheonji Church of Jesus in northern part of South Korea. The government then shut down nursing homes and community centres and banned public rallies in Seoul.

---

9 English Source : *The Sun*, "Coronavirus chaos as 300,000 people travelled out of Wuhan on trains in just one day before lockdown", www.thesun.co.uk/news/10809454/coronavirus-thousands-fled-train-wuhan/Chinese Source: *The Paper*, "學術視角告訴你：500萬武漢人是'逃離'還是'正常離開'", www.thepaper.cn/newsDetail_forward_5654383

10 *The Paper*, "學術視角告訴你：500萬武漢人是"逃離"還是"正常離開"", www.thepaper.cn/newsDetail_forward_5654383

11 *New York Times*, "China's Ban on Wildlife Trade a Big Step, but Has Loopholes, Conservationists Say," February 27, 2020

Italy, the third highest, saw its cases surge overnight on 28 February from 655 to 888, exceeding Diamond Princess. Officials locked down 10 towns, closed schools and cancelled sporting and cultural events. Even with cases rising, Italy decided to leave its borders open whilst several European neighbouring countries advised their nationals to postpone their trips to Italy.

On 24 February, Iran had 61 cases and 12 deaths in less than a week. The source of spread in Iraq, Afghanistan, Bahrain, Kuwait, Oman, Lebanon, the United Arab Emirates and Canada were traced to Iran. The death toll in Iran surged quickly, with local officials reporting 50 cases on 25 February, raising concerns about things running out of control. Confirmed cases in Iran exploded by 10-fold in 4 days, reaching 593 on 29 February.

Figure 1.6   Countries of top-10 confirmed cases, as of 29 February 2020

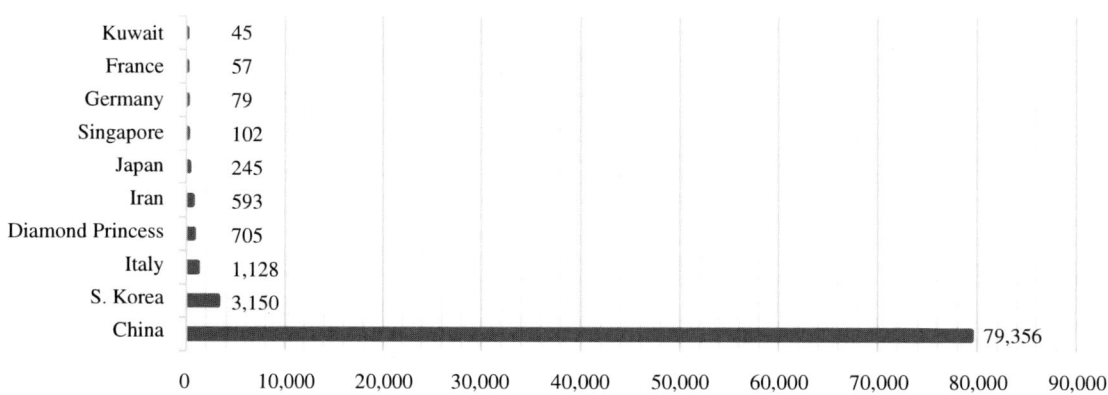

Source: Graph constructed with data from Johns Hopkins University

March 2020: Start of Global Spread

March was a critical month when the epicentre of the outbreak shifted from Asia and severely hit Europe and North America. Cumulative cases reached 807,614 as of 31 March, an 847% increase from the end of February. The number of deaths reached 38,719, a 12-fold increase to the death toll in February. The distribution of cases changed dramatically during March. The previous top country, China, ranked the fourth accounting for 12% of the total cases from top-10 list, while the U.S. became the first place with a 27% share. Italy and Spain ranked second and third with 15% and 14% shares respectively. The rest were no more than 10%. The total cases of top-10 took up about 85% of the global total.

The U.S. became the country hit the hardest with the virus with 188,744 cumulative cases and over 5,000 deaths at the end of March, after reporting its first case on 29 February. The cases surged in the middle of March. Daily deaths soared from nearly zero in mid-March to over 1,000 by end of March. Cumulative cases in the U.S. ranked the first globally on 26 March, surpassing Italy and China overnight. China's ranking drops from the top first place during January and February to the fourth with 82,279 cumulative cases by 31 March. According to the data mapping by Johns Hopkins University, the early outbreak in the U.S. took place mainly in the north-eastern coast, especially New York and New Jersey. In New York, the daily cases first reached over 1,500 on 18 March and then quickly exceeded 5,000 on 25 March. Daily cases in New Jersey also soared to over 1,000 from 25 March.[12]

Italy and Spain in the second (105,792 cases) and third places (95,923 cases) exceeded China's cumulative confirmed cases on 27 and 30 March respectively. Spain's first case emerged on 31 January: a German tourist who had recently visited China. Italy announced the first "red zone" "lockdown" areas in Europe on 9 March, affecting 16 million people, which was extended the very next day to a nationwide lockdown. The Italian Government announced a 25 billion euros plan to fight the virus.

Ranking the fifth after China, Germany had its first case on 28 January. It had 71,808 cases as of 31 March, 908 times of February. Iran, the sixth, had 44,605 cases which is 75 times that of February. The virus reached Europe on the 24 January in France, with 3 people who had travelled to Wuhan. France reported a total of 44,550 cases as of 31 March. U.K. (25,521), Switzerland (16,605) and Turkey (13,531) first entered the list of top-10.

Figure 1.7   Countries of top-10 confirmed cases, as of 31 March 2020

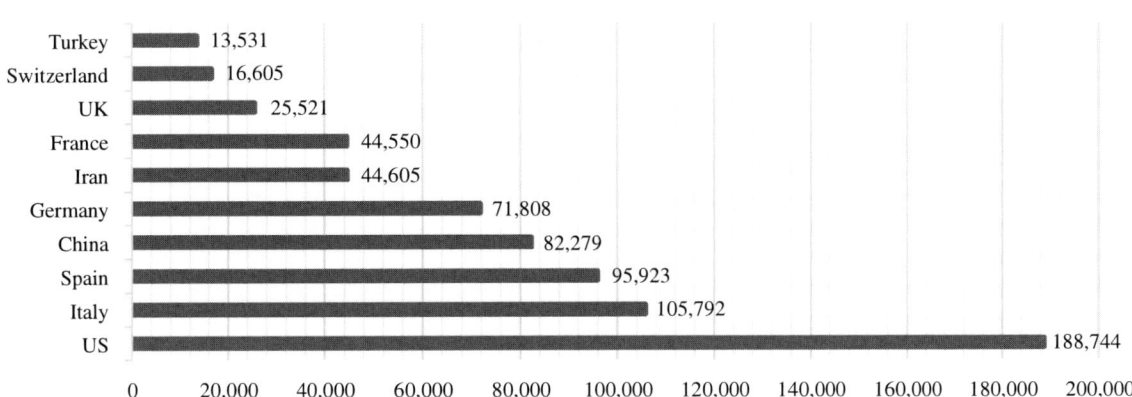

Source: Graph constructed with data from Johns Hopkins University

April 2020: Epicentre in Europe

By end of April, the global cumulative cases reached 3,138,126, an increase of 288% from end of March. Total death was 227,895, about six times of March. During this period, U.S. and Europe continued to see the spread of the outbreak. The first to sixth places on the top-10 list are all North American and European countries. The share of U.S., still the first place, in the top-10 total increased from 27% to 45%, with the rest of the countries all under 10%. Spain and Italy ranked the second both taking up about 9%. The U.K. and Germany followed with around 7%. The rest were no more than 5%. The top-10 countries shared about 75% of the global total.

The U.S. continued to be the country hit the hardest with 1,072,667 total confirmed cases as of 30 April. In 2 months since its first reported case on 29 February, the infection proliferated immensely,

---

12 "Daily confirmed new cases (3-day moving average). Outbreak evolution for the 50 STATES, D.C, AND PUERTO RICO," Coronavirus Resource Centre of Johns Hopkins University, 2020, https://coronavirus.jhu.edu/data/new-cases-50-states

about 109 times compared to the total cases at the end of January. It is worth noting that U.S. had confirmed cases more than five times that of Spain, at the second place, as of 30 April. The worst hit state at the time, New York, had its peaking daily new cases of 10,824 on 9 April, and New Jersey peaked at 3,972 on 4 April. Massachusetts also reached the highest daily number of 3,507 on 24 April. Louisiana which located in the south of U.S. had its first peak in April with 2,024 daily cases on 3 April. [13]

Spain's 213,435 cumulative cases was double that of the previous month. Italy, the third place, had 205,463 cases. The U.K. had its first case on 31 January. U.K.'s cases surged by almost 7-fold from 25,150 in March to 171,253, rising to the fourth from eighth place in the top-10. Germany followed with 163,009 cases. France has a cumulative number of 128,442, ranking the sixth. Turkey, from tenth to seventh, reported 120,204 cases as of 30 April. Russia first came into the top-10 list on the eighth place with 106,498 cases. Iran dropped by 3 places to ninth with 94,640 cases. Brazil had its first case on the 26th of February, which is also the first in Latin America. It ranked the tenth at the end of April with 87,187 confirmed cases. China dropped out of the top -10 list, with 83,944 cumulative cases.

Figure 1.8   Countries of top-10 confirmed cases, as of 30 April 2020

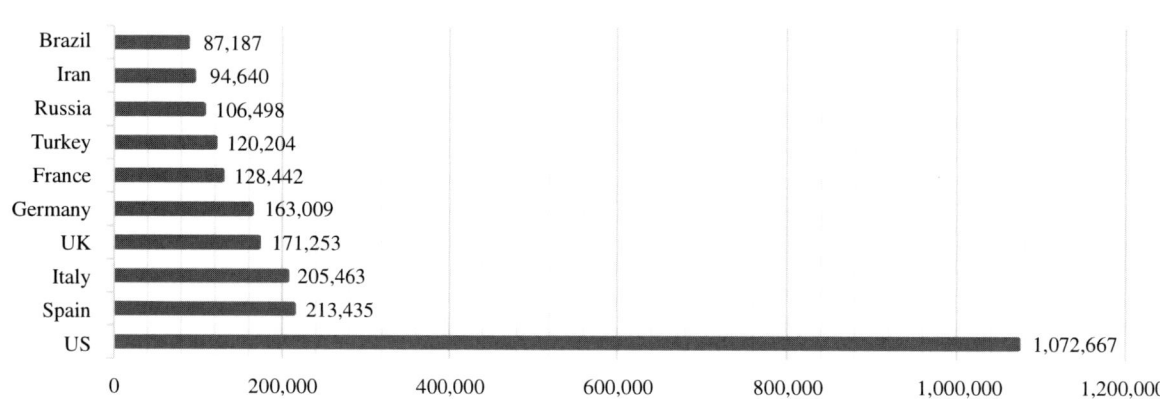

Source: Graph constructed with data from Johns Hopkins University

May 2020: Shift to the Americas

As of 31 May the global total confirmed cases reached 6,012,227, which has increased by 92% compared to April. Total death increased to 368,044 in total, and for the first time with a lower rate (61%). The global increase showed the first sign of slowing down. The outbreak largely left Asia and increasingly affected the Americas, with a dramatic nearly 6-fold surge in Brazil in a month and a second Latin American country, Peru, entering the top-10 list. U.S. took up 43% among the top-10 countries, a slight decrease. Brazil came at the second with 12%. The third was Russia with around 10% which also surged quickly compared to April. The rest were all under 7%. The top-10 list countries shared about 69% of the worldwide total, signalling a further spread of the outbreak among more countries globally.

The U.S. in the top place had 1,799,124 cases, doubling its end of April record. U.S. suffered its 100,000th death on 23 May. Resisting criticisms domestically and from abroad of its ineffective anti-

---

13 "Daily confirmed new cases (3-day moving average). Outbreak evolution for the 50 STATES, D.C, AND PUERTO RICO".

pandemic measures, President Trump deepened the blame-diplomacy and alleged the WHO for assisting China in covering up in the initial stages of the outbreak.

Brazil replaced China in 10th place on 30 April. However, by 22 May, it surpassed Russia with the second-highest count with 330,980 cases. As of the end of May, Brazil had almost 6 times of cases compared to that of 30 April. Russia in third place had 405,843 cases, 3.8 times of the previous month. European countries saw a flattening trend in May, either keeping the same rank or declining. In fourth place same as in April was the U.K. with 274,762 cases. Spain and Italy decreased the ranking. Spain had 239,479 cases and Italy 232,997 cases. India ranked seventh with 190,609. Germany followed with 183,410 cases from fifth in April to eighth as of May. Ninth was Peru, another South American country, with 164,476 cases and lastly Turkey with 163,942 cases.

Figure 1.9 Countries of top-10 confirmed cases, as of 31 May 2020

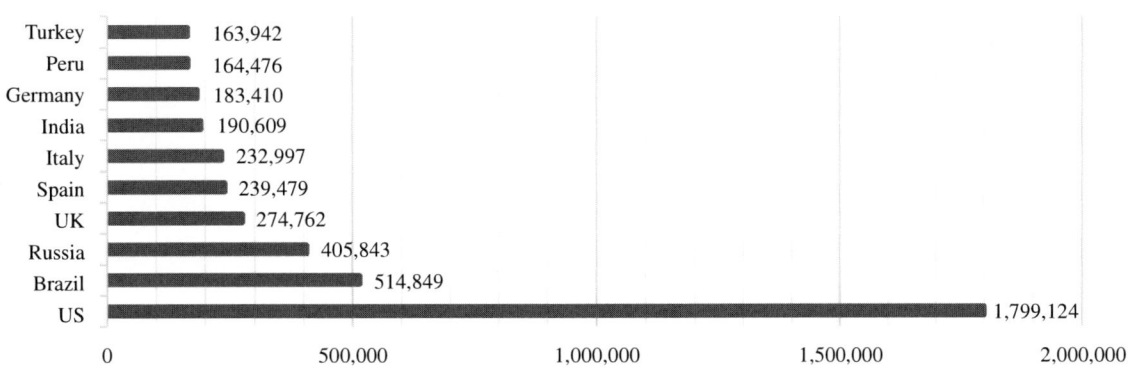

Source: Graph constructed with data from Johns Hopkins University

June 2020: Hitting BRICS

The BRICS countries (Brazil, Russia, India, China and South Africa), with the exception of China, began to be the hardest hit in June. Global total confirmed cases reached 10,245,215 as of 30 June with 502,122 deaths, a 70.5% increase from May and death increased by 36%. It continued to decline in terms of global case growth. The U.S. remained the most affected country with over 2 million total confirmed cases, about double of the second place, Brazil. Outbreaks in Brazil, India and Russia surged, making the second, third and fourth in the top-10 list. In comparison, the situation in Europe improved. The share of U.S. in the top-10 list decreased to 38%, followed by Brazil with about 20%. Russia and India, both taking up around 9%. The rest were below 5%. The top-10 countries shares around 67% of global total cases, decreasing further slightly.

The United States topped 2,000,000 cases and 100,000 deaths on 16 June, with 2,636,414 cases by 30 June. The trend of outbreak in the U.S. gradually shifted from north-east to the south and west. States such as Florida, California and Arizona began to report a much higher number of confirmed cases. The daily cases first surpassed 5,000 in Florida on 30 June. California reached over 5,000 daily cases on 22 June, and Arizona passed 2,500 on 21 June.[14]

---

14 "Daily confirmed new cases (3-day moving average). Outbreak evolution for the 50 STATES, D.C, AND PUERTO RICO".

Brazil followed the U.S. with 1,402,041 cumulative cases, 2.7 times that of the previous month. Brazil's death toll surpassed Italy to become the third highest in the world on the 5th of June. Russia came third with 646,929 cases. Russia topped its cases on the 11th of June. India came after with 585,481 cases as of 30 June, ranking from seventh to fourth of top-10. Doctors in India feared the virus had yet to peak there as Delhi hospitals struggled to find beds for patients. The U.K. came 5th with 312,654 cases.

Latin America registered 70,000 deaths by mid-June. Apart from Brazil, Peru and Chile were also hit severely with 1 in 300 infections per capita. Peru came sixth with 285,213 cases and Chile seventh with 279,393 cases. U.K. decreased by one rank to fifth as of 30 June, with 312,654. Spain came with 249,271 cases from fifth to eighth, and Italy with 240,578 from sixth to nineth. Last was Iran with 227,662 cases. France said that it had the virus under control. The epidemic in Europe was being contained as Germany, Turkey and France were not amongst the top-10 most affected countries anymore. The number of infected people passed 10 million and deaths reached 500,000 on 29 June.

Figure 1.10   Countries of top-10 confirmed cases, as of 30 June 2020

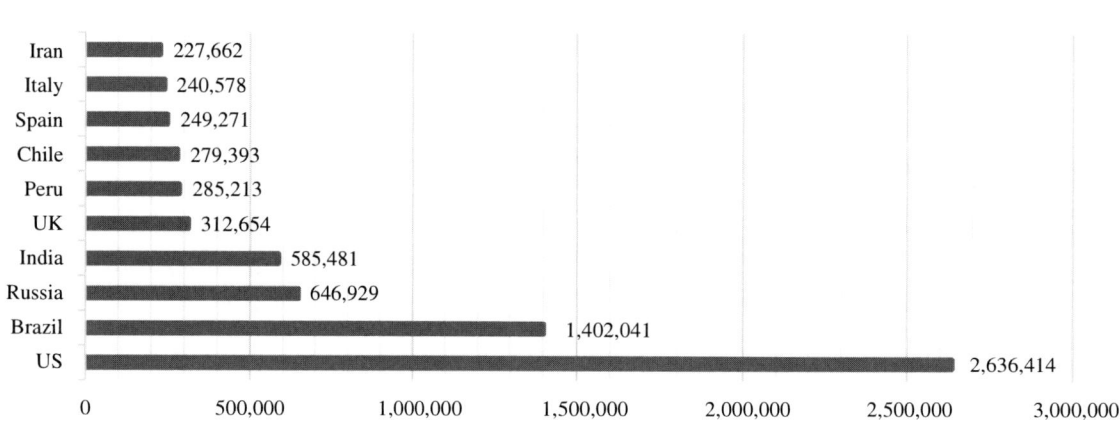

Source: Graph made by author based on data from Johns Hopkins University

July 2020: Escalation in the Americas

As of 31 July, the global total cases reached 17,298,367 (69% increase) and total death of 668,330 (33% increase). U.S. remains the hardest hit country and U.K. the only European country on the top-10 list, ranking the tenth. Cases surged in the Americas, in India, Russia, and Africa. The percentage of U.S. in the top-10 list stayed relatively consistent with 38%. The share of cases in Brazil moved slightly up to 22%. India surged quickly to 14% at the third place. The rest were all under 7%. The total cases within top-10 countries took up around 70%, which bounced back since June.

The U.S. reported 4,562,107 cumulative cases as of 31 July, almost double that of 30 June. July 16 was a record single day high with over 77,000 cases. Florida became the epicentre of U.S. in July, with a peaking daily confirmed number of 12,761 on 12 July. Arizona also reported a highest daily number of 4,300 on 1 July. California reached a peak of daily cases at 11,604 on 29 July.

Brazil came second with 2,662,485 cases, reaching over 90,000 deaths in total by the end of July. With a lack of testing the true figures were believed to be higher. With poverty and malnutrition, tackling the virus was a challenge. Indigenous communities were the worst affected. But the cases rose the fastest when it hit the cities such as Sao Paulo and Rio de Janeiro. The president of Brazil joined an anti-lockdown protest and repeatedly played down the risks, calling it the "little flu". Brazil passed the 80,000th death toll on 21 July.[15]

India announced 1,695,988 cases and overtook Russia to the third spot, after the U.S. and Brazil. Scientists claimed that India's peak may be reached in two months if there were strong public measures and precautions to be taken.[16] There were 13 deaths per 1 million people, compared to the U.S. with 400 and 320 in Brazil.[17] Russia had 838,461 cases.

South Africa rose to the fifth with 493,183 cases as of 31 July. It appeared on the 12th of July on the top-10 most hit countries, the first country in Africa. There are also signs that the pandemic is accelerating in Africa, especially in South Africa. According to the data of WHO, the Africa region had accumulated 303,986 confirmed cases and 6,155 deaths of which South Africa took 151,209 cases (49.7%) and 2,657 deaths (43.2%). By 28 July South Africa recorded 459,761 out of 734,783 total cases in Africa (62.6%) and 7,257 out of 12,476 total deaths (58.2%).[18]

Mexico appeared on the top-10 most hit countries on the 2nd of July and it ranked sixth as of 31 July with 424,637 cases. On 25 July, Mexico reported 8,400 new coronavirus cases in 24 hours, the highest number yet.[19] Peru ranking the seventh had 407,492 cases. Chile followed with 355,667 cases. Iran came after at ninth with 304,204.

The U.K. was the only European country to remain in the top-10 but dropped from the fifth to tenth place with 303,181 cases as of end of July. Prime Minister Boris Johnson admitted that the U.K. government did not understand the virus during the first few months of the outbreak. He agreed that the government could have done some things differently. More than 45,000 people died and almost 330,000 people tested positive with the virus in the U.K. as of 31 July.

Figure 1.11   Countries of top-10 confirmed cases, as of 31 July 2020

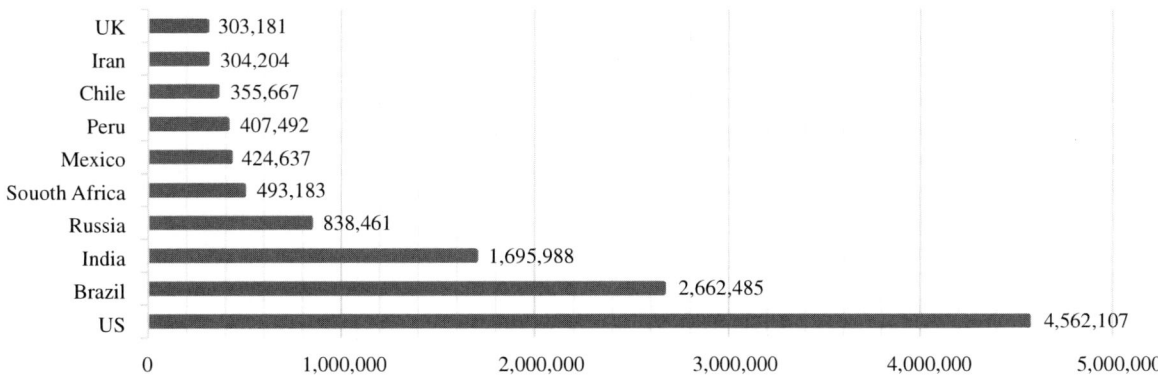

Source: Graph constructed with data from Johns Hopkins University

---

15 *BBC*, "In pictures: How coronavirus swept through Brazil," July 16, 2020.

16 *The Hindu*, "Coronavirus | Cases may peak in India as early as mid-September, says expert," July 19, 2020.

17 *Arab News*, "Why India coronavirus cases are rising to multiple peaks," July 11, 2020.

18 World Health Organization, "Situation reports, WHO African Region," www.afro.who.int/health-topics/coronavirus-COVID-19

19 *CNN*, "The latest on the coronavirus pandemic," July 25, 2020.

August 2020: Spread in South America

The top four in the world ranking of cases have not changed much up to end of August. The global total cases reached 25,275,799 with a 46% increase from July, compared to a 69% increase in July from June. Total death was 846,957 with 27% increase from July, compared to a 33% increase in July. Six out of ten countries in the top-10 are now American countries, of which four are in South America.

U.S. still ranked top of the list, with cases exceeding 6 million (6,030,587), which was about double of the second place, Brazil. U.S. also accounted for 34% of the total cases of the top-10 countries. Brazil led the most cases in South America (3,908,272) and India the third place led the most cases in Asia (3,691,166). Russia kept the fourth (992,402). The cases in Peru rose quickly, climbing from seventh to fifth place (647,166) with 59% increase from July. The ranks of several countries dropped: South Africa from fifth to sixth (627,041) and Mexico from sixth to eighth (599,560).

On 1 August, U.K. dropped out of the top-10 list since it first appeared at the eighth place in March. Then on 17 August Iran also dropped out of the list. Colombia and Argentina both entered the list for the first time, ranking seventh (615,094) and tenth (417,735) respectively. On 31 August, Argentina replaced Chile to be the last one in the list. Spain, the only country of Europe on the list, re-entered in August ranking the nineth (462,858). Europe had a second wave with cases rising in France, Germany, Poland, and Russia.[20]

Cases in Africa were also surging, with total cases exceeding 1.38 million as of 18 September which nearly doubled compared to two months previous; total death reached 33,430, double of two months ago (14,669). Within the continent, South Africa accounted for 655,572 cases (47%), while other countries mostly under 100 thousand, and 15,772 out of 33,430 total deaths (47%).

Figure 1.12   Countries of top-10 confirmed cases, as of 31 August 2020

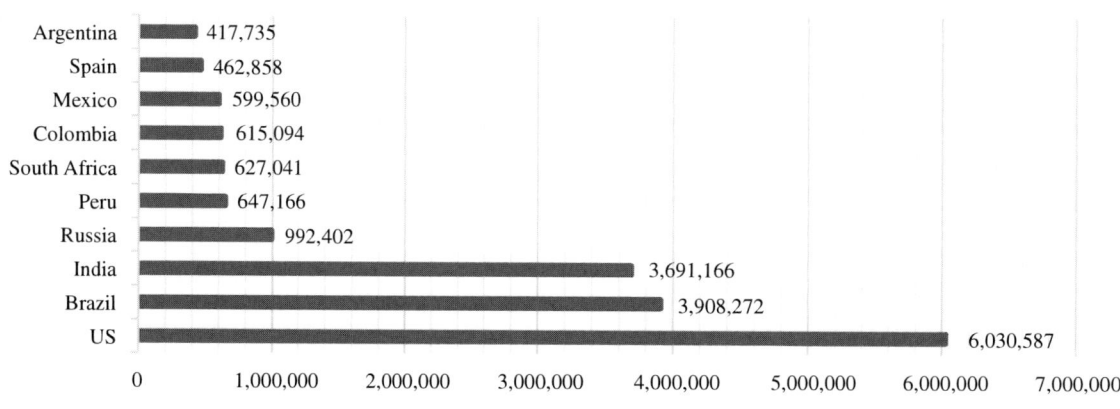

Source: Graph constructed with data from Johns Hopkins University

The global total cases surpassed 20 million on 11 August, reaching 20,086,237, with deaths exceeding 730,000. As of 18 September, total cases reached 30,232,252 and total deaths reached 946,778.

---

20 *The Guardian*, "Global report: France 'could lose control of COVID-19 at any time'," August 4, 2020,

Actions by International Institutions

World Health Organization[21]

On 11 February 2020, the disease previously known as "2019 novel coronavirus" was named officially by WHO as "coronavirus disease (COVID-19)", and on the same day the virus that caused the disease was named by the International Committee on Taxonomy of Viruses (ICTV) as "severe acute respiratory syndrome coronavirus 2 (SARS-CoV-2)" based on its genetic structure.[22]

The WHO has taken actions in mainly three aspects to support anti-epidemic work worldwide. First, they have worked to improve country preparedness and response. As of early August, WHO has shipped personal protective equipment to 148 countries, including 1 million goggles, 3.51 million gowns, 7.2 million face shields, 18.2 million respirators, 2.1 million gloves and 101.2 million medical masks. It also supported 15 countries in design and establishment of COVID-19 treatment centres. 125 technical guidance documents have been uploaded to the WHO Academy for sharing the knowledge to fight the virus. Second, WHO has accelerated research and development. WHO has supported 167 candidate vaccines, with participation of about 5,000 enrolled patients from 100 countries. Accessible online tools have been set up to facilitate research. To reduce misinformation, the WHO collaborated with IT companies and social media platforms, for example, Facebook, Google, WhatsApp and YouTube, to promote science-based health messages. Over 60 technical webinars have been held, with 287 panellists and more than 13,500 participants. The third kind of activity by the WHO is coordination across regions to assess, respond and mitigate risks. In total, 153 countries have joined the WHO partner platform on COVID-19. 180 emergency medical teams have been deployed worldwide.

WHO's actions on COVID-19 fall in three stages: (1) ringing early alarm in January and February, (2) roll-out of plans, tools and leadership during March to May, and (3) routinization of global pandemic management in June and July.

During January and February 2020, WHO's major role was to investigate the disease and alert the world of the risks, when cases were still largely contained within China and affected a number of South East Asian countries. The WHO strategic technical advisory group on infectious hazards held its first meeting on the outbreak during 10-12 January, and thereafter it published a comprehensive guidance on the management of outbreak of a new disease. During 20–21 January, the first WHO mission visited Wuhan and met Wuhan public health officials. On 3 February, the WHO finalised its Strategic Preparedness and Response Plan (SPRP), centred on improving the capacity to detect, prepare and respond to the outbreak, and translating the knowledge of virus into operational plans for countries and regions. On the next day, WHO suggested to the UN to activate the UN crisis management policy. On 16 February, the WHO-China Joint Mission, involving 25 national and international experts, began its work. Starting from 19 February, the Weekly WHO Member State Briefings began to share the latest knowledge on COVID-19.

The situation in March deteriorated as cases spread in countries in Europe and North America. The WHO announced COVID-19 a pandemic on 11 March, which means the epidemic of an infectious

21 Information sourced from official website of WHO for Coronavirus disease. World Health Organization, "Coronavirus disease (COVID-19) pandemic," 2020, www.who.int/emergencies/diseases/novel-coronavirus-2019

22 World Health Organization, "Naming the coronavirus disease (COVID-19) and the virus that causes it," www.who.int/emergencies/diseases/novel-coronavirus-2019/technical-guidance/naming-the-coronavirus-disease-(COVID-2019)-and-the-virus-that-causes-it

disease has spread to a large region, multiple continents or worldwide affecting huge number of people.[23] Since March through May, WHO shifted its focus to medical development and supplies of protective equipment, as the epicenter of the pandemic moved to Europe and the Americas. A real-time tracking platform was set up to support global collaboration of COVID-19 responses on 16 March. Then on 18 March, WHO launched the solidarity trial, an international clinical trial of medical treatments to collect data worldwide on the most effective treatment. The UN COVID-19 Supply Chain Task Force was launched on 8 April to coordinate and scale up the procurement and distribution of personal protective equipment, lab diagnostics and oxygen, so that the countries in most need of such resources can secure supplies. A month later on 5 May, a new COVID-19 Supply Portal facilitated supply requests from partner countries. On 18 and 19 May, the 73rd World Health Assembly adopted a landmark solution for global collaboration: "extensive immunization against COVID-19 as a global public good for health" and "equitable access to and fair distribution of all essential health technologies and products". Quickly, a WHO Foundation was established on 27 May to finance global public health needs. The COVID-19 Technology Access Pool (C-TAP) was set up on 29 May to provide a collaborative platform for 30 countries on vaccines, tests, treatments and other health technologies.

During June and July, there have been fewer initiatives from WHO but more updates and evaluations of existing mechanisms. On 5 June, guidance on mask wearing was updated. On 26 June, a press conference was held to detail the work by WHO's Access to COVID-19 Tools Accelerator in diagnostics, therapeutics, vaccines and the health system connector. It also called for 31.3 billion USD from the international community including governments, foundations, companies and individuals in the next 12 months for diagnostics, therapeutics and vaccines. Up until 26 June, the previous financing from various sources has reached 11 billion USD. On 9 June, the Independent Panel for Pandemic Preparedness and Response (IPPR) is delegated the task to evaluate the global response to the COVID-19 pandemic.

Figure 1.13   A summary of WHO COVID-19 mechanisms and departments

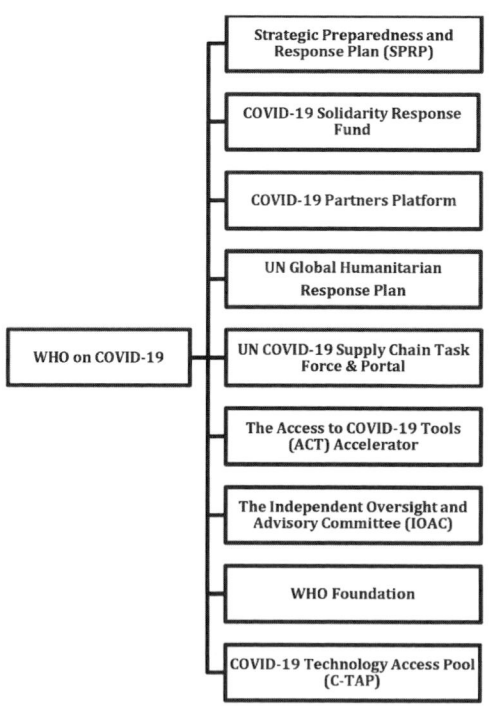

23   Miquel Porta, ed., *Dictionary of Epidemiology* (New York: Oxford University Press. 2008), p. 179.

WHO has conducted four visits to China, since the outbreak of the virus in January till the time of writing in September 2020, to investigate the context and source of the virus and understand China's approach to treatment of the epidemic. The earliest trip lasted for two days on 20 and 21 January to Wuhan, the venue of the initial outbreak, including visits to the Wuhan airport, a city hospital, Hubei provincial CDC, and a BSL3 laboratory under the national CDC.[24] A second visit was on 28 January, when a WHO delegation led by the Director General visited Beijing and met President Xi and other Chinese leaders. They discussed and agreed to continue collaboration to allow an international team of leading scientists to visit China and better understand the context, the overall response, and exchange information and experience.[25]

This pledge was followed up in a third visit. From 16 to 24 February, a WHO-China Joint Mission team visited Beijing, Guangdong, Sichuan and Wuhan. Then an official report was issued on 28 February jointly with the Chinese authority, with a Chinese version one day later.[26] The report detailed the findings on the virus and the transmission dynamics, and evaluated China's responses to the outbreak. China's containment efforts is described as the "most ambitious, agile and aggressive disease containment effort in history".

The role of WHO during the COVID-19 pandemic has become a subject of controversy amidst rising tension between China and U.S., and countries including Australia, Canada and EU, in 2020. In particular, WHO's evaluation of the Chinese response was criticised as overly in favour of Beijing. In May, President Donald Trump announced to end the ties between U.S. and WHO due to concerns over China's "control" over the WHO.[27] The World Health Assembly in late May unanimously called for a WHO mission to China to investigate the source of virus, a decision also supported by China, but details of this mission have been shrouded, with little transparency.[28] On 6 July, the spokesman for the UN Secretary of General confirmed US's notification of its withdrawal from the WHO.[29] On 16 July, German Health minister urged the WHO to hasten its review of its handling of the pandemic, with EU officials calling for a reform of the organization to improve its performance.[30]

When a fourth WHO trip was arranged in July, purportedly to follow up the May decision in the World Health Assembly, it subsequently raised more questions. First, it is not at all clear when the trip commenced and ended. Also, as of the end of August no report has been released to share its findings. A WHO statement released on 7 July says WHO experts would travel to China to work with Chinese experts and prepare for scientific plans to identify zoonotic source of the virus. No further details were released, whilst stressing that the mission would be an "evolving endeavour".[31] The trip was not reported

---

24 For a mission summary, see www.who.int/china/news/detail/22-01-2020-field-visit-wuhan-china-jan-2020

25 WHO, "WHO, China leaders discuss next steps in battle against coronavirus outbreak," 28 January, 2020, www.who.int/news-room/detail/28-01-2020-who-china-leaders-discuss-next-steps-in-battle-against-coronavirus-outbreak

26 Official reports in English and Chinese: World Health Organization, *Report of the WHO-China Joint Mission on Coronavirus Disease 2019 (COVID-19)* (2020), www.who.int/docs/default-source/coronaviruse/who-china-joint-mission-on-COVID-19-final-report.pdf; 中華人民共和國國家衞生健康委員會，《中國—世界衞生組織新型冠狀病毒肺炎（COVID-19）聯合考察報告》(2020), www.nhc.gov.cn/xcs/fkdt/202002/87fd92510d094e4b9bad597608f5cc2c.shtml

27 *Financial Times*, "Failure by WHO team to visit Wuhan sparks concerns over virus probe."

28 *South China Morning Post*, "WHO remains tight-lipped on experts sent to investigate coronavirus in China."

29 *BBC*, "Coronavirus: Trump moves to pull US out of World Health Organization," July 7, 2020, www.bbc.com/news/world-us-canada-53327906

30 www.reuters.com/article/us-health-coronavirus-eu-who-idUSKCN24H21X, accessed 25 September 2020.

31 WHO, "WHO experts to travel to China ," July 7, 2020, www.who.int/news-room/detail/07-07-2020-who-experts-to-travel-to-china

within China until 13 July.[32] On 3 August, the WHO Director General said during a media briefing that the team had concluded its mission to lay the groundwork for further joint efforts. However, when responding to media queries, it became clear that the WHO team had not visited the city of Wuhan, where COVID-19 had the first known confirmed case, during the reportedly 3-week stay in China. The effectiveness of the visit being cast into doubt, the WHO stressed this being an "advance team" only, whose duty was to make preparations for a forthcoming visit by a larger-scale, international mission. WHO also added that the advance team had remote conversation with the senior scientists in Wuhan Institute of Virology and both sides agreed that preliminary epidemiologist studies to the Wuhan market and earliest cluster of cases would be conducted within the coming weeks and months. However, weeks later, by late August it remained uncertain when the larger task team would be formed and whether it could visit Wuhan when the visit takes place.[33]

Figure 1.14   WHO's four visits to China

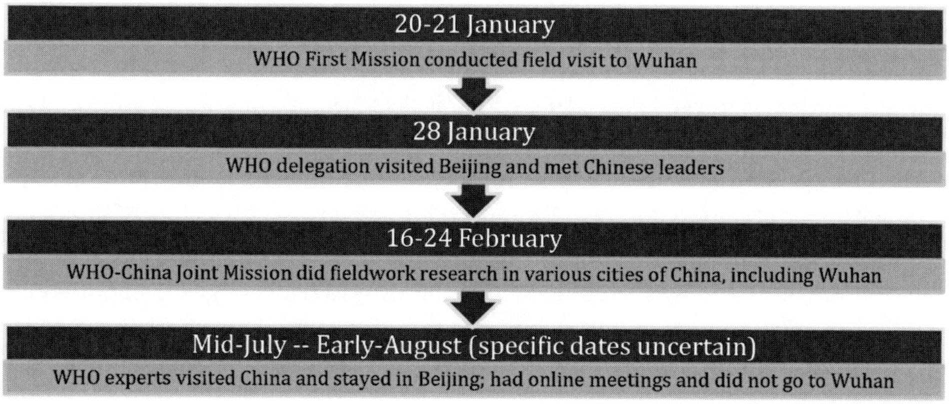

20-21 January
WHO First Mission conducted field visit to Wuhan

28 January
WHO delegation visited Beijing and met Chinese leaders

16-24 February
WHO-China Joint Mission did fieldwork research in various cities of China, including Wuhan

Mid-July -- Early-August (specific dates uncertain)
WHO experts visited China and stayed in Beijing; had online meetings and did not go to Wuhan

Source: WHO Timeline and media reports

International Monetary Fund (IMF)[34]

IMF mainly provides financial support and capacity building to mitigate the impact brought by COVID-19. Its help comes mainly in the following dimensions: emergency financing, grants for debt relief, enhancing liquidity, and adjusting existing lending arrangements. IMF has planned and prepared to source about one trillion USD to its member countries through quotas (440 billion USD), multilateral borrowing (196 billion USD) and bilateral borrowing (344 billion USD) arrangements. The assistance in relieving countries' burden in the pandemic has been rolling out since March when the one trillion USD goal was set.[35]

---

32 *South China Morning Post,* "WHO remains tight-lipped on experts sent to investigate coronavirus in China," 12 July, 2020, www.scmp.com/coronavirus/greater-china/article/3092861/who-when-where-no-word-who-experts-coronavirus-trip-china; *South China Morning Post*, "Coronavirus: China confirms WHO advance team in Beijing to pave way for origins search," July 13, 2020, www.scmp.com/news/china/society/article/3093007/coronavirus-china-confirms-who-advance-team-beijing-pave-way

33 *Financial Times*, "Failure by WHO team to visit Wuhan sparks concerns over virus probe," August 26, 2020, www.ft.com/content/f9dea077-66fb-4734-9d1d-076dc93568e1; Asia News, "WHO's international investigation in Wuhan not yet ready", www.asianews.it/news-en/WHOs-international-investigation-in-Wuhan-not-yet-ready-50891.html

34 Information sourced from official website of IMF for Coronavirus disease. International Monetary Fund, "The IMF and COVID-19 (Coronavirus)," 2020, www.imf.org/en/Topics/imf-and-COVID19

35 IMF, "The IMF is able to lend about $1 trillion to its member countries," March 16, 2020, www.imf.org/en/About/infographics/imf-firepower-lending

The IMF Managing Director and the President of the World Bank on March 25 called on official bilateral creditors to suspend debt service payments from the poorest countries. The G20 responded to this call by agreeing on a suspension of debt service on official bilateral credit worth about USD 11 billion from the poorest countries. On 9 April, IMF released a policy paper "Streamlining Procedures for Board Consideration of The Fund's Emergency Financing During Exceptional Circumstances Involving A Pandemic", facilitating to increase rapid financial support to the member countries.

Access to the two emergency facilities (the Rapid Credit Facility (RCF) and Rapid Financing Instrument (RFI)) has been doubled to meet the expected demand of about USD 100 billion in financing. Up until August, 80 countries have received financial assistance through various lending facilities.

Debt service relief to 29 countries has been offered under the IMF's revamped Catastrophe Containment and Relief Trust (CCRT). This enables the poorest and most vulnerable members to meet their IMF debt obligations for an initial phase over the next six months. Target has been set to increase the CCRT to USD 1.4 billion to provide two years of grant-based debt relief. IMF is also working to increase its capacity to provide concessional financing at zero-interest to low-income poorest countries under the Poverty Reduction and Growth Trust (PRGT) facility. A USD 17 billion target was set in new PRGT resources and is getting close to meeting its target through donations including from Japan, U.K., France, China, Spain, Australia and Canada.

To improve the liquidity of countries in pandemic, IMF has also approved the establishment of a Short-term Liquidity Line (SLL) to further strengthen economic stability and confidence, especially for members in need of short-term moderate balance of payments support.

For the existing lending capacity, IMF is expanding existing lending programs to accommodate urgent new needs due to the pandemic which enables existing resources to be channeled for the necessary spending on medical supplies and equipment and the containment of the outbreak. Other lending facilities are Stand-By Arrangements (SBAs), Standby Credit Facility (SCF), Extended Fund Facility (EFF) and Extended Credit Fund (ECF). They are tailored to help countries of different economic status to resolve problems in balance of payments.

Figure 1.15   A summary of major IMF facilities to fight COVID-19

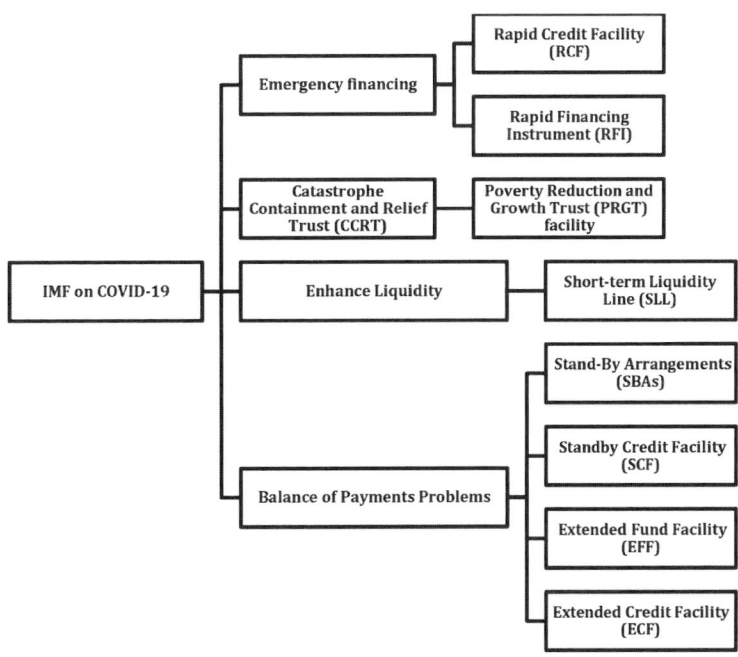

In total, 80 countries have received financial assistance through various channels. Table 1.1 shows the distribution of regions and the amounts on the financing. Cumulatively, 63,871.06 million Special Drawing Rights (approximately 50,907.2 million USD) are granted, out of the one trillion firepower proposed by IMF. Sub-Sahara Africa has the largest number of countries supported (32 countries). Countries in the Americas, mostly Central and South America, have received the largest amount in total, which is 37,085.1 million SDR (about 50,907.2 million USD). Within the total financing amount, 183.13 million SDR (251.24 million USD) are sourced through the pipeline of Catastrophe Containment and Relief Trust (CCRT) for 28 countries in the first tranche from 13 April to 13 October 2020.

Table 1.1   IMF assistance and debt service relief by region (Period from 13 April to 13 October 2020)

Lending facilities and relief by Region	Amount in Special Drawing Rights (SDR) (million)	Amount approved in USD estimated (million)	Number of countries
Asia and Pacific	1,342.30	1,844.53	8
Europe	4,419.10	6,118.63	7
Middle East and Central Asia	10,155.94	13,944.33	13
Sub-Sahara Africa	10,868.62	15,027.44	32
Americas	37,085.10	50,907.20	20
Total	63,871.06	87,841.52	80
Catastrophe Containment and Relief Trust (CCRT)	183.13	251.24	28

Source: Constructed based on data provided by IMF
Note: Chad is the 29th country under CCRT but is not listed in the first tranche period from 13 April to 13 October, 2020.

The Hard Questions the World Health Organization Must Answer in Its Coronavirus Inquiry[1]

Lai-Ha Chan and Pak K. Lee

If the World Health Organization (WHO) wants to maintain its legitimacy on the world stage, it must now answer some tough questions about the extent it has kowtowed to China during the coronavirus pandemic.

It has a chance to do so, after its members agreed to adopt a resolution for an inquiry into the global handling of the pandemic at a virtual meeting of the World Health Assembly (WHA), the decision-making body of the WHO, on May 19, 2020.[2] But there are still many other questions that need to be answered before it can restore its credibility.

We have studied China's engagement with global health institutions such as the WHO, China's compliance with global public health norms and how far it succeeds in creating and promoting its own norms around the world.[3] Amid the global crisis caused by the coronavirus pandemic, which has infected 37.0 million people and killed 1.07 million, according to Johns Hopkins University's Coronavirus Resource Center,[4] an understanding the relationship between China, where the outbreak began, and the WHO is crucial to the future of global public health.

Uncritical of China

The WHO's leadership has come under unprecedented scrutiny during the pandemic for giving the impression that it has been swayed by, and beholden to, China.[5] In late January 2020, in the early days of the outbreak, the WHO's director-general, Tedros Adhanom Ghebreyesus, heaped unqualified praise on

---

1   This article expands on an online essay entitled "The World Health Organization must answer these hard questions in its coronavirus inquiry," originally published on *The Conversation*, May 20, 2020, https://theconversation.com/the-world-health-organization-must-answer-these-hard-questions-in-its-coronavirus-inquiry-138959. The authors also update the key developments in the work of the WHO since the publication.

2   World Health Assembly, "COVID-19 Response," World Health Organization, May 19, 2020, https://apps.who.int/gb/ebwha/pdf_files/WHA73/A73_R1-en.pdf (accessed September 27, 2020).

3   Lai-Ha Chan, Pak K. Lee and Gerald Chan, "China Engages Global Health Governance: Processes and Dilemmas," *Global Public Health* 4, no. 1 (2009): 1–30; Gerald Chan, Pak K. Lee and Lai-Ha Chan, *China Engages Global Governance: A New World Order in the Making?* (Abingdon: Routledge, 2012), Chapter 7; Pak K. Lee and Lai-Ha Chan, "China Joins Global Health Governance: New Player, More Medicines, and New Rules?" *Global Governance: A Review of Multilateralism and International Organizations* 20, no. 2 (2014): 297–323.

4   Up to October 10, 2020. See the website of the Coronavirus Resource Center at: https://coronavirus.jhu.edu (accessed October 10, 2020). The crude mortality for COVID-19 is about 3% which is substantially higher than that for seasonal flu (below 0.1%), according to the WHO. World Health Organization, "Q&A: Influenza and COVID-19 – Similarities and Differences," March 17, 2020, www.who.int/emergencies/diseases/novel-coronavirus-2019/question-and-answers-hub/q-a-detail/q-a-similarities-and-differences-covid-19-and-influenza/ (accessed September 28, 2020).

5   Kate Kelland and Stephanie Nebehay, "Caught in Trump-China Feud, WHO's Leader Is under Siege," Reuters, May 15, 2020, www.reuters.com/investigates/special-report/health-coronavirus-who-tedros/ (accessed September 27, 2020).

China's COVID-19 policy measures and the leadership of Xi Jinping.[6] He commended the "seriousness" with which China was taking the outbreak, "the commitment from top leadership, and the transparency they have demonstrated".[7] His compliments were used by the Chinese government as part of its official propaganda.[8]

But non-transparency and censorship are pervasive in all levels of China's system of government.[9] Tedros had been warned by his aides of the potential repercussions of his effusive praise of China, but reportedly ignored them.[10] It appears that the WHO also took the initial information and data about the epidemic transmitted to it by China at face value.[11] In addition, a WHO policy advice was apparently used by China as an instrument of its diplomacy. Both China and the WHO were initially opposed to restricting international travel.[12] When countries such as the US, Russia, Italy and Australia imposed travel restrictions on visitors from China, beginning in late January 2020, China felt ostracized and used that WHO advice to delegitimize travel restrictions on Chinese people.[13] In early February 2020 Hua Chunying of China's Ministry of Foreign Affairs lamented over US over-reaction, which "certainly [ran] counter to WHO advice." [14] Qin Gang, China's Vice Minister of Foreign Affairs, criticized Italy of stopping flights without contacting China in advance.[15] In late March 2020, however, China no longer

---

6 Ministry of Foreign Affairs of the People's Republic of China, "Xi Jinping Meets with Visiting World Health Organization (WHO) Director-General Tedros Adhanom Ghebreyesus," January 29, 2020, www.fmprc.gov.cn/mfa_eng/zxxx_662805/t1737014.shtml (accessed September 27, 2020).

7 World Health Organization, "WHO, China Leaders Discuss Next Steps in Battle against Coronavirus Outbreak," January 28, 2020, www.who.int/news-room/detail/28-01-2020-who-china-leaders-discuss-next-steps-in-battle-against-coronavirus-outbreak (accessed September 27, 2020).

8 Xinhua, "WHO Chief Confident in China's Epidemic Prevention and Control Ability," January 28, 2020, www.xinhuanet.com/english/2020-01/28/c_138739356.htm (accessed September 30, 2020).

9 For two studies of the Chinese censorship programme, see Gary King, Jennifer Pan and Margaret E. Roberts, "How Censorship in China Allows Government Criticism but Silences Collective Expression," *American Political Science Review* 107, no. 2 (2013): 326–343; idem, "How the Chinese Government Fabricates Social Media Posts for Strategic Distraction, Not Engaged Argument," *American Political Science Review* 111, no. 3 (2017): 484-501.

10 Kelland and Nebehay, "Caught in Trump-China Feud".

11 A WHO tweet, dated January 14, 2020, said, "Preliminary investigations conducted by the Chinese authorities have found no clear evidence of human-to-human transmission of the novel #coronavirus (2019-nCoV) identified in #Wuhan, #China," https://twitter.com/WHO/status/1217043229427761152?s=20 (accessed September 27, 2020).

12 When the WHO declared the outbreak as a public health emergency of international concern (PHEIC) in late January 2020, it at the same time did "not recommend any travel or trade restriction based on current information available." World Health Organization, "Statement on the Second Meeting of the International Health Regulations (2005) emergency Committee Regarding the Outbreak of novel Coronavirus (2019-nCov)," January 30, 2020, www.who.int/news-room/detail/30-01-2020-statement-on-the-second-meeting-of-the-international-health-regulations-(2005)-emergency-committee-regarding-the-outbreak-of-novel-coronavirus-(2019-ncov) (accessed September 30, 2020).

13 See, e.g. White House, "Proclamation on Suspension of Entry as Immigrants and Nonimmigrants of Persons Who Pose a Rise of Transmitting 2019 Novel Coronavirus," January 31, 2020, www.whitehouse.gov/presidential-actions/proclamation-suspension-entry-immigrants-nonimmigrants-persons-pose-risk-transmitting-2019-novel-coronavirus; Aerospace Technology, "Coronavirus: Italy and Israel Ban All Flights from China," January 31, 2020, www.aerospace-technology.com/news/italy-israel-ban-flights-china/; Minister for Foreign Affairs, Australian Government "Updated Travel Advice to Protect Australians from the Novel Coronavirus," February 1, 2020, www.foreignminister.gov.au/minister/marise-payne/media-release/updated-travel-advice-protect-australians-novel-coronavirus (all accessed September 30, 2020).

14 Ministry of Foreign Affairs of the People's Republic of China, "Foreign Ministry Spokesperson Hua Chunying's Daily Briefing Outline on February 3, 2020," www.fmprc.gov.cn/mfa_eng/xwfw_665399/s2510_665401/t1739548.shtml (accessed October 1, 2020).

15 Sandip Sen, "How China Locked Down Internally for COVID-19, But Pushed Foreign Travel," *Economic Times* (India), April 30, 2020, https://economictimes.indiatimes.com/blogs/Whathappensif/how-china-locked-down-internally-for-covid-19-but-pushed-foreign-travel/ (accessed September 28, 2020).

pay heed to that WHO advice by suspending almost all entry to it by foreigners for fear of the second wave of infection.[16]

In late March, Japan's deputy prime minister, Taro Aso, quipped that the WHO should be renamed the "Chinese Health Organization".[17] The US president, Donald Trump, went further – criticising the WHO of being too "China-centric" in handling the pandemic and of an "alarming lack of independence" from China.[18]

Investigation Battlefield

The WHO now needs to restore its global credibility. The call for an independent, comprehensive review of the COVID-19 pandemic quickly became a battlefield between China and Western countries, especially Australia and the US.[19] What was eventually adopted by the World Health Assembly on May 19, 2020 without objection was a compromise resolution, submitted by the European Union and endorsed by more than 100 other countries.[20]

The resolution does not refer to China,[21] but asks the WHO to work with the World Organization for Animal Health and the Food and Agriculture Organization, now led by the Chinese scientist Qu Dongyu, to: "Identify the zoonotic source of the virus and the route of introduction to the human population, including the possible role of intermediate hosts."[22] The resolution also looks forward, pointing to potential intellectual property right issues surrounding a new vaccine.[23]

Speaking at the World Health Assembly the day before the resolution was adopted, Xi framed China as a staunch supporter of multilateral global health governance and committed US$2 billion over two years to the international campaign to combat COVID-19. He promised that Chinese vaccines would be "global public goods", directly confronting fears of a rise in vaccine nationalism in the West.[24] But China's moves were principally aimed at improving its tarnished reputation. Initially China had not signed

16   Ibid.; Jun Mai, "Coronavirus: Beijing's Ban on Foreign Travellers Comes into Force Months after It Criticised Other Countries for 'Isolating China'," *South China Morning Post*, March 27, 2020, www.scmp.com/news/china/society/article/3077355/coronavirus-beijings-ban-on-foreign-travellers-comes-force-months (accessed September 28, 2020).

17   Emma Colton, "Japanese Deputy Prime Minister Says WHO Should Be Renamed China Health Organization," *Washington Examiner*, April 2, 2020, www.washingtonexaminer.com/news/japanese-deputy-prime-minister-says-who-should-be-renamed-china-health-organization (accessed September 27, 2020).

18   "Coronavirus: Trump Attacks 'China-Centric' WHO over Global Pandemic," *BBC News*, April 8, 2020, www.bbc.co.uk/news/world-us-canada-52213439; Donald J. Trump's tweet, dated May 19, 2020, https://twitter.com/realDonaldTrump/status/1262577580718395393 (all accessed September 27, 2020).

19   Karen DeYoung, "U.S., Australia Call for Global Investigation of Pandemic Response; Pompeo Says WHO Funding Freeze Could Be Permanent," *Washington Post*, April 24, 2020, www.washingtonpost.com/national/coronavirus-death-toll-who-trump/2020/04/23/d5c37400-8580-11ea-ae26-989cfce1c7c7_story.html (accessed September 27, 2020).

20   Patrick Wintour and Julian Borger, "Member States Back WHO after Renewed Donald Trump Attack," *The Guardian*, May 19, 2020, www.theguardian.com/world/2020/may/19/member-states-back-who-after-renewed-donald-trump-attack (accessed September 27, 2020).

21   China claimed that the resolution adopted was "completely different" from the one proposed by Australia, which was, according to Beijing, politically motivated. Ibid.

22   World Health Assembly, "COVID-19 Response".

23   Ibid.

24   Xinhua, "Full Text: Speech by President Xi Jinping at Opening of 73rd World Health Assembly," *Global Times*, May 18, 2020, www.globaltimes.cn/content/1188716.shtml. For a study of "vaccine nationalism", see Adam Kamradt-Scott, "Why 'Vaccine Nationalism' Could Doom Plan for Global Access to a COVID-19 Vaccine," *The Conversation*, September 7, 2020, https://theconversation.com/why-vaccine-nationalism-could-doom-plan-for-global-access-to-a-covid-19-vaccine-145056 (all accessed September 27, 2020).

up to the COVID-19 Vaccines Global Access Facility (COVAX) by its September 18, 2020 enrolment deadline. COVAX is co-led by Gavi, the Coalition for Epidemic Preparedness and Innovations (CEPI) and the WHO; it aims at equal access to available COVID-19 vaccines by up to 3% of all participating states' populations.[25] China made a U-turn on October 9, 2020 when its Foreign Ministry spokeswoman Hua Chunying wrote on Twitter that China has joined it without saying how it would contribute.[26] One may speculate that China did this about-turn in order to shed its negative international image as a result of its misstep in handling the outbreak of the pandemic. Three days before this unexpected announcement (October 6), Pew Research Center released the results of a new 14-country survey about their changing views of China in recent years. The findings conclude that negative views of China have reached "historic highs" in many of the 14 industrialized countries in the past year. A clear majority of the respondents opines that "China has done a bad job handling COVID-19", and their confidence in Xi Jinping has fallen substantially as well. A median of 78 per cent of interviewees across all 14 advanced economies expressed no confidence in Xi's actions in managing international affairs.[27]

In addition, in a race with the U.S. over rolling out vaccines, China was seeking the WHO's help to assess the four experimental vaccines Chinese pharmaceutical companies were producing.[28] The safety and effectiveness of Chinese vaccines has been a matter of concern since Chinese health officials disclosed in August 2020 that they began inoculating some health workers and employees of state-owned enterprises with an experimental vaccine in late July, even though it did not pass through the standard clinical trial process. In August 2020 Papua New Guinea refused the entry of a group of Chinese miners who received an unapproved experimental COVID-19 vaccine before leaving China.[29]

Tasks for the Inquiry

With the resolution adopted, the battle now centres on the inquiry. In July 2020 the WHO announced a review panel, the Independent Panel for Pandemic Preparedness and Response (hereafter referred to as

25   Peter Beaumont, "'Landmark Moment': 156 Countries Agree to Covid Vaccine Allocation Deal," *The Guardian*, September 21, 2020, www.theguardian.com/global-development/2020/sep/21/landmark-moment-156-countries-agree-to-covid-vaccine-allocation-deal (accessed October 9, 2020); *Euronews* with AP, "Coronavirus Vaccines: US, China and Russia Absent from WHO's Equal Access COVAX Coalition," *Euronews*, September 22, 2020, www.euronews.com/2020/09/22/coronavirus-vaccines-us-china-france-and-germany-absent-from-who-s-equal-access-covax-coal; Simone McCarthy, "Coronavirus: Why China Has Left Its Options Open for WHO's Global Vaccine Plan," *South China Morning Post*, September 23, 2020, www.scmp.com/news/china/diplomacy/article/3102572/coronavirus-why-china-has-left-its-options-open-whos-global. Founded by the Bill and Melinda Gates Foundation and other partners, Gavi is a vaccine alliance. It was formerly known as the Global Alliance for Vaccines and Immunization (http://www.gavi.org).

26   Lily Kuo, "Covax: Covid Vaccine Global Effort Gets China's Support," *The Guardian*, October 9, 2020, www.theguardian.com/world/2020/oct/09/covax-vaccine-global-effort-gets-chinas-support ; Tom Mitchell, "China Joins WHO Vaccine Initiative in Diplomatic Push," *Financial Times*, www.ft.com/content/f4c6b81c-3014-4bbd-b4bd-02dd75f03fad. China's Global Times reported that on October 8 (2020) China signed an agreement with Gavi to join COVAX officially. Leng Shumei and Li Xuanmin, "China Join COVAX, to Provide Vaccines to Developing Countries First," *Global Times*, October 9, 2020, www.globaltimes.cn/content/1202940.shtml. See also a website of Gavi at www.gavi.org/sites/default/files/covid/pr/COVAX_CA_COIP_List_COVAX_PR_09-10-2020.pdf (all accessed October 9, 2020).

27   Laura Silver, Kat Devlin and Christine Huang, "Unfavorable Views of China Reach Historic Highs in Many Countries," Pew Research Center, October 6, 2020, www.pewresearch.org/global/2020/10/06/unfavorable-views-of-china-reach-historic-highs-in-many-countries/ (accessed October 9, 2020).

28   Reuters, "China in Talks to Have WHO Assess Its COVID Vaccines for Global Use," *Nikkei Asia*, October 6, 2020, https://asia.nikkei.com/Spotlight/Coronavirus/China-in-talks-to-have-WHO-assess-its-COVID-vaccines-for-global-use (accessed October 9, 2020).

29   Eva Dou, "China Says It Began Public Use of Coronavirus Vaccine a Month Ago, Bypassing Clinical Trials," *Washington Post*, August 24, 2020, www.washingtonpost.com/world/asia_pacific/china-coronavirus-vaccine-bypass-clinical-trials/2020/08/24/1813779a-e5be-11ea-bf44-0d31c85838a5_story.html (accessed October 10, 2020).

the Panel), co-chaired by Helen Clark, former New Zealand Prime Minister, and Ellen Johnson Sirleaf, former President of Liberia and Nobel Peace Prize laureate. They have appointed 11 panellists, including two former heads of the Global Fund to Fight AIDS, Tuberculosis and Malaria, a former international president of Médecins Sans Frontières (MSF) and Chinese pulmonologist Zhong Nanshan.[30] Starting to conduct its review in September 2020, the Panel is set to submit interim findings to the World Health Assembly meeting in November 2020 and a final report in May 2021.

If this inquiry is to be genuinely independent, it must address unanswered questions about who was China's "patient zero" and when and how he or she was infected. Anecdotal evidence suggests that the outbreak might not take place at Huanan Seafood Market in Wuhan in December 2019. A paper published online in The *Lancet* on January 24, 2020 indicates that three out of the first four COVID-19 patients in Wuhan did not have exposure to the seafood market.[31] A real test would be whether the WHO-led delegation could meet, independently of Chinese authorities, some of the key figures involved in managing the initial stages of the country's COVID-19 outbreak. It would be enlightening for them to hear at first-hand from frontline doctors in Wuhan hospitals who treated the first batch of COVID-19 patients, such as Dr Ai Fen.[32] Others they may want to meet are the Wuhan Institute of Virology's Shi Zhengli, known as China's "bat woman"[33] and the heads of the genomics laboratories which were reportedly asked by the Hubei Provincial Health Commission to destroy the samples after testing.[34] Zhang Yongzhen of Fudan University in Shanghai would also be worth speaking to. Zhang has rarely appeared in Chinese official narratives, but his team concluded that the virus was of the coronavirus family, and their results were published in the journal *Nature* in early February 2020.[35] It later emerged that his laboratory had

---

30 Peter Beaumont, "Covid-19 Pandemic Accelerating Says WHO as Review Panel Announced," *The Guardian*, July 9, 2020, www.theguardian.com/world/2020/jul/09/covid-19-pandemic-accelerating-says-who-as-review-panel-named. See the website of the Independent Panel for Pandemic Preparedness and Response, www.theindependentpanel.org/ (accessed September 27, 2020).

31 Chaolin Huang et al. "Clinical Features of Patients Infected with 2019 Novel Coronavirus in Wuhan, China," *The Lancet* 395, no. 10223 (2020): 497-506, published online January 24, 2020, www.sciencedirect.com/science/article/pii/S0140673620301835/ (accessed September 28, 2020). See also Josephine Ma, "Coronavirus: China's First Confirmed Covid-19 Case traced Back to November 17," *South China Morning Post*, March 13, 2020, www.scmp.com/news/china/society/article/3074991/coronavirus-chinas-first-confirmed-covid-19-case-traced-back; Donna Lu, "The Hunt for Patient Zero: Where Did the Coronavirus Outbreak Start?" *New Scientist*, April 1, 2020, www.newscientist.com/article/mg24532764-000-the-hunt-for-patient-zero-where-did-the-coronavirus-outbreak-start/; Mark Hodge, "Where Is She? Hunt for 'Patient Zero' Scientist Who 'Disappeared' from Wuhan Lab after Coronavirus Outbreak," *The Sun*, August 23, 2020, www.thesun.co.uk/news/12476233/patient-zero-scientist-wuhan-lab/ (all accessed September 27, 2020).

32 Stories about Dr Ai Fen abound. See, e.g. Lily Kuo, "Coronavirus: Wuhan Doctor Speaks out against Authorities," *The Guardian*, March 11, 2020, www.theguardian.com/world/2020/mar/11/coronavirus-wuhan-doctor-ai-fen-speaks-out-against-authorities; Elisabeth Bik, "Dr. Ai Fen, 艾芬, the Wuhan Whistle," *Science Integrity Digest*, March 11, 2020, https://scienceintegritydigest.com/2020/03/11/dr-ai-fen-the-wuhan-whistle/. For a Chinese interview with Dr. Ai Fen, see https://matters.news/@2020Era/%E5%8F%91%E5%93%A8%E5%AD%90%E7%9A%84%E4%BA%BA-bafyreihrpvzudkmtakoxvquhhw75ajqvhkn4oxb4pges3od5rqusa436ba (all accessed September 27, 2020).

33 Jane Qiu, "How China's 'Bat Woman' Hunted Down Viruses from SARS to the New Coronavirus," *Scientific American*, March 11, 2020 (updated June 1, 2020), www.scientificamerican.com/article/how-chinas-bat-woman-hunted-down-viruses-from-sars-to-the-new-coronavirus1/ (accessed September 27, 2020).

34 The Chinese genomics companies included BGI, formerly known as the Beijing Genomics Institute. Gao Yu et al. "How Early Signs of the Coronavirus Were Spotted, Spread and Throttled in China," *Strait Times*, February 28, 2020, www.straitstimes.com/asia/east-asia/how-early-signs-of-the-coronavirus-were-spotted-spread-and-throttled-in-china. The story was also published in Caixin Global, www.caixinglobal.com/2020-02-29/in-depth-how-early-signs-of-a-sars-like-virus-were-spotted-spread-and-throttled-101521745.html (all accessed September 27, 2020).

35 Fan Wu et al., "A New Coronavirus Associated with Human Respiratory Disease in China," *Nature* 579 (2020): 265-269, published online on February 3, 2020, www.nature.com/articles/s41586-020-2008-3.pdf (accessed September 27, 2020).

been ordered to close in early January 2020, with no reason given.[36]

Besides the inquiry into the origins of the virus, another key question is whether the WHO delayed declaring an international emergency after coming under pressure from China, a claim reported by *Der Spiegel* and *Newsweek* in May 2020. The *Der Spiegel* story says, "According to the BND [German Federal Intelligence Service], China has even urged the World Health Organization to delay a global warning. On January 21, China's head of state Xi Jinping during a phone call with WHO chief Tedros Adhanom Ghebreyesus asked to withhold information about a person-to-person transmission and to delay a pandemic warning. The WHO was silent for a week." [37] In response, the WHO issued a short statement to refute the story, but the statement only said that Tedros and Xi "did not speak on 21 January and they have never spoken by telephone" without directly clarifying whether China did attempt to sway the WHO to decide when to declare COVID-19 as a PHEIC.[38] According to WHO records, the International Health Regulations Emergency Committee (EC), convened by the WHO Director-General, failed to reach a conclusion on its meetings on January 22-23, 2020 whether the outbreak constituted a PHEIC. Upon returning from his trip to China, Tedros reconvened the EC on January 30, which decided that the outbreak had met the criteria for a PHEIC.[39] According to *Newsweek*, citing a CIA report, the delay allowed China to hoard essential medical supplies and personal protective equipment from abroad.[40] Australian mass media reported in March 2020 that Chinese property development companies in Australia sourced and shipped tonnes of medical supplies to Wuhan in January-February.[41]

WHO's Mission Impossible?

Although the WHO had made multiple visits to China since the start of the outbreak, its visit in July–August 2020 — the first after the adoption of the resolution by the WHA in May 2020 — garnered no new insight. In fact, the team of two experts, who according to the WHO were sent with the purpose of laying the groundwork for a full investigation of the origin of COVID-19, stayed in Beijing for

---

36 Zhuang Pinghui, "Chinese Laboratory That First Shared Coronavirus Genome with World Ordered to Close for 'Rectification', Hindering Its Covid-19 Research," *South China Morning Post*, February 28, 2020, www.scmp.com/news/china/society/article/3052966/chinese-laboratory-first-shared-coronavirus-genome-world-ordered (accessed September 27, 2020).

37 Georg Fahrion, "Die Schuldfrage (The Question of Guilt)," *Der Spiegel* (The Mirror), May 9, 2020, https://magazin.spiegel.de/SP/2020/20/170816271/index.html (accessed September 27, 2020).

38 World Health Organization, "WHO Statement on False Allegations in Der Spiegel," May 9, 2020, www.who.int/news-room/detail/09-05-2020-who-statement-on-false-allegations-in-der-spiegel (accessed September 27, 2020).

39 World Health Organization, "Timeline of WHO's Response to COVID-19," June 29, 2020 (updated September 9, 2020), www.who.int/news-room/detail/29-06-2020-covidtimeline (accessed September 27, 2020).

40 Naveed Jamali and Tom O'Connor, "Exclusive: As China Hoarded Medical Supplies, the CIA Believes It Tried to Stop the WHO from Sounding the Alarm on the Pandemic," *Newsweek*, May 12, 2020, www.newsweek.com/exclusive-cia-believes-china-tried-stop-who-alarm-pandemic-1503565 (accessed September 27, 2020).

41 Two Australian Chinese companies were reported to be involved in the shipment of medical supplies to Wuhan. They were Greenland Australia, a subsidiary of the Greenland Group which was majority-owned by the Shanghai government, and Risland Australia, a subsidiary of Country Garden Holdings, a large property developer in China. Kate McClymont, "Chinese-Backed Company's Mission to Source Australian Medical Supplies," *Sydney Morning Herald*, March 26, 2020, www.smh.com.au/national/chinese-backed-company-s-mission-to-source-australian-medical-supplies-20200325-p54du8.html; idem, "Second Developer Flew 82 Tonnes of Medical Supplies to China," *Sydney Morning Herald*, March 26, 2020, www.smh.com.au/national/second-developer-flies-82-tonnes-of-medical-supplies-to-china-20200326-p54e8n.html; Alex Turner-Cohen, "The Chinese Companies Stockpiling City's Medical Supplies," *The Chronicle*, April 6, 2020, www.thechronicle.com.au/news/staff-emailed-to-hoard-supplies-for-china/3989814/ (all accessed September 28, 2020).

duration of the visit and did not visit Wuhan.[42] Questions remain as to why they bothered going to and staying in Beijing for three weeks if they could only manage to have video conversations with senior, yet unidentified, scientists from the Wuhan Institute of Virology.[43] While the Chinese Ministry of Foreign Affairs argued that concerns about the credibility of the inquiry was "totally unjustified", it dodged questions about the itinerary of the WHO team as well as the access it was granted during the three-week visit.[44]

Some scientists were also concerned about whether the WHO had already bought into, without seeking further evidence, China's narrative that the virus jumped naturally from wildlife to human beings in the Wuhan wet market, as the WHO indicated that its team would only investigate the "zoonotic source" of the outbreak. Arguing that the Wuhan Institute of Virology was keeping samples of horseshoe bats which have been found to carry a virus (RaTG13) that is 96% genetic match with SARS-COV-2, they called for addressing the alternative possibility that the virus infected human beings through a laboratory accident or by cloning.[45]

Altogether these have further fuelled concern about Beijing's commitment to identifying the exact source of COVID-19 and whether the WHO is manipulated by China.

WHO sources told that the organization would soon invite member states to nominate experts for the larger mission to China, and the larger team would likely visit China, including Wuhan, later in 2020. However, whether the WHO full delegation would have unrestricted access to the country, especially Wuhan, remains to be seen. This will, in particular, require China to yield some measure of national sovereignty which it has, however, jealously guarded against encroachment.

Concluding Remarks

Like other United Nations organisations, the WHO cannot enforce its decisions and policies without the support of its member states. Its success relies on whether it can persuade politicians and officials to comply with its decisions or the ability to exert pull to compliance with, in particular, its policy advices as well as the consent-based International Health Regulations.[46] Our study has illustrated that China has

---

42   Peter Conradi, "Coronavirus: World Health Organisation Inquiry Will Not Visit Wuhan Laboratory," *The Sunday Times*, July 12, 2020, www.thetimes.co.uk/article/coronavirus-world-health-organisation-inquiry-will-not-visit-wuhan-laboratory-kqbvw0tw8; Christian Shepherd, Katrina Manson and Jamie Smyth, "Failure by WHO Team to Visit Wuhan Sparks Concerns over Virus Probe," *Financial Times*, August 27, 2020, www.ft.com/content/f9dea077-66fb-4734-9d1d-076dc93568e1; Sophia Yan, "WHO Goes on Three-Week Covid Mission to China – but without Visiting Wuhan," *Telegraph*, August 27, 2020, www.telegraph.co.uk/news/2020/08/27/covid-19-team-three-week-mission-china-does-not-visit-wuhan/ (all accessed September 28, 2020).

43   According to the *Telegraph*, the two experts were kept in quarantine in a hotel outside Beijing "for the best part of two weeks", although they had made multiple phone calls with their Chinese counterparts. Yan, "WHO Goes on Three-Week Covid Mission to China".

44   Shepherd, Manson and Smyth, "Failure by WHO Team to Visit Wuhan Sparks Concerns over Virus Probe"; Yan, "WHO Goes on Three-Week Covid Mission to China".

45   Conradi, "Coronavirus"; Shepherd, Manson and Smyth, "Failure by WHO Team to Visit Wuhan Sparks Concerns over Virus Probe". For an investigative report about RaTG13, see George Arbuthnott, Jonathan Calvert and Philip Sherwell, "Revealed: Seven Year Coronavirus Trail from Mine Deaths to a Wuhan Lab," *The Sunday Times*, July 4, 2020, www.thetimes.co.uk/article/seven-year-covid-trail-revealed-l5vxt7jqp (accessed September 28, 2020). In September 2020 Chinese virologist, Li-Meng Yan, who has fled to the US, claimed in a co-authored, non-peer-reviewed paper that the virus was made in a laboratory by using bat coronavirus. The paper was uploaded onto Zenodo, an open-access site, https://zenodo.org/record/4028830#.X3HtrmhKiUk (accessed September 28, 2020).

46   Thomas M. Franck, *The Power of Legitimacy among Nations* (Oxford: Oxford University Press, 1990).

not been cooperative with the WHO as its official narratives would lead us to believe and that the WHO has not been critical enough of Chinese narratives and action. The allegations that China holds undue sway over the WHO and the WHO leadership is beholden to China are not groundless. Maintaining its legitimacy and credibility in the eyes of member states and the world's population is crucial for the WHO to effectively tackle the current and future health crises that affect all of humanity. A properly conducted independent and comprehensive inquiry into the origin and the course of the pandemic is pivotal to the maintenance of the WHO's legitimacy.

GLOBAL

Linda Chelan Li, assisted by Xin Yan and Fanny Unterreiner

02.02–24.08 Total 127,703 cases / 28,131 deaths

08.02.2019

Coronavirus Cases

SCMP: Patient in Wuhan sought medical help for pneumonia like symptoms

31.12.2019

Landmark Events

NYT: Health officials in China claimed that they were monitoring the outbreak to prevent spread

01.01.2020

Landmark Events

WHO: South China Seafood Wholesale Market in Wuhan was closed for environmental disinfection

WHO

WHO: WHO activated its incident management support team (IMST) to ensure coordination of activities and responses across the three levels

02.01.2020

WHO

WHO: WHO informed Global Outbreak Alert and Response Network

partners about the cluster of pneumonia cases in China

Incident management system was activated across three levels of WHO (national office, regional office and headquarters)

05.01.2020

WHO

WHO: WHO shared detailed information about the cluster cases through IHR (2005) event information system to member states

WHO released its first disease outbreak news report to scientific and public health communities and global media: the number of cases, clinical status, the Chinese authority's measures in Wuhan, risk assessment and advice on public health measures

09.01.2020

Landmark Events

WHO: Chinese authorities determined that the outbreak was caused by a novel coronavirus

10–12.01.2020

Coronavirus Cases

NYT: First death in China caused by the virus

Landmark Events

SCMP: Shanghai laboratory where researchers published the world's first genome sequence of coronavirus was shut down for 'rectifications' on 12 January, one day after the publication

Medical Development

WHO: Global Coordination Mechanism for Research Development planned global strategy and preparedness plan to allow rapid activation of research and development activities during epidemics

SCMP: Professor Zhang Yongzhen's team at the Shanghai Public Health Clinical Centre published the genome sequence on open platforms on 11 January

WHO

WHO: Strategic technical advisory group on infectious hazards held its first meeting on novel coronavirus outbreak

WHO published comprehensive packages of guidance documents for countries

13.01.2020

Coronavirus Cases

WHO: Thailand reported its first case from a traveller from China, the first reported case globally outside of China

14.01.2020

Medical Development

WHO: In a WHO press briefing, it was stated that based on experience with respiratory pathogens, there was a possibility of limited human-to-human transmission in the 41 cases in China

16.01.2020

Coronavirus Cases

WHO: Japanese Ministry of Health informed WHO of a first confirmed case in Japan from a person who had recently travelled to Wuhan

WHO

WHO: Pan American health organisation/

The timeline is based on mainly the following three sources, otherwise specified:

1. WHO: www.who.int/news-room/detail/29-06-2020-COVIDtimeline
2. *SCMP*: www.scmp.com/yp/discover/news/global/article/3071167/coronavirus-timeline-outbreak-related-deadly-sars
3. *NYT*: www.nytimes.com/article/coronavirus-timeline.html

WHO regional offices in Americas issued the first epidemiological alert, with recommendations for international travellers, infection prevention, control measures and laboratory testingtailed infor

18.01.2020

Landmark Events

SCMP: Wuhan government hosted a banquet attended by 40,000 families in a bid to set a Guinness world record

19.01.2020

Medical Development

WHO: In a tweet, the Western Pacific Regional Office of WHO said that there was evidence of limited human-to-human transmission according to latest information available and WHO analysis

20.01.2020

Landmark Events

SCMP: Wuhan municipal government said it was distributing 200,000 free tickets to residents for festive new year activities

Singapore began temperature checks at airport

WHO

WHO: WHO published guide for home care for patients with suspected infections

21.01.2020

Coronavirus Cases

NYT: The first reported case in USA was a male in his 30s and resident of Washington State, who developed symptoms after returning from a trip to Wuhan.

SCMP: Death toll raised to 6 in China, cases rose to 300 and 15 medical workers were confirmed infected in Wuhan

Landmark Events

SCMP: Chinese aviation authority warned companies not to charge cancelling fees for people travelling abroad. Face masks were selling fast in China and Hong Kong.

North Korea banned foreign travellers

WHO

WHO: WHO paid its first visit to China on 20–21 Jan on the novel coronavirus and met with China's public health officials in Wuhan to learn about the response to the cluster of cases of novel coronavirus.

WHO tweeted that "it is now very clear" that there were "at least some" human to human transmission.

WHO convened the first meeting of the global expert network on infection prevention and control.

22.01.2020

Coronavirus Cases

SCMP: Macau reported its first case

HKFP:[1] First case reported in Hong Kong: a traveller from Wuhan

Landmark Events

SCMP: Chinese authorities urged people to avoid large crowds and public gatherings, warning the disease could mutate

Gao Fu, head of the Chinese centre for disease control shared that officials were working on assumption that the outbreak resulted from human exposure to wild animals traded illegally at the food market in Wuhan

WHO

WHO: WHO issued a statement that, based on its first mission to China, there was evidence of human-to human transmission, and urged for more investigation to understand the extent of the transmission.

IHR emergency committee in charge to advise WHO Director General of WHO was unable to reach conclusion on whether the outbreak constituted a public health emergency of international concern.

SCMP: Taiwan urged WHO to include Taiwan in its conduct of business.

23.01.2020

Landmark Events

NYT: Wuhan (11 mil habitants) started a lock down. At least 17 people have died and 570 infected in China and worldwide

National authorities in China are checking the number of active cases nationwide

WHO

WHO: WHO met again; decided to reconvene within next 10 days

24.01.2020

Coronavirus Cases

WHO: France reported 3 cases all with a recent travel history to Wuhan: first cases in Europe

SCMP: China confirmed two deaths outside of Hubei province

Medical Development

SCMP: China building a new hospital dedicated to treating people infected with the virus

WHO

WHO: PAN American health organisation urged American countries to be prepared to detect early, isolate and care for patients infected

25.01.2020

Coronavirus Cases

WHO: 1,320 cumulative cases confirmed glob-

---

1   *HKFP*: https://hongkongfp.com/2020/01/22/breaking-first-case-sars-like-virus-hong-kong-source/

ally, of which 1297 from China, 5 Hong Kong, 2 Macau, 3 Taipei. Of the 23 out-of-China cases, 21 had travelled to Wuhan.

SCMP: Nepal confirms first case

Landmark Events

SCMP: France began to bus nationals out of Wuhan to escape the virus

Medical Development

SCMP: More than 20 hospitals in Wuhan have posted public statements pleading for aid to meet shortage of personal protection equipment including masks and gloves

WHO

WHO: WHO's regional Director in Europe issued a public statement outlining the importance of being ready at the local, national levels for detecting cases, testing and clinical management.

26.01.2020
Medical Development

SCMP: Studies suggested that the virus has an infection index of 3.8 which was regarded as very high

Hospitals in Wuhan have been using anti-HIV drugs on patients

27–28.01.2020
Coronavirus Cases

SCMP: Mongolia, still virus free, closed its borders with China

Landmark Events

SCMP: Hong Kong and Malaysia banned the entry of people from Wuhan. Kazakhstan suspended its 72 hours transit visa for Chinese. The Philippines stopped issuing visas to Chinese nationals.

Socio-Economic Development

SCMP: China's National Development and Reform Commission allocated 300 million yuan (around US$43.25 million) for medical equipment purchase and the construction of Huoshenshan and Leishenshan hospitals which will be used for coronavirus patients in Wuhan.

Medical Development

SCMP: The US said it's developing a vaccine, but would take another three months to start initial trials.

WHO

WHO: WHO regional director in south-east Asia in a press release urged countries in the region to raise readiness for the rapid detection of imported cases to prevent further spread

WHO met the Chinese President and came to agreement that an international team of leading scientists should travel to China to better understand the context of the infection in China, the Chinese response and experience in fighting the disease.

29.01.2020
Coronavirus Cases

WHO: United Arab Emirates reported its first case, also the first in the WHO eastern Mediterranean region. It was from a family that visited Wuhan.

SCMP: Finland and Tibet confirmed their first cases.

Landmark Events

SCMP: British airways became the first major airline to announce a total suspension of flights to China.

Socio-Economic Development

WHO: In collaboration with the World economic forum, WHO established the Pandemic Supply Chain Network aiming at improving the market network and access to supplies in relation to the fight against the pandemic.

Medical Development

SCMP: University of Hong Kong researchers were developing a vaccine, through modifying a flu vaccine with part of the surface antigen of the novel coronavirus.

Australian scientists, in Melbourne, successfully replicated the virus for the first time outside of China.

China handed over the genome to Russia for help in developing a vaccine

WHO

WHO: WHO director general expressed deep concern over evidence of a human-to-human transmission outside China, that there was potential for a much larger outbreak outside China

WHO issued advice on the use of masks in home care and health care settings.

30.01.2020
Coronavirus Cases

NYT: 1000 new cases reported in China

Landmark Events

SCMP: US issued a level 4 "do not travel" (to China) advice; Germany suggested travellers to avoid Hubei Province.

Japanese officials said 13 of the 210 Japanese nationals evacuated from Wuhan had health issues. Two tested positive for the virus.

Lufthansa and Air France cancelled all flights to China.

Italy suspended flights to China after 2 confirmed cases were reported in Italy.

WHO

WHO: IHR reconvened, Director General accepted that the outbreak met the criteria for a PHEIC, and issued as temporary recommendations under the IH. Director General provided statement with an overview of the situation in China and globally.

NYT: WHO declared a global health emergency over the novel coronavirus outbreak.

31.01.2020

Coronavirus Cases

NYT: 9,800 cumulative cases worldwide and 213 deaths (in China) registered

SCMP: Britain announced its first two cases

Landmark Events

NYT: Trump administration banned entry of all foreign nationals who had been in China for past 14 days.

SCMP: Italy declared a state of emergency

Singapore closed its borders to all travellers who were in mainland China over the past 14 days

WHO

WHO: Regional director of WHO for Africa sent a guidance note to all countries in the region emphasising the importance of readiness and early detection of cases

01.02.2020

Coronavirus Cases

SCMP: Sweden and Russia reported their first cases

NYT: 1st death outside China – in the Philippines

Landmark Events

SCMP: United, Delta and American Airlines cancelled all flights to China

Britain pulled embassy staff and their families out of China.

Guatemala and El Salvador said they would turn back visitors who were in China in the last two weeks before arrival.

Medical Development

WHO: RT-PCR lab diagnosis kits shipped to WHO regional offices

03.02.2020

Socio-Economic Development

SCMP: At full capacity, China's factories were only able to produce around 20 million masks a day

Medical Development

SCMP: Hong Kong non-essential medical workers continued their strike to get the government to seal the borders with China

Medical experts warned case numbers might not reflect true scale of the outbreak as many patients may be undiagnosed.

WHO

WHO: WHO finalised a strategic preparedness and response plan on improving capacity to detect, prepare, and respond to the outbreak. Two foci: how rapidly to (1) establish international coordination; (2) scale up country preparedness and response operations and accelerated research and innovation.

04.02.2020

Coronavirus Cases

SCMP: Belgium reports first case

Landmark Events

SCMP: Macau closed its casinos to help stop the infection.

More Chinese cities, e.g Hangzhou and Wenzhou in Zhejiang Province of east China, were placed under lockdown, affecting 12 million more people

WHO

WHO: WHO director general asked UN secretary General to activate UN crisis management policy, and called for more studies on asymptomatic patients

05.02.2020

Coronavirus Cases

NYT: Diamond Princess cruise in Japan quarantined 3,600 passengers , of who 218 were tested positive: the largest numbers so far outside of China

06.02.2020

Landmark Events

SCMP: While a second newly built hospital was due to open in Wuhan, authorities are struggling to find hospital beds as numbers in Wuhan continued to surge.

Medical Development

SCMP: Britain scientists shared a breakthrough in

their search for a vaccine, and would start animal trials in the following week

07.02.2020

Socio-Economic Development

SCMP: The Asian Development Bank announced a plan to distribute US$2 million to strengthen measures to detect the virus in Cambodia, China, Laos, Myanmar and Vietnam.

Medical Development

SCMP: Chinese researchers shared that a virus found in pangolins is a 99 per cent genetic match to the novel coronavirus.

09.02.2020

WHO

WHO: WHO deployed an advance team to make preparations with the Chinese authorities for a WHO-China joint mission, to follow up the agreement reached with the Chinese President Xi during the end of Jan visit.

10.02.2020

Medical Development

SCMP: The number of people cured of the disease, cumulatively and worldwide, was three times of the deaths.

11.02.2020

Landmark Events

WHO announced that

the disease caused by the novel coronavirus would be named COVID-19. Following best practices, the name of the disease was chosen to avoid inaccuracy and stigma and therefore did not refer to a geographical location, an animal, an individual or group of people.

WHO

WHO: First meeting between WHO director general and UN secretary general

12.02.2020

Coronavirus Cases

NYT: 44,653 cumulative cases, of which 393 cases in 24 countries outside of China

Medical Development

SCMP: US health officials warned the government that the pharmaceutical industry was unable to produce drugs to fight the virus due to its dependence on ingredients supplied by China. In some cases, China has been the sole supplier of active ingredients of US drugs.

WHO

WHO: WHO published guidelines to support country preparedness and response.

Participants of the global research and innovation forum assessed the level of knowledge, identify the gaps to accelerate and fund priority research.

13.02.2020

WHO

WHO: WHO digital solutions unit convened a roundtable of 30 companies in Silicon Valley on COVID-19

14.02.2020

Coronavirus Cases

NYT: First death in Europe (in France)

WHO

WHO finalised guidelines for mass gatherings

15.02.2020

Coronavirus Cases

SCMP: Egypt had its first case, also the first in Africa

WHO

WHO: Munich Conference called for stepping up preparedness, adopting a whole-of-government approach guided by solidarity. There was a concern about the lack of urgency in funding the response

16.02.2020

Coronavirus Cases

SCMP: Taiwan reported its first death from COVID-19

WHO

WHO: The WHO-China joint mission began work to assess the severity of the disease, transmission, impact of China's control measures. The mission included international experts from 25 countries and visited Beijing, Guangdong, Wuhan and Sichuan between 16–24 Feb.

17.02.2020

Landmark Events

SCMP: Beijing Government asked everyone entering the city to self-quarantine for 14 days

Medical Development

SCMP: Chinese Centre of Disease Control and Prevention published a study of earlier cases of the disease. 80% of people infected had mild illness.

19.02.2020

Coronavirus Cases

NYT: A total of 621 people were infected on Diamond Princess cruise, off Japan. 443 passengers left the cruise after testing negative; those who shared rooms with infected passengers stayed aboard

Landmark Events

SCMP: Russia banned all Chinese nationals from entering the country.

Medical Development

SCMP: Experts commented that COVID-19 is not as deadly as SARS or MERS, but easy to catch. Men have a higher risk of dying of it. People's whose immune systems are compromised and medical staff are high risk groups.

WHO

WHO: Weekly WHO Member States Briefings on COVID-19 began, to share the latest knowledge and insight on the disease.

20.02.2020

Coronavirus Cases

SCMP: Two infected passengers from Diamond Princess cruise died in Japan

South Korea reported its first death, with 82 confirmed cases.

21.02.2020

Coronavirus Cases

SCMP: Israel reported its first case

Lebanon flags its first confirmed case

Italy flags its first death from COVID-19

Landmark Events

NYT: Secretive church in South Korea linked to the rise of cases (+200). To contain the outbreak, the government ordered shut down of kindergartens, nursing homes and community centers, and banned rallies in Seoul

SCMP: North Korea cancelled the Pyongyang Marathon scheduled for April.

WHO

WHO: WHO director general appointed special envoys on COVID-19 to provide strategic advice and high level political advocacy and engagement in different parts of the world

22.02.2020

Medical Development

SCMP: A recovered patient in China tested positive again 10 days after release from hospital for home self-isolation

23.02.2020

Landmark Events

NYT: Cases in Italy spiked to more than 150 cases from fewer than 5 reported cases days ago: the first major outbreak in Europe. Ten towns in the Lombardy region entered a lock-down.

WHO

SCMP: The WHO has not yet officially announced the disease a pandemic.

24.02.2020

Coronavirus Cases

NYT: Cases in Iraq, Afghanistan, Bahrain, Kuwait, Oman, Lebanon, the United Arab Emirates and one in Canada, were traced back to Iran, China public health experts warned. Iran had in less than one week 61 cases and 12 deaths.

Landmark Events

SCMP: Austria has blocked all trains from crossing into the country from Italy.

WHO

WHO: WHO-China joint mission on COVID-19

reported to media their main findings. It warned that much of the international community was not yet ready in their preparations, and made recommendations for fast top-level decision making, and implementation of non-pharmaceutical measures such as contact tracing, case detection and isolation, and community engagement.

WHO published operational considerations for managing COVID-19 cases and outbreaks on board ships, following the outbreak of COVID-19 in Diamond Princess cruise.

25.02.2020

Coronavirus Cases

SCMP: Norway, Greece, North Macedonia, Georgia and Pakistan, Romania, Croatia, Austria, Switzerland, Kuwait, Oman, Bahrain, Algeria and Afghanistan reported their first cases.

Landmark Events

SCMP: Local officials in Iran reported 50 cumulative deaths in total, raising doubts of a cover up.

26.02.2020

Coronavirus Cases

NYT: Latin America reports first case (Brazil) from a man travelled to Italy for business, Tracked

the other passengers on the same flight

SCMP: Denmark, Estonia, San Marino, Netherlands confirm their first cases.

Medical Development

SCMP: Medical workers in China were being infected at a high rate, whilst others were dying from exhaustion as the local health care sector in some cities was overwhelmed.

27.02.2020

Landmark Events

SCMP: In Europe, countries neighbouring Italy decided to keep their borders open despite the spread of the virus to Tuscany, Sicily and Liguria. But several governments encouraged their nationals to postpone trips.

NYT:[2] China announced a permanent ban on wildlife trade and consumptions, except for some specific purposes (fur, medicine or research).

WHO

WHO: Report of the WHO-China joint mission was issued to offer a reference for countries on measures to contain COVID-19

28.02.2020

Coronavirus Cases

SCMP: Qatar, Ireland, Ecuador, Luxembourg, reported their first cases.

29.02.2020

Coronavirus Cases

SCMP: Armenia, Czech, Dominican Republic, St Barth, Saint Martin reported their first cases

NYT: US reported the first death, Cases rose to 87,000 and Trump administration issued the highest level travel warnings

Medical Development

WHO: WHO published an interim guidance on quarantine of individuals in the context of containment (who should be quarantined and the minimum conditions for quarantine to avoid spread)

01.03.2020

Coronavirus Cases

SCMP: Andorra, Chile, Indonesia, Latvia, Morocco, Portugal, Saudi Arabia, Senegal, Tunisia reported their first cases.

Landmark Events

SCMP: Researchers in the US claim that the virus may have been circulating in Washington State for six weeks before detected

02.03.2020

Coronavirus Cases

SCMP: Argentina, Chile, Gibraltar, Liechtenstein, Ukraine, reported their first cases.

---

2   *NYT*: www.NYT.com/2020/02/27/science/coronavirus-pangolin-wildlife-ban-china.html

03.03.2020

Coronavirus Cases

SCMP: Faeroe Islands, Hungary, Poland, Slovenia, signalled their first infections

NYT: 90,000 cases and 3,000 deaths worldwide

WHO

WHO: WHO called for a 40% increase of production of personal protective equipment to meet global demand

04.03.2020

Coronavirus Cases

SCMP: Bosnia Herzegovina, Costa Rica, Martinique Palestine, South Africa flagged their first cases.

Medical Development

SCMP: Scientists in China said the virus had mutated into two different strains, making finding a cure more difficult.

05.03.2020

Coronavirus Cases

SCMP: Bhutan, Colombia, Cameroon, Peru, Serbia, Slovakia, Togo, Vatican City flagged their first cases.

Landmark Events

SCMP: A Hong Kong pet dog tested 'weakly positive' in swab test. Further blood tests would be done.

Medical Development

SCMP: A group of Chinese scientists found that one type, which they called the L type, was more

prevalent than the other, the S type, meaning it was more infectious. They also found that the L type had evolved from the S type, and that the L type was far more widespread before January 7 and in Wuhan.

06.03.2020

Coronavirus Cases

SCMP: Bulgaria, French Guiana, Maldives Malta, Moldova, Paraguay had their first cases

Hong Kong confirmed that a dog has caught COVID-19 from its owner

WHO

WHO: WHO published a roadmap that outlines research priorities in 9 key areas

07.03.2020

Coronavirus Cases

WHO: Cumulative count of COVID-19 cases exceeded 100,000 globally

SCMP: Albania and Bangladesh flagged their first cases

WHO

WHO: WHO issued a statement calling for action, contain, control, delay to reduce the impact of the virus

08.03.2020

Coronavirus Cases

SCMP: Brunei, Burkina Faso, Channel Islands and Cyprus flagged their first cases

Landmark Events

SCMP: Saudi Arabia put about half a million people in lockdown

North Korea began evacuating foreign diplomats from Vladivostok in Russia

Italy put around 16 million people in lockdown in Lombardy and other northern provinces

09.03.2020

Coronavirus Cases

SCMP: Bolivia, DRC, Jamaica, Mongolia, Panama and Turkey reported their first cases

Landmark Events

SCMP: Italy placed the whole country on lockdown

WHO

WHO: WHO and World Bank established a monitoring board to monitor global preparedness for health emergencies

10.03.2020

Coronavirus Cases

SCMP: Cuba, French Polynesia, Honduras, Ivory Coast, Reunion, St Vincent Grenadines reported their first cases

Iran reported its highest daily death toll at 54, bringing its total to 291

WHO

WHO: WHO, UNICEF and the International Federation of Red Cross and Red Crescent Societies (IFRC) issued guidance outlining

critical considerations and checklists to keep schools safe with tips for parents and caregivers as well as children and students

11.03.2020

Coronavirus Cases

SCMP: Ghana, Guyana and Trinidad and Tobago recorded their first cases

Landmark Events

NYT: Trump blocked travellers from continental Europe

Socio-Economic Development

SCMP: Italian Government put up 25 billion Euros to fight the virus

WHO

WHO: WHO declared COVID-19 a pandemic, sent important warnings to all countries and asked countries to "detect, test, treat, isolate, trace, and mobilize their people in the response"

12.03.2020

Coronavirus Cases

SCMP: Antigua Barbuda, Aruba, Cayman Islands, Curacao, Ethiopia, Gabon, Guadeloupe, Guatemala, Guinea, Kazakhstan, Kenya, Mauritania, Saint Lucia, Sudan, Suriname, Seychelles, Uruguay and Venezuela reported their first cases

Landmark Events

SCMP: China said the peak of its outbreak had passed

13.03.2020

Coronavirus Cases

SCMP: Equatorial Guinea, Eswatini, Mayotte, Namibia and Rwanda reported their first cases

SCMP[3]: China's first confirmed COVID-19 case, according to government record, could be traced back to November 17 in 2019, but "patient zero" was not yet confirmed.

Landmark Events

NYT: Trump declared national emergency, USD 50 billion were made available to combat the virus

SCMP: Asian markets fell after the US and European markets lost 10 per cent

Socio-Economic Development

WHO: Europe became new epicentre with more reported cases and deaths than the rest of the world combined, apart from the cases in China

Medical Development

WHO: UN foundation raised more than $70m for frontline workers, patient treatment and to advance research and vaccines

14.03.2020

Coronavirus Cases

SCMP: Bahamas, Central African Republic, Congo, Uzbekistan reported their first cases

16.03.2020

Coronavirus Cases

SCMP: Barbados, Gambia and Montenegro reported their first cases

Italy saw an overnight death toll of 349

Benin, Greenland, Somalia and Tanzania recorded first cases

Bahrain recorded its first death

Landmark Events

NYT: Latin America imposed restrictions on citizens, such as national wide quarantine in Venezuela, countrywide lockdown in Ecuador and Peru, borders shut to non-residents in Colombia, and borders closed in Costa Rica.

SCMP: South Africa declared national emergency and closed its borders

France went on full lockdown

Daily Mail[4]: US President Donald Trump released a series of coronavirus guidelines called '15 Days to Slow the Spread', which advised closing of restaurants and schools

to stop the spread of the virus. His guideline would be revisited after the initial 15-day proposal.

Socio-Economic Development

SCMP: World markets continued to plunge

WHO

WHO: WHO launched a COVID-19 partners platform as an enabling tool for all countries - real time tracking to support the planning, implementation and assessment of country preparedness and response activities

17.03.2020

Coronavirus Cases

SCMP: Bermuda, Djibouti, Kyrgyzstan, Mauritius, Montserrat, New Caledonia, Sint Maarten and Zambia reported their first cases

Landmark Events

NYT: European leaders voted to close off at least 26 countries to nearly all visitors from the rest of the world for at least 30 days.

WHO

WHO: WHO, IFRC, International Organization for Migration (IOM) and United Nations High Commissioner for Refugees (UNHCR) published guide on scaling

up COVID-19 outbreak readiness and response operations in camps and camplike settings

18.03.2020

Coronavirus Cases

SCMP: Chad, El Salvadore, Fiji, Isle of Man, Nicaragua and Niger reported their first cases

WHO

WHO: WHO launched Solidarity trial, an collaborative international clinical trial which is to generate robust data around the world to find the most effective treatment for COVID-19 (accelerated process)

WHO published guide on mental health considerations

19.03.2020

Coronavirus Cases

NYT: China reported 0 cases from the previous few days

SCMP: Angola, Cabo Verde, Haiti, Madagascar, Papua New Guinea and Zimbabwe reported their first cases

20.03.2020

Coronavirus Cases

SCMP: Eritrea, Timore Leste and Uganda reported their first cases

---

3   *SCMP*: www.scmp.com/news/china/society/article/3074991/coronavirus-chinas-first-confirmed-covid-19-case-traced-back

4   *Daily Mail*: www.dailymail.co.uk/news/article-8118415/Donald-Trump-tells-America-lockdown-15-days-stop-coronavirus.html

21.03.2020

Coronavirus Cases

SCMP: Dominica, Grenada, Mozambique and Syria reported their first cases

Landmark Events

SCMP: Lockdowns began across Africa. 41 of 54 nations reported infections

Medical Development

WHO: Member states faced shortfall in testing capacity

WHO

WHO: WHO published recommendation for labs

22.03.2020

Coronavirus Cases

SCMP: Belize, Myanmar, Nicaragua and Turks and Caicos Islands reported their first cases.

23.03.2020

Coronavirus Cases

SCMP: Laos and Libya reported their first cases

Landmark Events

Guardian[5]: UK went in lockdown. People were ordered to stay at home except for food and medicine

Medical Development

SCMP: Boots pharmacies in Britain limited the number of paracetamol to one pack per customer

24.03.2020

Landmark Events

SCMP: Tokyo Olympics originally scheduled to start in July 2020 was delayed until 2021. Delays only happened previously due to war

NYT: India went on lockdown for 21 days

25.03.2020

Coronavirus Cases

SCMP: Anguilla reported its first case

Landmark Events

SCMP: China suspended entry of foreigners to stop imported infections.

WHO

WHO: WHO updated its operational planning guidelines to help countries balance the demands of responding to COVID-19

26.03.2020

Coronavirus Cases

NYT: USA became the country hardest hit with 81,321 cases and 1,000 deaths cumulatively

Socio-Economic Development

WHO: Global education coalition set up to enhance learning opportunities for children and youth in COVID-19 context

WHO

WHO: G20 summit leaders said they would unite to fight the virus and strengthen health system globally

27.03.2020

Coronavirus Cases

SCMP: Italy's death toll spiked to 969 in 24 hours

Landmark Events

South Africa entered a 3-week lockdown

Socio-Economic Development

NYT: Trump signed law with 2 trillion USD program to respond to the US spread

WHO

WHO: WHO published a manual on how to set up and manage a severe acute respiratory infection treatment centre and a severe acute respiratory infection screening facility in health care facilities to optimise patient care.

29.03.2020

Coronavirus Cases

SCMP: Botswana reported its first case

Medical Development

SCMP: British hospitals began rationing ventilators, prioritizing patients with a reasonable chance of recovery.

300 people in Iran died after drinking ethanol believing it will cure the virus

30.03.2020

Coronavirus Cases

SCMP: Sierra Leone and Burundi reported their first cases

Landmark Events

NYT: Most US states issued a stay-at-home directive

Medical Development

WHO: WHO shipped 2 million individual items of protective gear to 74 countries in need

WHO

WHO: WHO's Director-General called for countries to work with companies to increase production, ensure free movement of essential health products for equitable distribution

31.03.2020

Coronavirus Cases

SCMP: Caribbean Netherlands reported its first case

Medical Development

WHO: Medical Product Alert warned consumers and health authorities about the false medical products

SCMP: China reported more than 1,300 asymp-

---

5   *The guardian*: www.theguardian.com/politics/live/2020/mar/23/uk-coronavirus-live-news-latest-boris-johnson-minister-condemns-people-ignoring-two-metre-distance-rule-in-parks-as-very-selfish

tomatic coronavirus cases. This first report of asymptomatic cases followed public concern over people tested positive but not showing symptoms.

WHO

WHO: Scientific Brief published on the off-label use of medicines for COVID-19

02.04.2020

Coronavirus Cases

SCMP: Malawi reported first case

North Korea said it is virus free

Landmark Events

SCMP: Hong Kong International Airport and Heathrow in Britain closed one runway as travel was low

Socio-Economic Development

NYT: 10 million Americans were out of work in just a few weeks. 6.6 million applied for employment benefits

Medical Development

WHO: In a situation report, WHO reported there was evidence on transmission from symptomatic, pre-symptomatic and asymptomatic people.

03.04.2020

Coronavirus Cases

SCMP: Global cases exceeded 1 million and recorded 54,197 deaths

04.04.2020

Coronavirus Cases

SCMP: Western Sahara reported its first cases

Medical Development

SCMP: Britain held a virtual Grand National. The world famous horse race brought in US$3.2 million for the national healthcare system

05.04.2020

Coronavirus Cases

SCMP: Saint Pierre Miquelon and South Sudan reported their first cases

A tiger, Nadia, at Bronx zoo tested positive after developing a dry cough.

06.04.2020

Coronavirus Cases

SCMP: Sao Tome and Principe reported its first case

WHO

WHO: WHO advised decision makers on masks use

07.04.2020

Landmark Events

WHO: World heath day celebrated the health workers

WHO

WHO: WHO issued document for health systems to address COVID-19 and violence against women

Practical considerations for religious leaders and faith-based communities finalised

08.04.2020

Medical Development

WHO: Supply chain task force launched to scale up distribution of medical equipment

09.04.2020

Coronavirus Cases

WHO: 100 days since the virus was identified

10.04.2020

Medical Development

NYT: Moscow's health system pushed to limits with 12,000 cases reported

11.04.2020

Landmark Events

SCMP: The African Union expressed its "extreme concern" about the situation in Guangzhou and called on Beijing to take immediate corrective measures after reports of racism

Medical Development

WHO: WHO drafted a landscape of the candidate vaccines

13.04.2020

Landmark Events

SCMP: Guinean President Alpha Conde made mask wearing compulsory

14.04.2020

Coronavirus Cases

SCMP: Taiwan reported no new cases of the virus

Landmark Events

SCMP: Africans battled stigma and discrimination in China over the pandemic, after a cluster of cases in the Nigerian community was reported in Guangzhou

Austria opened shops under strict conditions, the first country in Europe to ease restrictions following 4 weeks of lock down

Socio-Economic Development

NYT: IMF warned the worst economic downturn since the Great Depression. World economy was expected to contract by 3%

Medical Development

WHO: Strategy was updated for countries in transition from a widespread transmission to a low-level to no transmission.

WHO

WHO: WHO launched a Facebook messenger chatbox offering instant, accurate and multilingual information and guidance

15.04.2020

Landmark Events

SCMP: Denmark reopened school

WHO

WHO: WHO finalised guidelines on public health advice for social and religious practices during Ramadan

16.04.2020

WHO

WHO: WHO issued guidance in adjusting public health and social measures, largescale movements restriction (lockdown)

17.04.2020

Coronavirus Cases

SCMP: Global virus death toll surged past 150,000

Landmark Events

SCMP: Serious death tolls in long-term care homes were reported in Montreal, Canada.

NYT: Trump encouraged protests against some state restrictions

Medical Development

SCMP: Hospitals in Japan were increasingly turning away people with suspected COVID-19 symptoms as the country struggled with surging infections and its emergency medical system on the brink of collapse. Some emergency rooms in hospitals even refused to treat people of strokes, heart attacks and external injuries.

WHO

NYT:[6] WHO failed to tell Syrian Kurds of their first death from coronavirus. WHO knew the death 11 days before informing local authorities. WHO attributed it to internal procedural problems and miscommunications.

19.04.2020

Medical Development

SCMP: Ebola returned to the Democratic Republic of Congo, with six cases reported in the week

20.04.2020

Coronavirus Cases

SCMP: Europe logged more than 1 million cases

Medical Development

WHO: The resolution was adopted by the WHO General Assembly, entitled "International cooperation to ensure global access to medicines, vaccines and medical equipment to face COVID-19"

21.04.2020

Landmark Events

NYT: California reported two deaths on Feb 6 and Feb 17 due to the virus, making them the earliest known victims of the pandemic in the United States.

24.04.2020

Medical Development

WHO: Virtual event with President of France, President of European Commission and Bill Gates Foundation to accelerate the development, production and equitable access to vaccine, diagnostics and therapeutics

WHO issued a Scientific Brief on "immunity passports" – but the risk-free certificate may increase the risk of continued transmission

26.04.2020

Coronavirus Cases

NYT: Global death surpassed 200,000

27.04.2020

Coronavirus Cases

SCMP: Hong Kong reported no new infections

Landmark Events

SCMP: Almost 2 million people in Australia downloaded a new app designed to make virus contact tracing easier

Medical Development

SCMP: The US Center for Disease Control and Prevention (CDC) added six new symptoms to the COVID-19 symptom list

28.04.2020

Coronavirus Cases

SCMP: Brazil passed 5,000 deaths

29.04.2020

Landmark Events

SCMP: Singapore battled a resurgence of cases

30.04.2020

Coronavirus Cases

SCMP: Comoros Islands reported its first case

Landmark Events

NYT: Airlines announced rules on wearing face masks

WHO

WHO: IHR Emergency Committee convened for a third time, with an expanded membership

WHO accepted the Committee's advice that WHO would work to identify animal source of the virus through international scientific and collaborative missions

01.05.2020

Socio-Economic Development

SCMP: More than 30 million laid-off workers in the US applied for unemployment benefit, a record high since the 1930s.

02.05.2020

Medical Development

SCMP: Madagascar shipped its herbal virus remedy to Guinea-Bissau. Named "COVID Organics" the tea was made from artemisia plant, which is effective in treating malaria, and other herbs

---

6   *NYT*: www.NYT.com/2020/04/17/world/coronavirus-news-updates.html

03.05.2020

Landmark Events

NYT: Australia, Britain and Germany called for an inquiry into the origin of the virus

04.05.2020

Coronavirus Cases

SCMP: Western Sahara and Saint Pierre and Miquelon reported their first cases

Landmark Events

SCMP: Iran reopened mosques in 132 countries

WHO

WHO: Director General addressed leaders from 40 countries. An emphasis was placed on equal distribution of prevention, detection and treatment tools to ensure health for all

SCMP: Taiwan raised the issue of its membership with WHO again

05.05.2020

Landmark Events

SCMP: Afghanistan found one third of 500 people randomly tested in Kabul were positive

NYT: French doctor traced suspected first cases of the virus in France to December 2019. It raised a question if the virus

07.05.2020

Socio-Economic Development

WHO: UN launched an update to the global humanitarian response plan for 6.7 billion USD to help 63 low and middle income countries

Medical Development

SCMP: South Korea found false positives, but could not effectively differentiate between active and inactive virus

08.05.2020

Medical Development

SCMP:[7] the approved number of manufacturers making industry-standard masks in China dropped to 14 from 86, according to FDA documentation.

Some authorised sample products failed to meet expected performance meaning that it allowed tiny particles in.

The FDA was increasing surveillance of respirators imported from China which would be subject to random testing

10–14.05.2020

Coronavirus Cases

SCMP: Wuhan in China had a new case after a month with no infections

Hong Kong recorded a new local case, breaking a 23-day streak of no local infections

The Kingdom of Lesotho recorded its first case

Landmark Events

SCMP: Seoul shut down night clubs after a spike in cases in South Korea

The US's top virus doctor, Anthony Fauci, warned against opening schools in the US in autumn as scientists still did not know everything about the virus.

WHO

WHO: WHO issued interim guidance on contact tracing

4 annexes were published on the considerations in adjusting public health and social measures for school, workplace, mass gathering and public health criteria

NYT: WHO official claimed that the virus may never go away

WHO issued advocacy brief advising countries to incorporate a focus on gender in order to ensure that public health policies and measures to curb the pandemic account for gender inequality

15.05.2020

Coronavirus Cases

SCMP: A Rohingya refugee camp in Bangladesh reported a first case

WHO

WHO: A Scientific Brief entitled "Multisystem inflammatory syndrome in children and adolescents with COVID-19" was published

17.05.2020

Socio-Economic Development

NYT: Japan and Germany entered recession

18–19.05.2020

WHO

WHO: 73rd World Health Assembly adopted resolution to fight COVID-19, including intensification of efforts to control the pandemic and equitable access to and fair distribution of all health technologies and products

Oversight committee for WHO finalised the interim review on WHO's response from January to April

20.05.2020

Socio-Economic Development

IMF:[8] IMF would help countries address economic impacts of coronavirus through:

1/ Emergency financing: The fund has doubled the access to its emergency facilities (rapid credit facil-

---

7   *SCMP*: www.scmp.com/news/china/article/3083416/us-regulator-pulls-approval-dozens-companies-making-masks-china

8   IMF: www.imf.org/en/About/Factsheets/Sheets/2020/02/28/how-the-imf-can-help-countries-address-the-economic-impact-of-coronavirus

ity and rapid financing instruments) at a total value of $100bn. 100 countries have benefitted.

2/ Grants for debt relief: This provides grants to fund the poorest and most vulnerable members to cover their IMF debt obligations. 29 countries have benefitted.

3/ Calls for suspension of debt service: fast-acting initiative that frees up scarce money that can instead be used to safeguard lives and livelihoods. G20, World bank and IMF have called for private sectors to participate in this debt relief, it would add USD7bn.

4/ Enhancing liquidity: Approved the establishment of a short term liquidity line to strengthen economic stability and confidence. For member countries with strong policies and in need of short-term moderate balance of payments.

5/ Adjusting existing lending arrangements to accommodate urgent needs arising from the virus (medical supplies, necessary spending, equipment for the containment of the outbreak)

21.05.2020

Socio-Economic Development

WHO: A new agreement was signed with the UN refugee agency for supporting ongoing efforts to protect some 70 million people forcibly displaced from COVID-19

22.05.2020

Coronavirus Cases

NYT: Brazil exceeded Russia with second highest count of infections in the world, exceeding 330,000 total cases.

NYT: Peru and Chile ranked among hardest hit countries in terms of infection per capita (1 in 300)

Ecuador suffered one of the world's worst outbreak, whose death toll was 15 times of the government reported number according to an analysis of mortality data by NYT.

USA remained the epicentre with 1.6 million cumulative cases

27.05.2020

Coronavirus Cases

NYT: The United States recorded its 100,000th death

29.05.2020

Landmark Events

NYT: India eased restrictions after 2 months of severe lockdown. But cases continue to rise (160,000 known cases).

Trump claimed China was responsible for the 100,000 deaths in US

Medical Development

WHO: 30 countries launched the COVID-19 technology access pool, an initiative to make vaccines, tests, and treatment's and other technologies to fight COVID-19 accessible for all

WHO

NYT: US announced to leave WHO after claiming that WHO helped China cover up the early days of the pandemic

31.05.2020

Landmark Events

NYT: Massive Black Lives Matter protests in at least 75 US cities raised concerns for new infections

02.06.2020

Medical Development

WHO: Executive Director of WHO said that COVID-19 was placing a major burden on global health systems

04.06.2020

Coronavirus Cases

NYT: the number of known cases in the world increased faster than ever with more than 100,000 new infections recorded daily

WHO

WHO: In Global Vaccine Summit, funding commitments were made to help maintain immunization in lower-income countries.

The Summit also highlighted how important a safe, effective and equitably accessible vaccine will be in controlling COVID-19.

WHO published a guidance on the use of masks: who should wear one, when it should be worn, and what it should be made of.

05.06.2020

Coronavirus Cases

SCMP: Brazil's death toll surpassed Italy to become the third-highest in the world.

Landmark Events

SCMP: France said it has the pandemic under control

Socio-Economic Development

SCMP: US President Trump announced an unexpected gain of 2.5 million jobs.

09.06.2020

Landmark Events

NYT: Moscow ended lockdown as it reported 1,000 daily new cases

10.06.2020

Landmark Events

SCMP: Sweden's softer lockdown led to one of the world's highest death rates, relative to population

An EU Commission report blamed China and Russia for spewing false and misleading online information on COVID-19

11.06.2020

Coronavirus Cases

SCMP: Russian cases topped 500,000

Latin America logged 70,000 deaths

SCMP: WHO said the pandemic was accelerating in Africa, with South Africa accounting for a quarter of all the continent's cases

NYT: WHO said it took 98 days for Africa to reach 100,000 cases but only 18 days for it to double, maybe due to increase in testing but can also be due to community transmission

Landmark Events

SCMP: Beijing reported a case linked to a wholesale food market

Medical Development

SCMP: Doctors in India feared the virus had yet to peak there as Delhi hospitals struggled to find beds for patients.

13.06.2020

Coronavirus Cases

WHO: Chinese officials reported a cluster of COVID-19 in Beijing.

16.06.2020

Coronavirus Cases

SCMP: The United States topped 2,000,000 cases and 100,000 deaths

Landmark Events

SCMP: Europe was planning to open internal travel next month, but tourists from other continents including Asia were excluded for now

The UK began easing social distancing measures

India, already overwhelmed with COVID-19, was about to face its deadly monsoon season, which brings dengue fever and malaria

New Zealand reported its first case in 25 days

NYT:[9] So far, 25,523 meatpacking workers have tested positive and 89 have died. 129,000 tons of pork produced in America were exported to China since January 2020. The industry publicly lobbied the Trump administration to intervene with state and local officials or risk major meat shortages across American grocery stores. Analysts said the meat shortages have subsided, with most plants having reopened, though many are operating at slower speeds.

Socio-Economic Development

SCMP:[10] Oxford scientists found a low-cost and widely available drug, Dexamethasone, to reduce death rate. Deaths reduced by 1/3 for patients on ventilators. 1/5 for those on supplemental oxygen. No benefits to those who do not require respiratory aid.

Medical Development

WHO: WHO welcomed initial trial results from the UK (Oxford U) that showed that dexamethasone could be lifesaving for critically ill COVID-19 patients.

17.06.2020

Coronavirus Cases

NYT: 77 nations worldwide were still on an upward trend and only 43 registered a decline trend

Socio-Economic Development

SCMP: New Zealand entered a recession

Medical Development

WHO: Evidence showed that hydroxychloriquine did not reduce mortality for hospitalised COVID-19 patients

18.06.2020

Socio-Economic Development

SCMP:[11] Half of the world's undergoing vaccine tests were developed by Chinese scientists.

China adopted a different approach – inactivated viruses,

same method used for hepatitis A, polio, influenza.

This involved growing virus in lab and using heat to destroy the ability to replicate. Body reacted by making antibodies against the virus. Immunity could be limited though (and this was why countries were reluctant to develop this method). High risk of adverse reaction was also another issue.

Medical Development

SCMP: German scientists claimed that a person's blood group might affect the severity of the virus, with A type being most at risk and O type being safest

19.06.2020

Coronavirus Cases

SCMP: Brazil totalled 1 million cases

Landmark Events

SCMP: Governors in California and North Carolina and mayors from a string of cities across the US made mask wearing in public mandatory

---

9   NYT: www.NYT.com/2020/06/16/business/meat-industry-china-pork.html

10   SCMP: www.scmp.com/news/world/europe/article/3089315/dexamethasone-can-help-save-lives-very-ill-coronavirus-patients

11   SCMP: www.scmp.com/news/china/science/article/3089356/can-china-win-COVID-19-vaccine-race-old-school-technology

20.06.2020

Landmark Events

NYT: Southern USA states saw sharp rise in cases

SCMP: Turkey shut down the entire country for six hours

21.06.2020

Coronavirus Cases

SCMP: WHO recorded the largest ever growth in daily cases with 183,020 being reported, with Brazil reporting the most at 54,771 cases and the US recording 36,617 to take second place.

22.06.2020

Coronavirus Cases

SCMP: India reported 15,000 new cases in 24 hours, with a death toll of 14,000

Landmark Events

NYT: Pilgrimage to Mecca would only welcome very limited numbers

WHO

WHO: WHO warned of an "accelerating" pandemic

24.06.2020

Socio-Economic Development

The Guardian:[12] The global economy would take $12tn hit from coronavirus. It would take two years for world output to return to levels at the end of 2019. They also warned governments to be cautious about removing financial support to their fragile economies. G7 members and leading developing nations revised down their growth projection.

Medical Development

BBC:[13] Imperial College, London tested on 300 people. Oxford University also tested. Imperial College London used synthetic strands of genetic code (RNA) mimicking the virus which aimed to train the immune system to recognise and fight coronavirus without having to develop COVID-19.

25.06.2020

Landmark Events

SCMP: The EU planned to reopen their shared borders by July 1

Medical Development

SCMP: World leaders called for vaccines to be a public good, but many countries have been making deals with medicine makers to be first in line.

26.06.2020

WHO

WHO: ACT Accelerator's four pillars of work : diagnostics, therapeutics, vaccines and health system connector and cross cutting workstream was consolidated for investment case

27.06.2020

Coronavirus Cases

SCMP: India passed 500,000 infections

Landmark Events

NYT: Even with high cases, Egypt reopened mosques and cafes

Medical Development

NYT:[14] The spread of the virus could be with people who were healthy or not yet developed symptoms. This meant that everyone wearing masks could help contain the spread. 30-60% of the spreading occurred when people had no symptoms. In the Diamond Princess ship, about 1/3 of the infected passenger and staff had no symptoms. Researchers in Hong Kong estimated that 44% of COVID-19 transmission occurred before symptoms began. A British study estimated the figure to be 50%.

28.06.2020

Coronavirus Cases

SCMP: India reported nearly 20,000 cases in one day

The number of people who have been infected with COVID-19 passed 10 million and 500,000 deaths worldwide

Landmark Events

SCMP: China imposed a strict lockdown on nearly half a million people near Beijing to contain a fresh virus outbreak there

30.06.2020

Landmark Events

NYT: EU reopened to other countries on 1 July but not to USA, Brazil or Russia

01.07.2020

Landmark Events

NYT: Iran shut down 8 more red zone provinces (total 11 provinces shut)

SCMP: Greece opened islands for tourism

02.07.2020

Landmark Events

SCMP: New Zealand's health minister, David Clark, resigned following a series of personal blunders during the coronavirus pandemic.

New Zealand's anti-COVID-19 response had won global praise.

Kazakhstan announced lock down 2.0 from July 5

---

12   *The guardian*: www.theguardian.com/business/2020/jun/24/global-economy-will-take-12tn-hit-from-coronavirus-says-imf

13   BBC: www.bbc.com/news/health-53061288

14   *NYT*: www.NYT.com/2020/06/27/world/europe/coronavirus-spread-asymptomatic.html

NYT:[15] Australia thought the virus was under control. The virus got spread because security guards shared a cigarette lighter. Later on, it circulated in the low-income neighbourhoods in Melbourne. Flare-ups were inevitable even in countries that have largely supressed the virus as restrictions on people's movement were loosened. Racism surged against Asian communities and then migrants and ethnic groups - prejudice that these groups did not need public health advice.

Socio-Economic Development

SCMP: Cases rose rapidly in South Africa, while economy went down in lockdown.

02.07.2020

Coronavirus Cases

SCMP: The US recorded 57,683 new cases in 24 hours

Landmark Events

Guardian[16]: England published list of 59 countries travellers can go to without being quarantined on return, added by 14 British overseas territories

(US, China, Thailand and Portugal not included)

04.07.2020

Landmark Events

SCMP: UK opened pubs

BBC:[17] Medical misinformation about masks continued to circulate about the impacts of wearing a mask.

WHO

SCMP:[18] WHO revised coronavirus timeline that it was alerted by its own office in China, not by Chinese authorities, to the first case of "viral pneumonia" on December 31 on a Wuhan health commission website. After two requests, Chinese authorities provided information on January 3.

05.07.2020

Coronavirus Cases

SCMP: Hong Kong entered a new third wave of outbreak with 17 new cases in the last 24 hours. 1,286 cumulative cases were reported since January.

Medical Development

SCMP: More than 200 scientists accused WHO for ignoring aerosol transmis-

sion: the virus could hang in the air for long periods and float, making poorly ventilated rooms and confined spaces (buses) dangerous

Masks worn properly and having ultra violet light in ceiling units can help reduce spread of virus

NYT:[19]

Countries around the world set up their own factories to provide supplies with this pandemic and outbreaks of the future.

Those factories might struggle to survive as China laid some groundwork to dominate the market for protective and medical supplies for the years to come. Once the vaccine emerged, factories would close but China would still have low costs and be the best positioned for the next outbreak. American companies were reluctant to make big investments as they were worried the mask demand might be temporary. Industrial policy advisor in the USA pushed federal governments to buy American-made pharmaceuticals and medical supplies.

06.07.2020

Coronavirus Cases

SCMP: India overtook Russia with 700,000 cumulative cases and took third spot of the world's hardest hit nations behind the US and Brazil

NYT: US deaths surpassed 130,000 and 50,000 new daily cases

Landmark Events

SCMP: Australia prepared to seal off Victoria from the rest of the country in next day's night in a drastic move to quell the virus

WHO

BBC[20]: Spokesman for the UN Secretary of General confirmed US's notification of its withdrawal from the WHO

07.07.2020

Coronavirus Cases

SCMP: Bermuda joined the list of counties with no active cases

Landmark Events

NYT: Brazil's president tested positive after denying seriousness of the virus

SCMP: Dubai opened for tourists

15   *NYT*: www.NYT.com/2020/07/02/world/australia/melbourne-coronavirus-outbreak.html

16   *The guardian*: www.theguardian.com/world/2020/jul/03/england-publishes-list-of-countries-travellers-can-go-to-without-being-quarantined-on-return

17   BBC: www.bbc.com/news/53266431

18   *SCMP*: www.scmp.com/news/china/science/article/3091820/who-revises-coronavirus-timeline-clarify-its-china-office-raised

19   *NYT*: www.NYT.com/2020/07/05/business/china-medical-supplies.html

20   BBC: www.bbc.com/news/world-us-canada-53327906

Australia locked down Melbourne's more than 5 million residents, ordering them to stay at home

Beijing reported zero new cases over the last 24 hours

08.07.2020

Coronavirus Cases

SCMP: Africa's combined cases exceeded half a million

WHO

SCMP: WHO headed to China to search for COVID-19 origins

09.07.2020

Coronavirus Cases

SCMP: The US reported 65,000 new cases in the last 24 hours

Landmark Events

SCMP: China's embassy in Kazakhstan reported a significant increase in pneumonia cases in the country

10.07.2020

Landmark Events

Hong Kong announced school closures as third wave hit

SCMP: China announced it would suspend imports of shrimps from Ecuador after it finds the virus in a shipment

Kazakhstan dismissed a report from the Chinese embassy that it was facing an outbreak of pneumonia

Sierra Leone said it would re-open mosques and churches

BBC:[21] Iran had rapid surge in numbers recently. The packed city transports, banks and offices were a major contributing cause. People were ignoring the social distancing rules.

Medical Development

SCMP: South Africa was running low on oxygen as hospitals are flooded with virus patients

11.07.2020

Landmark Events

SCMP: South Africa reimposed curfew and a ban on alcohol as cases spike to almost 500 new cases an hour

Arabnews:[22] Health Ministry in India was doing relatively well as they have 13 deaths per 1

million people, compared to USA with 400 and 320 in Brazil.

13.07.2020

Medical Development

SCMP:[23] King's College London found that after 90 days several patients had no detectable antibodies in their bloodstream.

WHO

SCMP: China confirmed WHO team was in Beijing to search for the origin of the virus

14.07.2020

Landmark Events

BBC:[24] Florida became US's epicentre. It had 10,000 new cases per day in the last week. On July 12 it had 15,300 cases. On July 14, 4,400 died of the virus. The Republican governor downplayed the severity of the outbreak.

Medical Development

NYT:[25] Baby was infected with coronavirus in the womb

WHO

SCMP: Research found that even after recovering

from the virus, people continued feeling the symptoms and had difficulties breathing or continuous fatigue

15.07.2020

Medical Development

SCMP:[26] Radiation therapy was found to result in faster recovery and shorter hospital stays, better incubation rates and improved lung conditions.

16.07.2020

Landmark Events

BBC:[27] In Brazil, there were more than 74,000 deaths and testing was insufficient. The true figures were believed to be higher. The outbreak started in Manaus. With poverty and malnutrition, tackling the virus was a challenge. Indigenous communities were the worst affected. But the cases raised the fastest when it hit the cities such as Sao Paulo and Rio Janeiro. The president of Brazil joined himself an anti-lockdown protest and repeatedly played down the risks calling it the "little flu".

---

21   BBC: www.bbc.com/news/52959756

22   *Arabnews*: www.arabnews.com/node/1703001/world

23   *SCMP*: www.scmp.com/news/world/europe/article/3093021/coronavirus-immunity-may-not-last-more-few-months-study-finds

24   BBC: www.bbc.com/news/world-us-canada-53357742

25   *NYT*: www.NYT.com/2020/07/14/health/coronavirus-pregnancy-COVID-19.html?searchResultPosition=2

26   *SCMP*: www.scmp.com/news/world/united-states-canada/article/3093315/x-ray-study-elderly-coronavirus-patients-could-pave

27   BBC: www.bbc.com/news/world-latin-america-53429430

SCMP:[28] people's immune system response could be a matter of life or death. Doctors might need to tailor a different treatment for those who release the "helper" immune type.

BBC:[29] Most African countries were experiencing community transmission. This made it hard to track down the source of the outbreaks. South Africa and Egypt were the hotspots in Africa.

NYT: It is reported that the employees at state-owned enterprises were among the first in China to take a coronavirus vaccine raising ethical concerns.[30] It was later reported on 26 September that thousands in China, such as government officials and vaccine company staff, were further injected with the unproven vaccines (Phase 3 trial not completed yet), with risks unknown.[31]

Socio-Economic Development

SCMP:[32] China avoided recession after economy grew by 3.2% in the second quarter of 2020. The world's second largest economy shrank by 6.8% in the first three months. Data suggested that China would be the first economy to achieve positive economic growth even though USA, Europe and Japan still struggled to reopen.

Financial Times:[33] IMF took measures to help its member states. Many countries were hesitant to apply for the IMF loans. The ideal solution would be to tailor special allocation of SDR's to the needs of the IMF members. By doing so, it would avoid larger portions of the SDR allocation going to richer countries.

Medical Development

The Guardian:[34] Oxford team aimed to begin tests in volunteers. The vaccine was already tested in phase-one involving 1,000 volunteers. 10,000 people would be recruited in the UK, Brazil, South Africa and USA for phase-three. The expected results were to show that there were no serious side-effects from the vaccine.

17.07.2020

Socio-Economic Development

Asian Review:[35] Japan's Minister of Economy revealed plans to subsidise companies shifting manufacturing out of China to Southeast Asia or Japan. 87 companies would receive $653 million in total to move production lines.

BBC:[36] UN made an appeal for $10.3bn to help fight the virus. The money would be used for low income and fragile countries. Wealthy countries threw away the financial rule book to protect their economies and poorer nations should do the same. However, millions would go into starvations.

Medical Development

BBC:[37] People appeared to have multiple coronavirus infections in a short space of time. The scientific consensus was that problem lied in unreliable testing.

18.07.2020

Socio-Economic Development

Financial Times:[38] EU leaders attempted to agree on a 750bn euros recovery package to overcome the effects of coronavirus. Difficulties were found when deciding how much each country would get.

28 *SCMP*: www.scmp.com/news/world/article/3093500/coronavirus-immune-response-could-be-difference-between-life-and-death

29 BBC: www.bbc.com/news/world-africa-53181555

30 www.nytimes.com/2020/07/16/business/china-vaccine-coronavirus.html

31 www.nytimes.com/2020/09/26/business/china-coronavirus-vaccine.html?referringSource=articleShare

32 *SCMP*: www.scmp.com/economy/china-economy/article/3093371/china-gdp-economy-avoids-recession-second-quarter-growth-32

33 *Financial Times*: www.ft.com/content/e7efef20-3960-46e7-922b-112dba8f2def?accessToken=zwAAAXNqGe3YkdPn7-8gOWBG59OSKxEtuo8t7w.MEQCIB5BA_IXIKtX6bk3g3P5vGFTLR9MVdkXkwJ1oZni_Ad_AiBjjytkRa83FjRDnyC4tSas1kGj2YESvCuKsC5r8MiUA&sharetype=gift?token=4b9608c9-1909-4b2c-87c9-33fc1c5a5b45

34 *Theguardian*: www.theguardian.com/science/2020/jul/16/coronavirus-vaccine-oxford-team-volunteers-lab-controlled-human-challenge-trial?CMP=Share_iOSApp_Other

35 *Asian Review*: https://asia.nikkei.com/Economy/Japan-reveals-87-projects-eligible-for-China-exit-subsidies

36 BBC: www.bbc.com/news/world-53439535

37 BBC: www.bbc.com/news/health-52446965

38 *Financial Times*: www.ft.com/content/52d64224-736b-49a1-b62a-03fc5dcb43f3?accessToken=zwAAAXNqGaOgkc9S1kIkc2tJodO2KgP8XctD8w.MEQCICjjsB2usyajvtZqctNroF029rrIJZxlYQJ9CNnvg7XLAiAyUlcRmxeDUTIX_03hL41R886KBi6wiWHcgVYBjYkPdA&sharetype=gift?token=37ee540e-5e72-4080-9315-065845dd3497

19.07.2020

Landmark Events

BBC:[39] Hong Kong reported biggest one-day increase. Non-essential civil servants must work from home and testing would increase. Authorities closed bars, gyms, clubs and barred restaurants from allowing dinners to eat past 6pm.

Thehindu:[40] India's peak might be reached in two months if there were strong public measures and precautions taken. Different places in India would peak at different times.

BBC:[41] Studies showed men were unlikely to wear a mask. Men saw wearing a mask as shameful, weak and not cool. Death rates were higher with men. Men were also less compliant towards hygiene measures to help prevent the spread of the virus.

Socio-Economic Development

Financial Times:[42] G20 fell short to support the world's poorest countries. No countries asked for private creditors for special treatment, despite encouragement to do so. World Bank data showed that 73 countries were eligible for the G20's debt service.

41 countries applied for it. This, however, went at odds with G20's statement that 42 countries applied worth $5.3bn out of which $2bn was for China alone. More transparency and compatible treatment was required.

BBC:[43] EU leaders had conflict over the previously proposed €750 billion economic recovery package plans on an EU summit in Brussels. Some thought it should come as loans rather than grants. The third day of talks in the summit followed a record one-day rise in new infections worldwide (260,000 in 24 hours). The virus still remained a threat to Europe.

20.07.2020

Landmark Events

BBC:[44] Masks were mandatory in France. Anyone without a mask would be fined $154. Many European countries had been forced to re-impose lockdowns or national measures as cases rose. North-eastern region of Catalonia in Spain asked citizens to stay at home as hospitals were overwhelmed. Infections were rising in the Balkans with almost 300 new cases a day. Serbia, Albania and Montenegro reported 195 cases per 100,000 residents, the highest number in the region.

The Guardian:[45] Masks were made compulsory in Australia and Hong Kong.

Medical Development

Science Focus:[46] Oxford's vaccine suggested a safe immune reaction from the preliminary results. It caused few side effects. There was still some work to be done before giving it to the wider public. The vaccine should protect for a minimum of 6 months and reduce onwards transmission of the virus to contacts. Phase three trials in UK, Brazil and South Africa would confirm whether it was effective or not.

21.07.2020

Coronavirus Cases

The Guardian:[47] Belgium saw 66% jump in new infections, South Africa's death passed 5,000, Brazil passed 80,000 death toll. France reported 500 virus clusters, but there were no signs of second wave. Columbia's cases exceeded 200,000. Global cases passed 14.5 million.

39 BBC: www.bbc.com/news/world-asia-china-53462362

40 *The hindu*: www.thehindu.com/news/national/coronavirus-cases-may-peak-in-india-as-early-as-mid-september-says-expert/article32123282.ece

41 BBC: www.bbc.com/news/world-53446827

42 *Financial Times*: www.ft.com/content/e0673a53-7fee-4ef7-baaf-66cc97ee3296?accessToken=zwAAAXNqGk-AkdPgZzpTf-5O99O6r2bMl-4ylg.MEUCIFESL1CJ5w9lm2MkBP-HaAW2yW_30zgVRRHUnuy5fDDSAiEAgId9LVm gLvmROJM9I4cx3pWiKOKsLqlNUpowLRP-zQs&sharetype=gift?token=3064d90f-a4b1-4ec5-9daf-4b49c2841657

43 BBC: www.bbc.com/news/world-europe-53461738

44 BBC : www.bbc.com/news/world-europe-53471497

45 *The guardian*: www.theguardian.com/world/2020/jul/20/global-coronavirus-report-masks-made-mandatory-in-hong-kong-france-and-melbourne

46 *Science Focus*: www.sciencefocus.com/news/coronavirus-oxford-vaccine-shows-strong-antibody-and-t-cell-immune-response/

47 *The guardian*: www.theguardian.com/world/live/2020/jul/20/coronavirus-live-news-trump-says-fauci-alarmist-as-hong-kong-makes-masks-mandatory-indoors

Russian cases rose to more than 777,000.

Landmark Events

SCMP:[48] EU adopted region-wide standard to ensure a safe return to workplaces where commercial buildings were likely to look like hospitals. Quarantine room in buildings would have to be hospital grade, in an isolated part of the building with restricted access so that anyone with medical requirement was safely and securely handled. Hygiene needed to be improved in the common areas.

Socio-Economic Development

Euronews:[49] The frugal group countries (Austria, Denmark, Germany, Sweden and the Netherlands) reduced the grants from 500 billion to 360 billion euros. The total amount was also reduced from 750 billion to 672.5 billion euros. Eastern Europe leaders opposed attaching rule of law conditions, while south-ern European countries were rejecting demands from the so-called frugal five. There was a potential addition of a rule of law conditionality to assessing the funds. Poland and Hungary would be the most impacted and were the ones who wanted to veto the decision.

23.07.2020

Landmark Events

CNN:[50] Counties that were predominately Latino accounted for a disproportionate number of COVID-19 cases in most regions of the United States, with the exception of the South, and structural racism was in part to blame, according to a new study.

NYT:[51] China's national health commission demanded imported livestock and poultry to be virus-free before processing in Chinese plants. Chinese plants needed to have complete traceability mechanism, records of inspection, tests for coronavirus with nucleic acid. Animals that were slaughtered should come from non-epidemic areas.

Socio-Economic Development

UNDP:[52] Temporary Basic Income estimated that it would take $199 billion per month to provide a guaranteed basic income to the 2.7 billion people living below or just above the poverty line in the 132 developing countries. The people hardest hit by the pandemic were those not covered by social insurance programmes, like informal workers, low-waged, women and young people, refugees and migrants, and people with disabilities. Workers not covered by social protection could not stay at home without income. A Temporary Basic Income would give them the means to buy food and pay for health and education expenses. It was also financially within reach: a six-month Temporary Basic Income. One way for countries to pay for a Temporary Basic Income would be to repurpose the funds they would use this year to service their debt. For example, the government of Togo distributed over $19.5 million in monthly financial aid to over 12 percent of the population through its cash transfer programme, mostly to women who worked in the informal sector.

24.07.2020

Coronavirus Cases

The Guardian:[53] US was still the hardest hit nation. 70,000 new positive cases and 1,000 deaths were recorded.

CNN:[54] Mexico reported 8,400 new coronavirus cases in 24 hours, highest daily number yet.

Landmark Events

The Guardian:[55] Norway imposed a 10-day quarantine to travellers from Spain. France advised not to travel to the north-eastern region of Catalonia.

---

48 *SCMP*: www.scmp.com/business/companies/article/3093899/offices-resemble-hospitals-part-european-building-standard-being

49 *Euronews*: www.euronews.com/2020/07/20/eu-summit-deadlock-see-talks-stretch-into-sunday

50 CNN: https://edition.cnn.com/world/live-news/coronavirus-pandemic-07-24-20-intl/h_d4a50d5510deb8fed5f34fe1819d8a8b

51 *NYT*: www.NYT.com/reuters/2020/07/23/world/asia/23reuters-health-coronavirus-china-meatprocessing.html

52 UNDP: www.undp.org/content/undp/en/home/news-centre/news/2020/Temporary_Basic_Income_to_protect_the_worlds_poorest_people_slow_COVID19.html

53 *The guardian*: www.theguardian.com/world/live/2020/jul/25/coronavirus-live-news-close-watch-on-victoria-australia-and-record-infections-globally?CMP=Share_iOSApp_Other

54 CNN: https://edition.cnn.com/world/live-news/coronavirus-pandemic-07-24-20-intl/h_d4a50d5510deb8fed5f34fe1819d8a8b

55 *The guardian*: www.theguardian.com/world/live/2020/jul/25/coronavirus-live-news-close-watch-on-victoria-australia-and-record-infections-globally?CMP=Share_iOSApp_Other

BBC:[56] Boris Johnson admitted that the UK government did not understand the virus during the first few weeks and months of the outbreak. More than 45,000 people died and almost 330,000 people tested positive with the virus in UK.

CNN:[57] A total of 300 new novel coronavirus cases were detected in the south-eastern Australian state of Victoria. Of the 300 cases, only 51 were from a known source with connections to previous cases. Only 25 percent of the people tested positive were contacted for tracing interview, others unable to contact. To ensure tracing interviews, 28 teams of Australian Defence Force would be dispatched to go from door-to-door with health officials, if a first try of telephone contact failed.

Socio-Economic Development

CNN:[58] Chinese foreign minister announced $1billion loan to Latin America and Caribbean for COVID-19 vaccines access.

25.07.2020
Coronavirus Cases

The Guardian:[59] Brazil registered an additional 1,211 deaths from COVID-19, as well as a further 51,147 confirmed infections.

Israel: 60,000 people have tested positive for the virus.

Landmark Events

Business Insider[60]: Florida reported cumulatively over 414,000 cases, surpassing New York to be the second highest number state in the US.

26.07.2020
Landmark Events

The Guardian:[61] North Korean leader convened a state of emergency after a person suspected to have corona returned after crossing the border of South Korea illegally. North Korea received coronavirus kits from Russia and other countries and imposed strict border closures.

04.08.2020
Landmark Events

Guardian[62]: UN Secretary General Antonio Guterres warned of the largest disruption of education in history, caused by the pandemic, with schools closed in more than 160 countries in mid-July affecting more than a billion students.

Many parts of Europe risked a second wave, as social distancing measures eased. France and Germany saw sharp increases in new cases.

24.08.2020
Landmark Events

CNN[63]: Dr. Anthony Fauci warned against the notion of early emergency use authorization for a potential coronavirus vaccine, explaining that such a step could damage efforts to develop other vaccines. His warning came as White House officials raised the possibility of an early emergency authorization before late-stage trials were finished.

25.08.2020
Landmark Events

CNN[64]: Oxford coronavirus vaccine could be put before regulators by end of 2020 to collect data through clinical trials.

03.09.2020
Medical Development

NYT:[65] The first vaccine safe to try on humans started in March. Researchers had been testing 37 vaccines in clinical trials on humans, and at least 91 preclinical vaccines were under active investigation in animals. Only 3 vaccines had been approved for early or limited uses, and zero for full use. China and Russia approved vaccines without waiting for the results of Phase 3 trials, which

56   BBC: www.bbc.com/news/uk-politics-53525450
57   CNN: https://edition.cnn.com/world/live-news/coronavirus-pandemic-07-24-20-intl/h_d4a50d5510deb8fed5f34fe1819d8a8b
58   CNN: https://edition.cnn.com/2020/07/23/americas/china-billion-vaccine-latin-america-coronavirus-intl/index.html
59   *The guardian*: www.theguardian.com/world/live/2020/jul/25/coronavirus-live-news-close-watch-on-victoria-australia-and-record-infections-globally?CMP=Share_iOSApp_Other
60   *Business Insider*: www.businessinsider.com/florida-becomes-2nd-hardest-hit-us-state-surpassing-new-york-2020-7
61   *The guardian*: www.theguardian.com/world/live/2020/jul/25/coronavirus-live-news-close-watch-on-victoria-australia-and-record-infections-globally?CMP=Share_iOSApp_Other
62   www.theguardian.com/world/2020/aug/04/global-report-france-could-lose-control-of-COVID-19-at-any-time?CMP=Share_iOSApp_Other, accessed 10 August 2020.
63   CNN: https://edition.cnn.com/2020/08/24/politics/fauci-coronavirus-vaccine-emergency-use-authorization/index.html
64   CNN: https://edition.cnn.com/world/live-news/coronavirus-pandemic-08-25-20-intl/index.html?tab=Vaccines
65   *NYT*: www.NYT.com/interactive/2020/science/coronavirus-vaccine-tracker.html

were warned by scientists of serious risks.

04.09.2020

Medical Development

SCMP: After satisfactory trial tests, Sanofi, a French pharmaceutical giant, announced it would start human trials of the potential vaccine it was developing with GSK from Britain.

09.09.2020

Medical Development

SCMP: AstraZeneca suspended vaccine trial after unknown sickness

Boston Magazine[66]: Alina Chan, a Canadian molecular biologist at the Broad Institute, of Harvard University and MIT, reported her study that the possibility that COVID-19 was originated in a laboratory could not be ruled out.

10.09.2020

Medical Development

SCMP: China National Biotec Group reported

none of the recipients of its two coronavirus shots has shown any obvious negative reaction or infection

14.09.2020

WHO

SCMP: WHO delivered warning to Europe as infections hit new high.

15.09.2020

Landmark Events

The Washington Post[67]: A poll of 13 nations released by Pew Research Center suggested that the international reputation of the United States has dropped to a new low in the face of a disorganized response to the novel coronavirus.

Socio-Economic Development

NYT[68]: Protections like wearing masks were becoming more widespread in Europe, helping people get on with their lives with calculated risk.

17.09.2020

Landmark Events

SCMP: The world passed the 30 million infections mark.

News.com.au[69]: Chinese defector virologist Dr Li-Meng Yan published report claiming COVID-19 was lab-made

26.09.2020

Landmark Events

Asian Review:[70] Speaking to UN General Assembly, Australian Prime Minister reiterated the call for an inquiry into the origin of COVID-19 so that the world can better prepare to pre-empt a future pandemic.

28.09.2020

Coronavirus Cases

CNN[71]: More than 1 million people worldwide have died of Covid-19.

Medical Development

WHO[72]: Global partnership to make available 120 million affordable, quality COVID-19 rapid

tests for low- and middle-income countries

29.09.2020

Coronavirus Cases

CNN[73]: India's vice president tested positive for Covid-19.

Russia signed deal to supply Sputnik-V vaccine to Nepal.

02.10.2020

Landmark Events

NYT[74]: The US President Donald Trump tested positive, was hospitalized in Walter Reed National Military Medical Center and received an experimental drug for treatment.

Medical Development

NYT[75]: President Trump received a dose of an experimental antibody cocktail being developed by the drug maker Regeneron, in addition to several other drugs, including zinc, vitamin D and the generic version of the heartburn treatment Pepcid.

---

66 *Boston Magazine*: www.bostonmagazine.com/news/2020/09/09/alina-chan-broad-institute-coronavirus/

67 *The Washington Post*: www.washingtonpost.com/world/2020/09/15/global-views-united-states-trump-coronavirus-pew-poll/

68 www.nytimes.com/2020/09/15/world/europe/coronavirus-europe.html?referringSource=articleShare

69 News.com.au : www.news.com.au/lifestyle/health/health-problems/chinese-defector-virologist-dr-limeng-yan-publishes-report-claiming-covid19-was-made-in-a-lab/news-story/36decb0c2bca253b696dec0cb665c970

70 *Asian Review*: https://asia.nikkei.com/Spotlight/Coronavirus/World-needs-to-know-origins-of-COVID-19-Australia-PM-tells-UN

72 www.who.int/news-room/detail/28-09-2020-global-partnership-to-make-available-120-million-affordable-quality-covid-19-rapid-tests-for-low--and-middle-income-countries

73 www.cnn.com/world/live-news/coronavirus-pandemic-09-29-20-intl/index.html

74 *NYT*: www.nytimes.com/live/2020/10/02/world/covid-19-coronavirus/trump-joins-other-world-leaders-who-have-contracted-the-virus

75 *NYT*: www.nytimes.com/live/2020/10/02/world/covid-19-coronavirus/trump-joins-other-world-leaders-who-have-contracted-the-virus

TIME[76]: About 80% of deaths in the U.S. from COVID-19 occurred in those 65 or older, according to CDC.

03.10.2020
Medical Development

SCMP[77]: Vaccine developers sought to help group hit hardest by Covid-19: the elderly.

05.10.2020
Coronavirus Cases

SCMP[78]: Solomon Islands reported first case.

India recorded the highest number of daily cases globally, also had a low fatality rate of 1.56 percent, which was nearly half the global figure.[79]

Socio-Economic Development

Pope Francis said on Sunday that the COVID-19 pandemic was the latest crisis to prove that market forces alone and "trickle-down" economic policies had failed to produce the social benefits their proponents claim.[80]

Medical Development

CNN[81]: Trump was given a five-day course of the antiviral drug remdesivir and the corticosteroid drug dexamethasone on Saturday after his oxygen level transiently dipped.

06.10.2020
Medical Development

China in talks to have WHO assess its COVID vaccines for global use.[82]

07.10.2020
Coronavirus Cases

34 White House staffers and other contacts had been infected with the coronavirus in recent days.[83]

09.10.2020
Landmark Events

China joined a WHO-backed effort to distribute vaccines for the novel coronavirus, boosting a major public health initiative the White House pointedly rejected.[84]

10.10.2020
Coronavirus Cases

Trump delivered White House remarks in first public event since testing positive for COVID-19.[85] WHO reported new daily record, as India neared 7 million cases.[86]

11.10.2020
Medical Development

Covid survivors said brain fog was impairing their ability to work and function normally.[87]

15.10.2020
Coronavirus Cases

About 80% of European countries were seeing growth in Covid-19 cases, WHO official said.[88]

Medical Development

WHO study reviewed Remdesivir and three other repurposed drugs: hydroxychloroquine, lopinavir/ritonavir and interferon. None of them helped patients live any longer or get out of the hospital any sooner. WHO study found Remdesivir had "little or no effect on mortality" of hospitalized Covid-19 patients.[89]

19.10.2020
Landmark Events

Anticipating coronavirus vaccines, UNICEF planned to stockpile more than half a billion syringes.[90]

76   https://time.com/5895439/trump-covid-19-coronavirus-age/
77   www.scmp.com/news/china/science/article/3104038/vaccine-developers-seek-help-group-hit-hardest-covid-19-elderly
78   www.scmp.com/news/asia/article/3104097/coronavirus-india-records-75829-cases-crowds-flood-melbourne-beaches
79   https://hosted.ap.org/article/05e09934282e2f2e0c9f244c4e4a97e0/latest-australian-state-worried-about-mall-outbreak
80   www.reuters.com/article/us-pope-encyclical/pope-says-free-market-trickle-down-policies-fail-society-idUSKBN26P0E1
81   www.cnn.com/politics/live-news/trump-covid-19-updates-monday/index.html
82   http://asia.nikkei.com/Spotlight/Coronavirus/China-in-talks-to-have-WHO-assess-its-COVID-vaccines-for-global-use
83   www.businessinsider.com/leaked-fema-report-34-people-trump-orbit-coronavirus-2020-10
84   www.washingtonpost.com/world/asia_pacific/coronavirus-vaccine-china-covax-who/2020/10/08/cf4e1e96-09d2-11eb-8719-0df159d14794_story.html
85   www.usatoday.com/story/news/politics/elections/2020/10/10/trump-holds-first-white-house-event-since-testing-positive-covid-19/5952907002/
86   www.scmp.com/news/asia/south-asia/article/3104965/who-reports-daily-record-high-new-coronavirus-cases-india
87   www.nytimes.com/2020/10/11/health/covid-survivors.html?referringSource=articleShare
88   www.cnn.com/world/live-news/coronavirus-pandemic-10-15-20-intl/index.html
89   www.cnn.com/world/live-news/coronavirus-pandemic-10-15-20-intl/index.html
90   www.nytimes.com/2020/10/19/world/anticipating-coronavirus-vaccines-unicef-plans-to-stockpile-more-than-half-a-billion-syringes.html

Medical Development

Long-term heart damage likely in some Covid-19 survivors, review found.[91]

20.10.2020

Medical Development

Volunteers in London were to be infected with coronavirus early next year, in the world's first Covid-19 "human challenge trials".[92]

China promised preferential access to its Covid-19 vaccines to countries across Asia, Africa and Latin America, as Beijing used inoculations as a new tool to bolster its ties with nations neglected by the US.[93]

21.10.2020

Socio-Economic Development

China, Taiwan and Vietnam were the only major trading economies whose exports had recovered strongly, with all three reporting strong growth in the third quarter of 2020, according to research by the United Nations Conference on Trade and Development (Unctad).[94]

Taiwan was singled out as the "most effective and least disruptive of any country" in the world on pandemic preparedness.[95]

Medical Development

Older people, women and those with a wide range of symptoms in the first week of their illness appeared to be most likely to develop "long Covid," according to a preprint paper posted online by researchers at King's College London on Wednesday.[96]

25.10.2020

Coronavirus Cases

European nations returned to restrictions as virus surged.

Spain's second wave of infections prompted the return to a state of emergency.[97]

Medical Development

Rush for results could lead to inferior Covid vaccine, said scientists.[98]

28.10.2020

Coronavirus Cases

France and Germany announced new restrictions as cases surge in Europe.[99]

29.10.2020

Coronavirus Cases

Europe at the "epicenter" of Covid-19 pandemic again, WHO said. The number of coronavirus cases in Europe exceeded the 10 million mark since the beginning of the pandemic, with more than 1.5 million cases confirmed last week alone.[100]

30.10.2020

Coronavirus Cases

WHO warned that the pandemic reached "an alarming juncture" in the Middle East region.

Spain announced new restrictions on Friday.

Belgium locked down in a "last chance" bid to keep its hospitals from collapse.[101]

31.10.2020

Coronavirus Cases

England would enter a second national lockdown in the coming days, British Prime Minister Boris Johnson announced. The decision came hours after the UK passed the grim milestone of one million coronavirus cases.[102]

Slovakia to test all adults for SARS-CoV-2.[103]

06.11.2020

Medical Development

SCMP: Fosun, one of China's biggest private-sector conglomerates, aimed to launch BioNTech and Pfizer's Covid-19 vaccine in China at the same time as US and Europe.[104]

91   www.cnn.com/world/live-news/coronavirus-pandemic-10-19-20-intl/index.html

92   www.ft.com/content/6f9e6270-db88-41bc-aacb-7d384cf2f6fe

93   www.ft.com/content/ce9a4c98-49b5-4c24-9ff2-ed1c6a3f3412

94   www.scmp.com/economy/china-economy/article/3106403/china-taiwan-and-vietnam-successfully-contained-coronavirus

95   www.stuff.co.nz/national/health/coronavirus/123144103/what-nz-can-learn-from-taiwan-about-pandemic-preparedness?cid=app-iPhone

96   www.cnn.com/world/live-news/coronavirus-pandemic-10-21-20-intl/index.html

97   www.nytimes.com/live/2020/10/25/world/covid-19-coronavirus-updates

98   www.theguardian.com/world/2020/oct/25/rush-for-results-could-lead-to-inferior-covid-vaccine-say-scientists?CMP=Share_iOSApp_Other

99   www.nytimes.com/live/2020/10/28/world/covid-19-coronavirus-updates?referringSource=articleShare

100 www.cnn.com/world/live-news/coronavirus-pandemic-10-30-20-intl/index.html

101 www.nytimes.com/live/2020/10/30/world/covid-19-coronavirus-updates

102 www.cnn.com/2020/10/31/europe/uk-lockdown-coronavirus-europe-intl/index.html

103 www.thelancet.com/journals/lancet/article/PIIS0140-6736(20)32261-3/fulltext

104 www.scmp.com/business/companies/article/3108801/fosun-hopes-launch-biontech-and-pfizers-covid-19-vaccine-china

07.11.2020

Medical Development

CNBC: Pfizer and BioN-Tech announced their coronavirus vaccine was more than 90% effective in preventing Covid-19 among those without evidence of prior infection.[105]

10.11.2020

Coronavirus Cases

CNN: More than 50 million cases of Covid-19 had been recorded worldwide, as countries hit new records globally. The US surpassed 10 million cases.[106]

17.11.2020

Medical Development

SCMP: Coronavirus hunters picked up another piece of the trail in Italy. New research suggested the pathogen infected people across Italy months before it was detected in China. Antibodies specific to the coronavirus were found in blood samples from lung cancer screening tests going back to September last year.[107]

105 www.cnbc.com/2020/11/09/covid-vaccine-pfizer-drug-is-more-than-90percent-effective-in-preventing-infection.html

106 www.cnn.com/world/live-news/coronavirus-pandemic-11-10-20-intl/index.html

107 www.scmp.com/news/china/science/article/3110088/covid-19-virus-hunters-pick-another-piece-trail-italy

COVID-19 in Cambodia:
Managing a Crisis with Limited Resources

Oum Socheat

Cambodia's responses to the COVID-19 pandemic have been well-informed, swift and decisive. Applauded by the WHO, the multiple strategies including cooperation with neighbouring countries, travel restrictions, lockdown, legislative initiatives, financial aid to individuals, health support budget measures, and post-pandemic economic recovery plans have provided opportunities for strengthening community solidarity and mutual trust.

COVID-19: The Cases

As of 10 August 2020, the cumulative number of confirmed COVID-19 cases in Cambodia stood at 251 cases out of a population of 16,486,542. There had been no deaths, and a total of 219 cases had completely recovered from the virus (see Figure 2.1). How Cambodia achieved this remarkable result—one that earned the Kingdom the plaudits of the World Health Association (WHO)—is the subject of this chapter.

Figure 2.1 Daily confirmed cases, deaths, and recovered cases from 23 January to 10 August 2020

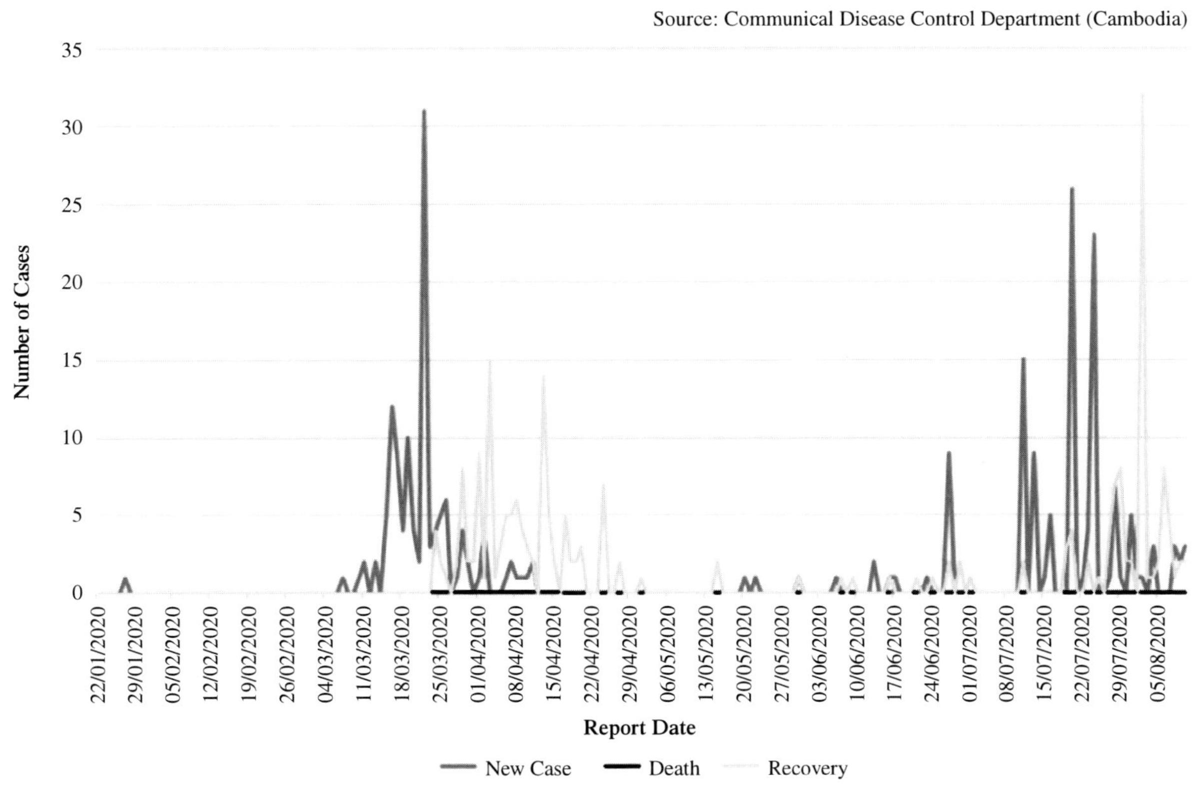

Source: Communical Disease Control Department (Cambodia)

Source: www.cdcmoh.gov.kh/479-update-on-covid-19

The Challenges and Community Response

Cambodia's remarkable response to the pandemic is even greater in light of the general view that the country's public health system is antiquated, without modern equipment, competent medical staff, or adequate facilities. However, the system and its medical staff, with enlightened support from the government and its citizens, brought the country through what would otherwise have been a catastrophe. Despite its success in stopping the spread of the virus, Cambodia's economy was hit hard by the global lockdown, plunging its three pillars of economic growth—tourism, construction, and garment and textile exports—into a deep recession.[1] The tourism sector showed the first sign of a slowdown in Siem Reap Province at the end of 2019. There was a sudden decline in the numbers of Chinese arrivals at the tourist hotspot, quickly followed by a decrease in the number of tourists from other countries. Without tourists, hotels, restaurants, and travel agencies crumbled, followed by that of related sectors. As the most important tourism draw, Siem Reap was one of the worst hit regions. Despite the fact that at the time Siem Reap was still open to international travelers, its hospitality sector, which mostly employs staff from vulnerable groups and poor households, came to a halt.[2] The entire sector was predicted to drop by 50 to 90 percent in 2020;[3] the first two months of 2020 alone witnessed a 25.1 percent decrease in tourist arrivals compared to the same period in 2019.[4] To understand the impact, in 2019, the tourism industry generated US$5 billion in revenue with 6 million international arrivals.

The construction sector accounts for the largest share of the Kingdom's economy, a total of 35.7 percent of GDP. Prior to the onset of COVID-19, the sector was booming, with investments of US$8 billion in 2018 and US$11 billion in 2019.[5] As it ground to a halt, the World Bank recorded a 47 percent drop in imported steel for construction projects and a 40 percent decline in direct foreign investments in the first quarter of 2020. The International Monetary Fund (IMF) projected that Cambodia's GDP, in real terms, will decline by 1.6 percent in 2020.

Similarly, the withdrawal of the "Everything But Arms" preferential trade policy by the European Union and the spread of COVID-19 have severely affected the garment and textile export sector, with 130,000 jobs lost, affecting millions of people who indirectly benefit from the sector.[6] Some workers rejoined their farming families, while others struggled to survive in the cities.

During the crisis, well-planned government responses were vital in preventing prevent the country from becoming the next COVID-19 epicenter. Initially, these measures focused on cooperation across sectors, dissemination of early warnings, health prevention measures, and restrictions to preserve security and social order.

As the effects of the virus began to be felt, unsubstantiated rumors in social media spread fears, causing panic buying and market chaos. Counterfeit goods, especially masks and sanitizers, proliferated.

---

1 WB, www.worldbank.org/en/country/cambodia/publication/cambodia-in-the-time-of-covid-19-coronavirus-economic-update-may-2020

2 VOA, www.voacambodia.com/a/siem-reap-tourism-reliant-residents-are-struggling-financially/5421521.html

3 Abiad, Abdul, Rosa Mia Arao, and Suzette Dagli. "The economic impact of the COVID-19 outbreak on developing Asia." (2020).

4 Ly, Sodeth, Claire Honore Hollweg, Sokbunthoeun So, Donna Louise Andrews, Khy Touk, and Sokunpanha You. Cambodia Economic Update: Cambodia in the Time of COVID-19-Special Focus: Teacher Accountability and Student Learning Outcomes. No. 148887. The World Bank, 2020.

5 CBRE, www.b2b-cambodia.com/news/cambodias-construction-sector-in-q1-2020/

6 *The Cambodia Daily*, https://english.cambodiadaily.com/business/covid-19-over-256-cambodian-factories-suspended-130000-workers-affected-164917/

However, the joint efforts of the provincial courts, prosecutors, and government departments, including the Ministries of Commerce, Information, Health and Foreign Affairs and International Cooperation, stopped these antisocial activities swiftly and decisively. Vendors who imported counterfeit protective products were charged and detained, while legal action was taken against sellers who over-priced face masks and sanitizers. Shortages of everyday necessities disappeared as supply chains were expedited; the sale of pharmaceutical drugs and medical equipment were better regulated; the identities of those in contact with COVID-19-positive patients were traced and tested; and foreign visitors were informed in advance about arrival procedures, testing, and quarantining.

In any country, the combined efforts of individuals and their local communities are the key to a successful response to COVID-19. Cambodia has an edge over other countries in that trust in community leadership is an important part of Cambodian culture, a trust that joins everyone behind clearly defined goals and objectives. As a consequence of wars over the past decades, Cambodians are prepared to be self-reliant and are used to making do with less in difficult times. Thus, in the response to COVID-19, the cooperation with medical personnel and government measures was almost universal. In April, 90,000 Cambodian migrant workers returned home from Thailand where they had either lost their jobs, were fearful of the virus, or both. The danger of community infections led to measures designed to keep both communities and returning workers safe.[7] Local communities took on the job of closely monitoring the health of their returned countrymen, and none were infected. Another factor that made a difference was the Cambodian lifestyle, as homes are gathered in smaller locations across the country. Those who commute generally do so in private vehicles, limiting the exposure that public transport would entail, even if it were widely available. In the countryside, transport is often by ox-cart or bicycle, both of which limit exposure to others.

One consequence of COVID-19 was a renewed faith in the country's public health system. For years, upper- and middle-class citizens had derided the system for what they perceived as a lack of modern medical equipment, under-funded and outdated facilities, and incompetent staff, choosing instead to travel to Singapore, Thailand, Vietnam, and the Philippines for their medical treatment. However, the poor and vulnerable relied on in-country public hospitals for their treatment, but did not entirely trust it. Because of COVID-19, there was a fear that perhaps the Cambodian health system might not be up to the task of stopping the spread of the virus. However, as events proved, these fears were unfounded. In fact, the stellar performance of the health system proved that the country's health system was not only up to the task, but had was in many ways superior to systems in other parts of Southeast Asia.

Decisions made by Prime Minister Hun Sen and the Ministry of Health on medical advice provided the key to stop the virus. Over US$100 million was gathered for a super fund for hospital improvements, equipment, drugs, and other benefits for frontline medical staff. Before June 2020, all COVID-19-positive patients, including foreigners, received standard treatment free of charge. The performance of the public health system under incredible pressure not only resulted in remarkable figures for cases of COVID-19, but it won the hearts of the Cambodian people while burnishing its reputation globally.

---

7   www.khmertimeskh.com/722847/about-14000-migrant-workers-in-battambang-cleared-of-covid-19/

The First and Second Waves

On 10 January, the Ministry of Health issued an advisory warning health professionals of a previously unknown respiratory disease, one with as-yet unknown cause and symptoms. The first case of COVID-19 in Cambodia was a Chinese man who boarded a direct flight from Wuhan with his family and landed in Preah Sihanouk Province on 23 January. He had a mild fever but later developed symptoms now associated with COVID-19. He was tested and on 27 January was confirmed positive.[8] Everyone who had contact with him, including his family, airport officials, a taxi driver, and staff at the hotel where he stayed, were closely monitored by the provincial health authority. Two weeks later he was discharged after twice testing negative. The arrival of the cruise ship MS Westerdam in mid-February became a major humanitarian event. The ship left Hong Kong for Yokohama, but was refused entry by Japanese authorities who feared the ship and its 1,455 passengers and 802 crew members were carrying the virus. Earlier, another cruise ship, the Diamond Princess, reported more than 600 cases of COVID-19, at the time the biggest virus cluster outside of China. After being rejected by Taiwan, Guam, Thailand, and the Philippines, was allowed to dock at Sihanoukville. Before disembarking, all on board were tested. When the test results showed they were negative, passengers were allowed to take flights to return home. The story of the MS Westerdam was hailed as an example of Cambodia being "a small country with a big heart".

The third week in March, however, saw a double-digit spike in cases. Those affected included French tourists on a Viking Mekong cruise ship, Malaysians who had traveled to Kampong Cham Province for a religious ceremony, and Cambodians returning from a religious observance in Malaysia. Precautionary measures held firm, however, and there were no new cases. The COVID-19 figures stood at 122, with only 1 community case.

Air traffic restrictions were eased in early May, but on 20 May a 26-year-old Cambodian who traveled from the Philippines and transited in South Korea tested positive at Phnom Penh International Airport. This sparked fears that a second wave of infection was imminent. The number of confirmed COVID-19 cases grew, with most involving Cambodians returning home from abroad. As of 8 August 2020, 246 new cases of COVID-19 had been recorded. Air routes connecting Malaysia, Indonesia, and the Philippines to Cambodia were subsequently suspended due to the increase of COVID-19 infected patients arriving on direct and connecting flights.

The Treatment Approach

The treatment approaches have never been revealed in Cambodia until a senior official wrote an article about his treatment journey. He is a senior diplomat who returned from France to Cambodia, discharged from Khmer-Soviet hospital after three weeks of treatment, provided a mixed treatement by Cambodia medics.[9] He was suspected of being infected by COVID-19 because a few of his cohort who joined the seminar in France were tested positive. Soon after he arrived in Phnom Penh, he rented an isolated apartment nearby the outskirt of Phnom Penh for a 14-day self-quarantine. His story began from mild symptom on the 2ND day including breathing problems and diarrhea. His conditions became more severe and typical of COVID-19 on the 7TH day. He suffered from strong fever, throat burn, sweating,

---

8   CDC, http://cdcmoh.gov.kh/?start=55
9   Freshnews, www.freshnewsasia.com/index.php/en/opinioneditorial/154624-2020-04-07-12-49-22.html

fatigue, and muscle pain. After that, the medics took his sample and confirmed that he tested positive for COVID-19. He was then sent to quarantine center. Overwhelmed by fear, he consumed a lot of food and conducted an intensive exercise in an attempt to improve his immunity. Unfortunately, his condition worsened because his body could not absorb all he had consumed, resulting in stomach ache and diarrhea. His throat became tight and itchy ("like insects roaming inside throat"). Later on, he was sent to ICU for ventilator breathing because of his severe respiratory condition. He escaped death and returned to normal quarantine routine. In his section of the quarantine center, he was placed with a couple of locals and foreigners. He observed that everyone's symptoms varied. Only he and one of the foreigners had a severe respiratory condition. The symptoms of the rest seemed less noticeable (only mild fever, difficult to sleep, and stomach pain). The samples for infected patients were taken twice or thrice a day. If a patient tested negative twice, the medic would transfer the patient to other sections of the quarantine center.

This account also commented on the patients' psychological condition. Stress and fear made the situation unpredictable. Some foreign nationals were worried about no connecting flight to return home. A foreigner uncontrollably shouted regardless of being not severely sick, and another was crying every day. Some complained that they were kept at the center too long even after they were tested negative. Some people with religious belief managed their emotions better than others by praying.

For drug treatment, the medicines that have been prescribed to patients are the cocktails of Kaletra, Chloroquine and Doliphrane and other supplements depending on the specific health conditions of the patients. Kaletra used to cures HIV, Chloroquine cures malaria and prevents lounge burning, and Doliphrane reduces fever and diarrhea. For less acute conditions of infected patients, doctors prescribed only Kaletra. However, if the symptom includes acute respiratory syndrome, doctors would add Choloquine to the prescribed list. A ten-day dose of Choloquine is used to prevent severe respiratory disease.

Government Measures

A wide range of government measures have been enacted in the wake of the first COVID-19 case, including strategies for local and regional cooperation, travel restrictions, including provincial lockdowns, suspension of public events, legislative initiatives, and budgetary measures to support health care and financial aid to individuals.

In early February, Prime Minister Hun Sen traveled to China with his prior plan to visit Cambodian students who were stranded in lockdown in Wuhan. But this visit cannot be done due to biosecurity arrangements, He only visited Beijing. He urged the students to remain calm and show solidarity and moral support between Cambodia and China in a time of crisis. On 12 February, one day after the WHO named the new disease COVID-19,[10] the government came out in support of its assessment that COVID-19 as "a Public Health Emergency of International Concern and issued a set of Temporary Recommendations". From mid-February, public schools, private education institutes, sports facilities, hair salons, prison visits prison, national exams, public buses, water-taxis, and entertainment venues businesses (including karaoke clubs and casinos) were ordered to close to contain the virus. However, public markets, grocery stores, factories, and restaurants continued their operations.

---

10 www.who.int/emergencies/diseases/novel-coronavirus-2019/technical-guidance/naming-the-coronavirus-disease-(covid-2019)-and-the-virus-that-causes-it

In March, the government stepped up health measures on international travel, including restrictions on travel in and out of Cambodia, revised bio-security guidelines, and limitations on visa procedures, all of which were strictly reviewed by government agencies. The ban on entry of foreigners from Iran, Italy, Spain, Germany, France, and the United States came into force on 14 March. However, this travel ban did not target some Asian countries, including China. Following the entry ban, visa exemptions, tourist visas, e-visas, and visas on arrival to all foreigners were suspended on 28 March. Foreigners and Cambodians allowed to enter Cambodia were, and still are, required to self-isolate for 14 days upon arrival.

In early April, the traditional Khmer New Year reunion and Royal Ploughing Ceremony were canceled. A ban on inter-provincial travel was also issued, but this was later relaxed to allow people who lived in adjacent or nearby provinces to continue to commute. Civil servants, private office staff, and factory workers who had traveled prior to or after the decision was issued were required to conduct self-quarantine or enter a quarantine center, as well as submit to COVID-19 testing. Anyone who did not comply with these restrictions faced penalties, such as losing social benefits and undergoing 14-days mandatory self-quarantine without salary and allowances.

On 14 April, the Prime Minister joined the ASEAN Special Summit on Public Health Emergencies. From the Summit, ASEAN leaders established nine priority interventions ranging from shared incident management, planning and surveillance, and risk assessment to points of entry and operational logistics. The Prime Minister threw his strong support behind the establishment of a COVID-19 ASEAN Response Fund. The Prime Minister also reiterated that they should prepare strategies to restore and promote the economy post-COVID-19.[11]

Cambodia found itself sealed off after Vietnam unilaterally closed its border on 19 March, followed by similar notifications from Thailand and Laos. The Ministry of Justice began drafting a National Emergency Law in March and sent it to the National Assembly and Senate for approval in mid-April. After approving it, the law was sent to the Constitutional Council for review. After the council found that the law was constitutional, it was signed into law by Acting Head of State Samdech Say Chhum on 30 April. Internationally, human rights groups decried the law, saying that the law violated the rights to privacy, free speech, and peaceful assembly. Cambodian officials held news conference to not only explain the necessity of the law but its legality under the Cambodian Constitution.

On 20 May, extra entry requirements for foreign nationals were issued, including presenting a negative COVID-19 medical certificate and health insurance of at least US$50,000. To complement larger scale economic provisions, on 26 May the Ministry of Labor authorized cash aid for workers in the garment and tourism industries who were unemployed due to the pandemic. On 12 June, a sub-decree created a relief program to provide monthly cash payments worth US$25 million to over 560,000 needy Cambodian families. The payments helped lift the financial burdens these families carried and provided them with much needed daily necessities.

The government's approach to education has embraced many modern and innovative approaches. As all schools were closed, distance education and e-learning was encouraged and adopted. Teachers were given assistance in adapting their teaching approaches to the new format, working with the private sector to provide free data and online class scholarships. A new mobile app for distance learning was launched, and courses were provided to train teachers to create digital educational content. Even the annual entry and year-end exams went digital. On 21 July, it was announced that schools would open in three phases

---

11   ASEAN, https://asean.org/storage/2020/04/FINAL-Declaration-of-the-Special-ASEAN-Summit-on-COVID-19.pdf

in September, with the first cohort being the 20 schools having the highest safety standards, followed by those with moderate safety and then the minimum safety schools.

As the COVID-19 pandemic has stabilized in the country, casinos were allowed to reopen to give the economy a much-needed stimulus. Strict safety procedures were established for this reopening. A similar approach in Phnom Penh allowed restaurants, clubs, and entertainment venues to reopen provided that strict social distancing, temperature checks, and frequent disinfection protocols were carried out. On 15 July, the government announced a five-day holiday to make up for the canceled Khmer New Year celebration. Following the announcement, the Ministry of Health issued instructions urging individuals and local authorities to be extra-vigilant in preventing the spread of COVID-19 during the holidays.

Tough as they were, the actions taken by the Cambodian government were well-received by its citizens and lawmakers. The cabinet reshuffle in early April demonstrated the government's deep commitment to absorb the shocks to the economy caused by the COVID-19-induced global recession. The value-added tax on daily necessities was also relaxed, while the hotel and tourism industry has received a four months tax break. Furthermore, garment workers' loan payments have been rescheduled, interest rates have been lowered, and there are plans to dollarize.

In the meantime, mega public infrastructure projects have been suspended, as have exports of rice to ease food security. The government also launched an emergency reserve fund between US$800 million to US$2 billion to stabilize post-pandemic economic recovery. Together, these initiatives are the spear-heads of the government's response to the embattled economy. During the COVID-19 pandemic, Cambodia has been shown to be resilient, utilizing voluntary donations from civil servants, private sectors, and international communities to support their efforts to stop the spread of the virus. The collective response of both the community and the government have helped keep Cambodians safe and have highlighted this country as a role model in their response to COVID-19.

CAMBODIA

Oum Socheat
22.01–26.08 Total 273 cases / 0 deaths

22.01–20.02 (1 / X)

Public Health Policies

27.01 A Chinese man confirmed positive of Covid-19. Everyone in contact with him, including his family members, airport officials, a taxi driver and receptionists at two hotels where he stayed, were quarantined.

05.02 Working Visit of Prime Minister of the Kingdom of Cambodia to the People's Republic of China

13.02 MS Westerdam cruise ship with 1,455 guests and 802 crew members on board allowed to dock in Sihanoukville after rejected by five countries due to fears over the spread of COVID-19. Blood and other samples from the passengers were taken and any ill passengers were given a thorough check up before allowing all crew and passengers to leave the ship.

20.02–01.03 (1 / X)

Public Health Policies

20.02 Sihanoukville authority suspended the business activities of Chinese hospital Thay Khang without a license and released inaccurate information related to COVID-19 inciting fear and social unrest.

26.02 Phnom Penh Municipal Court charged and detained an online face mask vendor for cheating six people of more than $40,000 in exchange for imported protective face masks amid the COVID-19 outbreak.

The Cambodian People's Party (CPP) issued a statement supporting the announcement by World Health Organization which considered COVID-19 as an emergency and international concerns needed to tackle seriously.

28.02 More than two weeks after docked at Sihanoukville Port, MS Westerdam, along with crew members on board, finally left Cambodia.

29.02 ASEAN-US summit was put on hold as fears of a worldwide epidemic of the COVID-19.

01.03 Information Ministry asked national police to take measures against several Facebook accounts which have allegedly accused Cambodia contracting COVID-19.

Socio-Economic Policy Packages

21.02 The Ministry of Economy and Finance relaxed the tax over food for daily consumption.

24.02 Prime Minister announced a four-month monthly tax break for hotels and guesthouses in Siem Reap to facilitate businesses because they lost visitors out of fears of the Covid-19.

26.02 The government decided to exempt the 4 percent stamp tax on all residential properties valued less than $70,000 until January.

02.03–30.03 (108 / X) (Three major confirmed cases led to huge increase of infected patients and there was no case related to MS Westerdam cruise)

a. 29 tourists and two Cambodians being quarantined at a hotel in Preah Sihanouk province's Sihanoukville tested positive for the virus after coming into contact with two COVID-19 patients, raising the tally to 84

b. The Health Ministry recorded two more cases of COVID-19 in Kampong Cham and Koh Kong provinces, raising the tally of infection to 86.

c. 04 passengers of the Viking Cruise Journey tested positive for COVID-19 after being quarantined in Kampong Cham province, raising the toll to 91

Sources:

- Communicable Disease Control Department: http://www.cdcmoh.gov.kh/479-update-oncovid-19
- Ministry of Foreign Affairs and International Cooperation: https://www.mfaic.gov.kh
- Ministry of Economy and Finance: https://www.mef.gov.kh
- *Khmer Times*: https://www.khmertimeskh.com/page/1/?s=Covid-19

Public Health Policies

02.03 Cambodia donated 300,000 masks and protective suits to China.

05.03 Government postponed all its construction projects in a bid to earmark the budget in preparation for fighting the possible COVID-19 outbreak. The government expenditure reduced by 50 percent to save money which could be used to finance efforts for the containment of COVID-19.

Siem Reap Provincial Governor ordered his officials to search for locations where the Japanese national stayed after Vietnamese media reported that he tested positive for COVID-19.

Ministry of Health officials claimed that no new cases of COVID-19 in Siem Reap. The officials tested up to 425 cases without positive detection of COVID-19.

07.03 The government ordered to temporally close all schools in Siem Reap city in order to prevent the spread of Covid-19 after the second case was confirmed (the first local case).

10.03 The Ministry of Commerce with related government bodies took legal action against business owners, such as shopkeepers and market traders who are pushing up prices to take advantage of the continuing COVID-19 situation

Vietnam requested medical declarations implemented for travelers from EU and Cambodia. It was reacted strongly by the PM.

11.03 Justice Minister instructed prosecutors at all municipal/provincial courts to come down strongly against those who are spreading fake news regarding the outbreak in Cambodia.

12.03 The Health Ministry yesterday urged journalists not to name or show pictures of COVID-19 patients because it violates their right to privacy.

14.03 Following the temporary closure of schools in Siem Reap town amid the coronavirus pandemic, the Ministry of Education, Youth and Sport launched e-Learning courses for the affected students.

The government announced an entry ban of foreigners from Italy, Germany, Spain, France, and the United States for a period of 30 days to prevent the possible spread of covid-19.

16.03 The government intervened in helping four Cambodian river cruise vessels which are stuck at Vietnam's water border as its authorities denied their docking due to fear of a COVID-19 outbreak.

17.03 Students were advised to learn remotely as all public and private academic institutes in

Cambodia temporarily close in response to the upswing in COVID-19 cases.

Foreign Affairs Minister ordered returning diplomats from overseas to self-quarantine for 14-days as a safety precaution.

19.03 The Information Ministry blacklisted nearly 50 Facebook pages and accounts which were allegedly spreading fake news about the COVID-19 outbreak.

The Health Ministry urged suspected COVID-19 patients to self-isolate to prevent possible coronavirus infections among family members.

The Vietnamese government unilaterally locked down its borders with Cambodia and imposed a month-long entry ban for any foreign traveler – except accredited diplomats – as the country adopts measures to contain the spread of the coronavirus.

20.03 The Ministry of Health appointed Her Excellency Ek Vandy, secretary of state and spokesperson.

The Ministry of Culture and Fine Arts announced the nationwide closure of museums for the foreseeable future in light of the coronavirus crisis.

Local authority warned businesses and individuals against distributing and selling counterfeit alcohol-based sanitizers or facing serious legal actions.

The Government shut down the border with Vietnam amid COVID-19 fears. "We will be closing down the border," PM said. "This is not a response to Vietnam's closure of its border with us."

Interior Minister urged all citizens not to discriminate against any group or race as COVID-19 fears mount in Cambodia.

Thailand informed Cambodian citizens who wish to travel to Thailand they must obtain a health certificate and insurance worth at least USD 100,000.

22.03 180 people were quarantined in Kampong Cham province and Sihanoukville after having contacts with seven Malaysians and two French nationals who tested positive of COVID-19.

23.03 The Cambodia found itself almost sealed off after Thailand and Laos closed their borders amid coronavirus fears.

Local authorities searched for hundreds of Cambodian migrant workers who have just returned from Thailand and had them self-isolated to contain COVID-19.

7 Chinese medical experts arrived in Phnom Penh to help the country in its fight against the coronavirus. The experts scheduled to stay in Cambodia for two weeks.

24.03 The Cambodian Muslim community called

for non-discrimination against Khmer-Muslim people following an upswing in coronavirus cases in the Kingdom, which saw a string of Khmer-Muslims infected.

Interior Minister ordered provincial authorities to seek out migrant workers who returned from Thailand and conduct checks on them for the Covid-19.

25.03 Sihanoukville officials searched to identify people who may have come across 31 French nationals who tested positive of COVID-19.

The Garment Manufacturers Association in Cambodia (GMAC) called for collaboration from all stakeholders in facing the critical situation caused by Covid-19 pandemic.

The government considered requesting King Norodom Sihamoni to place the country in a state of emergency amid the COVID-19 pandemic.

26.03 Dr Tedros Adhanom Ghebreyesus, WHO Secretary-General, praised Cambodia for allowing the Westerdam to dock. "This is an example of international solidarity we have been consistently calling for."

The government announced public markets, grocery stores, factories and restaurants will continue operations despite the COVID-19 outbreak.

PM said the government has reserved more than 3,000 rooms in anticipa-

tion to treat coronavirus patients across Cambodia.

Twenty-two former passengers of the Viking Cruise Journey left the Kingdom and flew to their home countries after testing negative twice for COVID-19.

General Department of Prisons announced a temporary suspension of inmate visitation rights in a bid to prevent a spread of the coronavirus in correctional facilities.

Svay Rieng Provincial Health Department quarantined 174 Chinese nationals to ensure they are not infected with COVID-19 upon their arrival in Bavet city.

The Phnom Penh Municipal Administration temporarily closed public city bus and water-taxi service linking the northern part of Phnom Penh to Takhmao city in Kandal province via the Mekong River.

27.03 The government reiterated its warning that it is considering taking legal action against traders, particularly pharmacy owners, who are selling surgical masks at unreasonably high prices. It could even include confiscating the protection-offering products and ordering chemists to shut down.

A man in Kandal province questioned by military police for allegedly promoting COVID-19 fake news.

Phnom Penh governor urged vendors to run their businesses at markets as usual after some raised their concern over COVID-19.

The government announced a ban on private tutor sessions while a teacher was arrested for allegedly attempting to meet a student amid COVID-19 fears.

Battambang provincial health department officials searched for people who have been in contact with a group of French nationals who tested positive for COVID-19 in Sihanoukville, as 22 people have been quarantined over the case in province.

A total of 174 Chinese nationals were placed under quarantine by the Svay Rieng provincial health department after high body temperatures were detected in two of them.

The Ministry of Health confirmed that its officials have tracked down 340 people who had indirect contact with a French tourist group.

28.03 The government suspended visa exemption policy and issuance of tourist visa, e-visa and visa on arrival to all foreigners for a period of one month.

29.03 All 174 Chinese nationals in a group, who were quarantined in Svay Rieng province tested negative for COVID-19.

Socio-Economic Policy Packages

10.03 The government will still increase the salaries of civil servants, military and police personnel and retired people next year even though it needs to save funds to fight COVID-19.

11.03 The government announced to prepare an emergency reserve fund of between $800million and $2billion to aid Cambodia's economic recovery in the wake of pandemic.

12.03 Garment workers whose jobs suspended, allowed to delay their loan repayments to the commercial banks and microfinance institutions.

17.03 Government launched a $50million special fund for SMEs to boost competitiveness, productivity and daily business operations amid the impact of the pandemic Covid-19 and a 20 percent withdrawal of EBA trade deal.

18.03 Cambodian Central Bank (NBC) announced three new measures to facilitate and urge financial institutions to have stronger liquidity and encourage the nation's financial institutions to continue lending to the private sector, amid the COVID-19 pandemic.

NBC decided to reduce the interest rate of reserve requirement to 7% for both local and foreign currencies.

20.03 The Ministry of Planning predicted COVID-19 will hinder a national development plan from upgrading Cambodia to become a higher middle income country. The economy of Cambodia is to suffer the effects of two hard blows EBA withdrawal and COVID-19.

The Ministry of Economy and Finance encouraged gradual approach on de-dollarization as medium and long-term goals.

Cambodian and Vietnamese senior officials have announced measures to re-open trade across the Bavet-Mộc Bài border crossing.

24.03 The Ministry of Commerce declared it is working to stop opportunistic food sellers 'price gouging (Panic buying has started across Phnom Penh as Cambodian border closures due to COVID-19 causes fear of food shortages in the country).

Local laptop producer KOOMPI has released a free online educational platform, exclusively designed for Cambodian students to continue their education at home amid the COVID-19 shutdown.

26.03 Electricity Authority of Cambodia (EAC) called for licensed private electricity distributors to receive cashless payments for electricity bills to prevent possible COVID-19 infections.

The combined 400 mega Watt (mW) supply of power plants proposed to run on heavy fuel oil outskirt Phnom Penh will not generate power as planned in the first part of this year because construction has been suspended by COVID-19.

27.03 The government issued income tax exemptions for the textile and garment, footwear and luggage sectors that produced export goods hit by the European Union's 20 percent Everything but Arms (EBA) tariff-free status withdrawal in February.

Cellcard Mobile company has announced that it will give free voice calls and SMS to doctors and key medical staff during the COVID-19 pandemic.

29.03 Owner of Sihanoukville Special Economic Zone, donated one million face masks to the Cambodian Red Cross for use in preventing the spread of COVID-19 pandemic in Cambodia.

30.03 Agriculture ministry reassured the public that there is no need to panic over potential food shortages amid the ongoing COVID-19 pandemic.

31.03–30.07 (13 / X)
Public Health Policies

31.03 PM issued additional measures for the seizure and destruction of unregistered COVID-19 rapid test kits and medicines being sold in the market.

PM ordered a stop to all exports of white rice and paddy from April 5 until further notice.

All casinos across the country shut down from April 1 to stem the coronavirus pandemic, a move which could cost about 20,000 Cambodian workers in the sector their jobs.

The government drafted a law to allow it to declare a state of emergency to fight COVID-19.

01.04 The National Police arrested more than a dozen suspects connected to the production and sale of unregistered COVID-19 test kits.

The state of emergency draft law forwarded directly to the National Assembly without the need of the Council of Ministers to approve amid COVID-19 outbreak.

The Ministry of Health strengthened regulation of the sale of pharmaceutical drugs, medical equipment and disinfectants, including prohibiting the sale of such products online.

02.04 Cabinet reshuffle: the National Assembly approved four new cabinet members for the four ministries, namely Ministry of Justice, Ministry of Posts and Telecommunications, Ministry of Cult and Religion, and Ministry of Civil Service.

03.04 The tough measures took by the Cambodian government are

widely appreciated.

Court placed two Chinese nationals in pre-trial detention after they were charged for allegedly selling COVID-19 test kits.

Many pharmacies ran out of medical equipment and supplies such as masks, gloves, hand-sanitizers and medication amid skyrocketing prices.

Two more people arrested for allegedly peddling medicines said to be able to treat COVID-19.

Ministry of Commerce's officials cracked down on the sale of 3,000 liters of counterfeit alcohol sanitizers.

The government decided that it extends visas for foreign tourists, who stranded in Cambodia due to COVID-19 outbreak, until they are able to return to their countries.

05.04 50,000 Cambodian migrants returned from neighboring countries were closely monitored for their health and place them under quarantine where possible.

The National Police directed all officers to make sure people do not celebrate the upcoming Khmer New Year at large gatherings to prevent any spread.

The Ministry of Health issued a directive on the Covid-19 at barbershop, beauty salon and related services.

06.04 12 Cambodian patients who were sequestered at a quarantine facility in Kandal province will be discharged after testing negative twice for coronavirus.

07.04 Over 400 people who came in contact with the French tourists who tested positive for COVID-19 were allowed to return home after getting the all-clear, provincial health departments of Sihanoukville and Siem Reap revealed.

Foreigners wished to enter Cambodia amid the global COVID-19 outbreak are now required to self-quarantine for two weeks after arriving in the country.

PM called on the public to take extra precaution amid the Covid-19 outbreak in the country, noting that Cambodia is still at "high risk".

Government decided to ban a flight carrying 150 Cambodians from Malaysia from entering Phnom Penh.

08.04 The government called on monks to observe cleanliness and proper hygiene as PM announced pagodas will not be closed.

Authority found and seized around three tones of counterfeit alcohol and hand sanitizers as well as other unregistered items at some business locations in Phnom Penh.

All people entering Cambodia, either by air or by land, including migrant workers needed be quar-

antined in designated quarantine areas to avoid the possibility of these people from contracting or spreading to others.

The government cancelled the celebrations of Khmer New Year, the biggest holiday of the year.

Cambodia Monk Committee asked all pagodas across the country to cancel the Khmer New Year celebrations to contain the pandemic.

09.04 The Ministry of Education, Youth and Sport postponed the secondary and high school exams.

The Cambodian Government ordered a temporary ban of all sports activities and gatherings in the country.

Ministry of Labor and Vocational Training (MoLVT) requested the workers on unpaid leave during the cancelled Khmer New Year will have to undergo mandatory 14 days self-quarantine if they breach the government's subdecree.

10.04 The leaders of 17 unions issued a joint statement urging garment workers to work as usual during Khmer New Year amid the coronavirus outbreak. Workers returning from home provinces after the festival will have to undergo 14-day mandatory self-quarantine.

The government ordered a week-long ban on all cross-district travels.

12.04 The Royal Ploughing Ceremony cancelled.

13.04 PM was due to attend the Special ASEAN Summit and Special ASEAN Plus Three Summit on the impact of COVID-19 tomorrow via video conference at the capital's Peace Palace.

The Senate's Permanent Committee met to discuss the implementation of the Law on the Management of the Nation in Emergencies after the National Assembly unanimously approved the draft law.

14.04 ASEAN Special Summit on Public Health Emergencies (The Government of Cambodia has also implemented social distancing to contain the spread of virus by instructing all public and private schools to start the vacation earlier than the schedule, while all mass gatherings such as entertaining club, cinema, concert, beer garden, casino, gym and religious gatherings countrywide are temporarily banned. The government placed the nine priority intervention areas: (1) Incident management and planning; (2) Surveillance and risk assessment; (3) Laboratory; (4) Clinical management and health care services; (5) Infection prevention and control; (6) Non-pharmaceutical public health measures; (7) Risk communications; (8) Points of entry; and (9) Operational logistics.

Minister of Interior called on local authorities

to continue imposing mandatory 14-day self-quarantine for all inbound passengers coming from abroad, particularly migrant workers returning from Thailand.

The Labour Ministry said more than 90 percent of garment factory workers reported for work on the first day of Khmer New Year.

Interior Minister called on authorities not to punish anyone who flouts the government's directive on a week-long travel restriction, saying they should instead be educated.

The Health Ministry expressed concerns toward possible cluster infections following the growing number of COVID-19 cases.

16.04 PM said, ASEAN needs to think more about strategically restoring and promoting combined economic growth now and after the end of the COVID-19 crisis.

Foreign nationals, mostly Chinese, continued to enter the Kingdom despite the government's restrictive measures amid the coronavirus pandemic.

The Senate's Commission on Legislation and Justice finished its study on the "The State of Emergency" and said it does not violate the Constitution or any laws in the country.

The Municipal Health Department took samples of about 40 people, suspected to have come in contact with a Vietnamese woman and her Canadian husband infected with COVID-19 in Boeng Keng Kang district.

The Senate expected to approve the "State of Emergency" draft law right after its Permanent Committee moved to place the draft for a special plenary session.

17.04 The government lifted an inter-provincial travel ban across the Kingdom to ease traffic jams after the Khmer New Year holidays came to an end.

Cambodian migrant workers were allowed to overstay and work in Thailand until November due to Covid-19 restrictions.

In an extraordinary session of members of the Senate voted in favour of the "State of Emergency" draft law, passing it to the final phase of becoming a legislation.

Note verbal of the Permanent Mission of the Kingdom of Cambodia to the United Nations Office and other International Organizations at Geneva addressed to the Office of the High Commissioner for Human Rights on the State of Emergency Law.

20.04 The Ministry of Commerce strongly urged businessmen and companies to refrain from distributing counterfeit alcohol in the market amid the pandemic. The call comes after relevant ministries and institutions

found more than 80 tones of methanol being sold across the country.

More than 10,000 garment workers who recently returned to Phnom Penh from various provinces after the Khmer New Year placed in mandatory quarantine.

21.04 A total of 1,423 of garment workers were screened in 10 designated health centers.

Justice Ministry slammed United Nations Special Rapporteur, in her recent statement, Rhona Smith, UN Special Rapporteur on the situation of human rights in Cambodia, warned that the government's state of emergency law in response to the COVID-19 pandemic risked violating the right to privacy, silencing free speech and criminalizing peaceful assembly.

23.04 After eight days of no Covid-19 positive cases, Cambodia was confident that the pandemic is under control but not certain about whether the curve has been flattened. The recovery rate after treatment is also high with 110 cases of recovery after admission to various hospitals in the country. The containment of the virus to just 13 provinces in the country shows that the authorities are capable of ensuring it does not become a nationwide pandemic.

The Constitutional Council of Cambodia

prepared to review the "State of Emergency" draft law's adherence to the Constitution, the Justice Ministry dismissed the criticisms made by UN Special Rapporteur, saying her remarks showed "double standards" and were politically motivated.

The announcement of the Ministry of Civil Service to temporally suspend all public official recruitment exams due to Covid-19.

24.04 The Labour Ministry reported nearly 3,000 workers who had returned from their home provinces after Khmer New Year were screened for coronavirus over the past four days. And 2,850 workers had come for checks and 2,703 were allowed to self-quarantine at home for 14 days.

Deputy Prime Minister lauded the fact that to date, there has been no cases of COVID-19 positive among returning migrant workers. He lamented that though they registered zero COVID-19 positive cases thus far, they also registered zero inward remittances, meaning their families are now impacted with a lack of sustainable income. Out of an estimated 86,000 workers who had returned back to Cambodia in the last four weeks.

27.04 The Constitutional Council of Cambodia unanimously approved the draft law on "State of Emergency", passing it to

the final phase of becoming law.

28.04 About 10,000 garment workers visited their home provinces during the Khmer New Year failed to return to Phnom Penh for fear of being quarantined, with some of them resorting to farming.

Telephone Conversation between H.E. Deputy Prime Minister PRAK Sokhonn and H.E. Wang Yi, State Councilor and Minister of Foreign Affairs of the People's Republic of China on joint efforts to response to Covid19.

29.04 The Cults and Religion Ministry told local authorities not to restrict small-scale religious gatherings of fewer than 10 people.

The government called on all employees to celebrate the International Labour Day on May 1 in their homes amid the coronavirus pandemic. The warning comes as Labour Day celebrations are typically met with protests and gatherings of unions.

30.04 Acting Head of State Say Chhum signed the draft law on "State of Emergency" into legislation after the Constitutional Council of Cambodia unanimously approved it earlier this week.

05.05 The World Health Organization warned Cambodia remains at high risk of a second wave outbreak of

COVID-19, although Cambodia has achieved a good response to the first phase of the coronavirus.

More regional airlines begun to slowly reinstate flights to Cambodia's international airports this month – under strict biosecurity guidelines.

18.05 The announcement of Ministry of Health (MoH) for owners of hotel and restaurants to comply with Ministry of Health's advice on Covid-19 including temperature checking and social distancing.

19.05 MoH advised the Ministry Culture and Fine Arts of the resumption of museum operation for local and international visitors.

MoH advised to all cities and provincial governors on advice on Covid-19 second wave preventions within the constituency.

20.05 Inter-Ministerial Announcement on Covid-19 Preventions:

- Allow all foreign nationals to enter Cambodia included Iranian, Italian, German, Spanish, French and US which previously banned.
- All travelers demanded to have health certificate (Notification of No-Covid-19 infection within 72 hours before their departure) with 50K insurance during their stay in the country.
- All travelers had to wait at waiting hall (await for Covid-19 results) before leave the airport.

22.05 MoH's ordinance on sanitary, food safety for all restaurants in 25 provincial locations.

Inter-Ministerial announcement on the relaxation of sport activities.

26.05 Civil aviation announcement on prevention measures of air travel.

27.05 A press conference on Covid-19 prevention measures for Khmer passport holders in every checkpoint (without the demand of Covid-19 free certificates).

08.06 MoEYS announced to allow education institute to hold student's exam via online platform.

08.06 Online summit of Belt and Road on Covid-19, participated by Cambodian Foreign Minister, Prak Sokhonn.

03.07 Government ordered KTV to transform to restaurant to secure labor market.

15.07 Government Decree of New Year replacement holiday (17-21 August 2020).

17.07 MoH announced the preventive measures of Covid-19 during upcoming holidays.

21.07 MoEYS announced the resumption operation of 20 high standard private education institutes.

25.07 The announcement of MoH to temporarily suspend all flights from Malaysia and Indonesia.

28.07 MoEYS allowed sport activities in public space and Olympic stadium.

31.07 Inter-ministerial announcement on the reminder of preventive measures of Covid-19 from all entries and checkpoint into Cambodia.

Meeting on tourism package to Siem Reap province and other tourist hotspots (aimed to recover this sector).

Socio-Economic Policy Packages

31.03 The government eased measures by disbursing special low-interest loans to specialized banks in a bid to shore up the embattled economy.

01.04 The World Bank released several urgent recommendations to Cambodia, stating governments need to act quickly, cooperatively and at scale to avoid serious financial shock and recession due to the COVID-19 outbreak.

The World Bank has predicted the Kingdom's real economic growth will slow to around 2.5 percent this year because of COVID-19.

The $800 million to $2 billion COVID-19 stimulus package announced by PM last month will only be given to those businesses that are legally registered.

02.04 Prince Holding Group donated USD 500,000 and pandemic prevention supplies to th government.

The government secured a stockpile of milled rice to ensure a sufficient domestic supply of the staple.

COVID-19 health measures and high levels of micro debt posed a serious concern for the approximately 2.4 million Cambodians with a combined outstanding debt of USD 8 billion.

The National Bank of Cambodia (NBC) affirmed that commercial banking and finances have strong capital and liquidity.

US State Department on issued a statement noting the US gave USD 2 million last month for the Kingdom's fight against COVID-19.

03.04 The government stated its commitment to making e-governance a priority during the COVID-19 outbreak to ensure services remain timely and available.

Establishment of multi-technical working group of bank and finance measures to mitigate the impacts from Covid-19 pandemic and EBA withdrawal.

Establishment of working group on fiscal policy financing, social assistance to monitor Covid-19 pandemic.

Establishment of working group on social assistance mechanism during Covid-19 pandemic.

Establishment of working

group on monitoring supply and price of strategic goods during Covid-19 pandemic.

Several ministers and senior government officials pledged to donate their salaries towards the country's fight against COVID-19, taking the cue from the PM.

06.04 The Agriculture Ministry issued measures for farmers to follow to boost crop cultivation during the upcoming rainy season and fill food reserves.

07.04 SMEs expected to apply for a loan from the newly formed SME Bank of Cambodia.

08.04 The Garment Manufacturers Association in Cambodia (GMAC) stated approximately 60 percent of its garment factories are severely affected by cancelled orders.

The government decided to provide USD 70 a month for each worker once their factories temporarily suspended their operations due to pandemic.

09.04 The government announced to cut USD918 million capital expenditure this year to inject into the health sector to assist the fight against the pandemic.

The European Branded Clothing Alliance asked the European Union (EU) to postpone withdrawing tariff preferences granted to Cambodia under the EU's Everything but Arms

(EBA) trade scheme.

09.04 Inter-ministerial announced to provide cash support for pregnant women and child under 2 years old.

10.04 Commercial banks and microfinance institutions applauded the government's initiative to disburse special low-interest loans to specialized banks in a bid to shore up the embattled economy.

Cambodia received 7 tons of medical and preventive supplies from China.

15.04 PM fully supported the establishment of a 'COVID-19 ASEAN Response Fund' to tackle the pandemic, and called for a united effort to fight the coronavirus regionally and globally.

16.04 Minister of Agriculture ministry planned to purchase $3.5 million's worth of potato seeds, in a project partnering with South Korea to produce potatoes in the Mondulkiri province.

17.04 Siem Reap province initiated collective rice farming to ensure food security, especially for the most marginalized, amid COVID-19 pandemic.

The government established technical working group on harmonization enlisting and monitoring database on social protection

20.04 Amrit, a financial institution in Cambodia, offered a helping hand to its customers by offering

a loan repayment grace period to 120,000 group-loan clients whose livelihoods have been affected by COVID-19 pandemic.

The National Bank of Cambodia requested all banks and financial institutions to reduce all service fees related to loan and reschedule the penalty period for outstanding loan.

EU provided Cambodia a €56 million ($66.7 million) grant to enhance the country's efforts to control the Covid-19 crisis and restore the economy.

23.04 A landed property (Lim Cheang Hak) developer joined finance institutions by offering a payment delay to ease customers' financial burdens in response to the virus crisis.

Maybank Cambodia is adding free financial advisory services to all its business clients in addition to its existing help.

PRASAC, financial institution participated "SME Co-Financing Scheme," an initiative of the government of Cambodia, aimed at providing low-interest loans to bolster and develop the small and medium sized enterprises in Cambodia.

The Garment Manufacturers Association in Cambodia (GMAC) has stated approximately 60 percent of its factories have been severely affected by cancelled orders of ready-made garment exports

29.04 US Agency for International Development committed a USD 1.5 million aid to the Ministry of Health to help in the efforts to mitigate the spread of Covid19. The donation is the latest COVID-19 assistance from the US to aid Cambodia currently amounting to over USD 3.5 million.

Australia committed AUD 40 million ($26 million) for the Cambodian Health Equity and Quality Improvement Programme (H-EQIP), pledging to provide a further AUD 10 million ($6.5 million) over the next two years.

30.04 The Ministry of Labour and Vocational Training's announced that a total of 130 garment factories applied to suspend operations, putting an estimated 100,000 workers out of work and affecting a further 400,000 who are dependents, as the Covid 19 continues to wreak economic havoc, concerns have been raised that social unrest could become a problem in the already struggling economic environment.

Approximately 84,776 poor pregnant women and children aged under 2 years received support from the government. Poor women receive in total USD 190 each since the start of the pregnancy until two years after delivery

05.05 Ministry of Tourism introduced new guidelines this month for business health standards for tourism-related businesses such as hotels, restaurants and resorts as the ministry aims to increase domestic tourism.

The governments new USD100 million Small and Medium Enterprise Co-Financing Scheme has yet to approve any applications, receiving only some inquiries pending approval.

08.05 The government reassessed the cost of assistance to laid-off garment workers affected by the COVID-19 pandemic as it braces itself to spend more on rising unemployment (nearly 200 factories suspended their operations because of the COVID-19 pandemic, wiping out 200,000 workers' jobs).

18.05 Ministry of Education and Youth and Sport (MoEYS) announced the online teaching and training.

19.05 A meeting between Minister of Economy and Finance (MoEF) with Australian Ambassador on the supports of Australian government to Cambodia.

21.05 MoEF announcement of US's relief fund to Cambodia (Covid-19 impacts).

25.05 Advised by the government to seek and build up database of poor and vulnerable families, led by Ministry of planning.

26.05 Ministry of Labor and Vocational Training (third round of disbursement relief funds for workers in garment and tourism sector whom have been suspended by operations by Covid-19)

A press conference held by the government on the extra measures for garment, tourism (employee and employers) from the impacts of Covid-19 and the post-covid-19 economic recovery.

3rd round of disbursement for workers in garment and tourism sector whom have been suspended by the pandemic.

28.05 Donation of 140 of white rice for poor families in Phnom Penh City.

MoU signed by MoEYS and IDP education Cambodia on online English class scholarship for undergrads.

09.06 Fourth round of funds for workers in garment and tourism sector whom suspended by operations by Covid-19.

16.06 The announcement of fifth and sixth round of funds for workers in garment and tourism sector.

23.06 Ministry of Tourism held a meeting regional tourism.

The announcement of seventh round of funds for workers in garment and tourism sector.

24.06 USD 25 million circulated to 560,000 poor families (each month).

MoEYS introduced Onlineplus platform for education institutes.

25.06 The announcement of seventh round of funds for workers in garment and tourism sector.

07–12.07 The announcement of 9th 10th 11th 12th round of funds for workers in garment and tourism sector.

15.07 The announcement of Mobile Free Data Distance Learning (Cellcard).

16.07 The announcement of 16th round of funds for workers in garment and tourism sector.

22.07 France granted 1,5 million Euro for Post-Covid-19 recovery for tourism sector.

24.07 The announcement of 15th, 16th, and 17th round of funds for workers in garment and tourism sector.

29–31.07 The announcement of 18th 19th 20th 21st 22nd round of funds for workers in garment and tourism sector.

01.08–26.08
Major cases increased from outbound travelers (direct and connecting flight from Malaysia, Indonesia and the Philippines) Total cases 251 and recovered 219 cases, as of 10 August 2020.

Public Health Policies

04.08 The announcement of relaxation of families (each month).

Khmer Passport holders to enter Cambodia.

05.08 A retreat meeting of MoEF on the resumption of education institute.

The relaxation measures on diplomatic passport holders (Visa type A and B).

10.08 MoEYS the resumed high school classes from September.

11.08 Government agreed with MoEYS to hold national exam.

MoH announced to temporarily suspended all flights from the Philippines.

14.08 MoH reminded public on health advice for the replaced upcoming holidays (replaced Khmer New Year) from 14-17 August.

25.08 MoEYS announced the 2nd phase reopening kindergarten, private primary and high school (Bak Tok high school is the first public allows to reopen).

Health advice for upcoming Pchum Ben Festival.

27.08 The signing to operate digital system for all high school in Cambodia.

28.08 MoH announced the security tighten at COVID-19 quarantine centers.

31.08 Health advice for upcoming Pchum Ben Festival (COVID-19 measures and food poisoning prevention) .

MoH announced the mechanisms for the reimbursement of the deposit of COVID-19 test from foreign travelers.

Socio-Economic Policy Packages

06.08 Technical supports from Swiss government to create online application.

18.08 MoEYS announced USD 95,000 research creativity and innovation fund 2020 (RCI Fund) including Digitalized for IR4.0; Applied agriculture research; and 21st Century Pedagogy Research.

21.08 World Tourism Organization applauded PM on COVID-19 health measures and promote local tourism.

22.08 The visit of Japan Foreign Minister to Cambodia to promote cooperation against COVID-19 pandemic.

26.08 The announcement of 25th and 26th round of funds for workers in garment and tourism sector.

COVID-19 in Mainland China: Anti-epidemic Social Mobilization under Comprehensive Management

Lanlan Xu and Yuqing Liang

As the original epicenter, China adopted a strategy of comprehensive control to deal with the pandemic. The centralized decision-making and command system efficiently allocated resources and applied strict control measures, including city-wide lock-downs, closures of most business activities, and severe restrictions on resident movements. This kind of "shock therapy" has had a rapid impact on infection control while raising questions internationally about social costs and sustainability. There has also been considerable diplomatic tension.

On 31 October 2020, the number of cumulative confirmed cases of COVID-19 in Mainland China reached 85,997, with 4,634 deaths and total of 81,004 recoveries (see Figure 3.1).[1] According to the reports from 31 provinces, autonomous regions, and municipalities directly under the Central Government and Xinjiang Production and Construction Corps, there were 24 new cases, 69 new asymptomatic patients, and 0 deaths (marking 200 days of zero COVID-19-related deaths between 15 April 2020 and 31 October 2020) (see Figure 3.2).

**Figure 3.1 Cumulative confirmed cases, cured and discharged cases,
and deaths from 20 January 2020 to 31 October 2020**

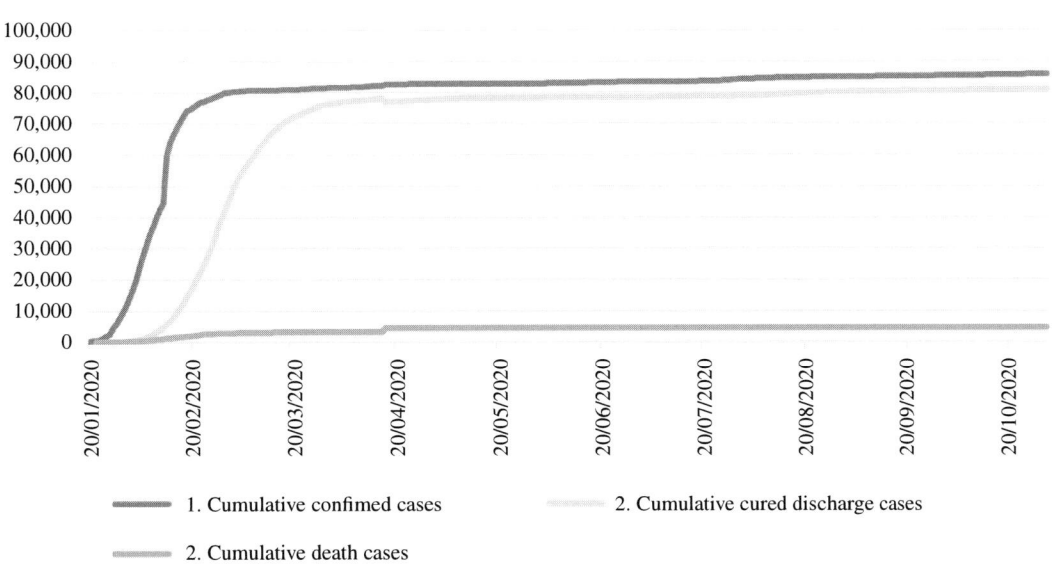

---

1   Most data are drawn from the Timeline (Mainland China). Other sources are individually specified.

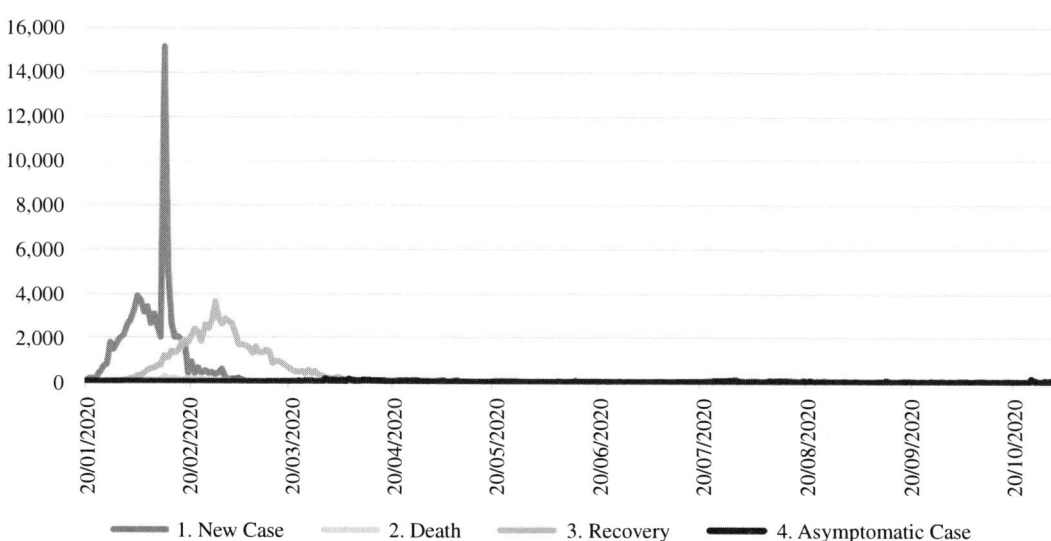

Figure 3.2 Daily new cases, deaths, recoveries, and asymptomatic cases from 20 January 2020 to 31 October 2020

Case Development

The first confirmed patient with COVID-19 in Mainland China dates back to 1 December 2019, as disclosed by an article in *The Lancet*. However, the earliest case officially reported was 8 December 2019. The response to the COVID-19 pandemic in China can be divided into four stages:

- Stage 1: the initial period (December 2019 to 19 January 2020);

- Stage 2: the outbreak period (20 January 2020 to the end of February 2020);

- Stage 3: the disruption period, which was characterized by the interruption of local transmission and imported overseas cases (March 2020 to April 2020); and

- Stage 4: the maintenance period, which focused largely on the normalization of epidemic prevention measures (beginning in May 2020).

Stage 1: Initiation (December 2019 to 20 January 2020)

The COVID-19 pandemic originated in Wuhan, the capital of Hubei Province. The number of the confirmed cases during this stage reached 291. At the beginning of December 2019, a cluster of patients with pneumonia of an unknown cause, all with travel records to the Huanan Seafood Market, aroused the attention of local doctors. In the following days, specimen samples were sent to gene laboratories in Guangzhou, Shanghai, Beijing, and other places for next-generation sequencing (NGS) testing. The test results showed that this virus was a new type of coronavirus similar to, but different from, the coronavirus responsible for severe acute respiratory syndrome (SARS). An alarm bell was rung by Wuhan authorities as well as those in Beijing.

On 30 December, Dr Li Wenliang, a doctor at Wuhan Central hospital, sent a message to a group of fellow doctors warning them about a possible outbreak of an illness that resembled SARS. On 31

December, a team of experts from the National Health Commission (NHC) in Beijing arrived in Wuhan to investigate. On the same day, the Wuhan Center for Disease Control and Prevention (CDC) and the Wuhan Health Commission notified the media that there was no obvious "human-to-human" transmission or infections within the medical sector in Wuhan. On 2 January, eight doctors, including Li Wenliang, who had issued an early warning to the public via social media, were accused by the government of making false statements and spreading rumors that disturbed public order. The accusation was publicly broadcast on television. At the same time, the new virus in Wuhan attracted the attention of the World Health Organization (WHO), which released its first statement on 6 January concerning the outbreak of unexplained pneumonia cases in China.

On 18 January, the officials of the Baibuting community in Jiang'an District, Wuhan City, organized a large number of citizens to participate in the Wanjia (literally "ten thousand households") Banquet to celebrate the upcoming Chinese Lunar New Year. The annual meetings of the Hubei Provincial People's Congress and Political Consultative Conference were also held as scheduled in the second and third weeks of January.

At that time, other provinces were mostly unaware of the disease outbreak in Wuhan. However, private discussions started to circulate in Shenzhen as they noticed that many Hong Kong citizens, their neighbor to the south, were starting to wear face masks in early January. Some doctors in Shenzhen hospitals also sent text messages to their relatives and friends in other parts of the country to tip them off to the possible risks, referring to suspicious cases in Shenzhen imported from other Mainland provinces.[2] On 18 January, nationally renowned respiratory expert Professor Zhong Nanshan of the Chinese Academy of Engineering, who earned international fame for managing the SARS outbreak in 2003, rushed to Wuhan to conduct an urgent investigation overnight. On 20 January, at a press conference organized by the NHC, Zhong confirmed that the new coronavirus could be transmitted from person to person. The whole country was immediately in an uproar. People rushed to snatch face masks off the shelves, and the prices of masks quickly soared. In many places they were simply out of stock. The sequence of the virus was soon published on an open-access database. Various speculations and rumors about the origin of the virus also started to spread within communities.

Stage 2: Outbreak (20 January to end of February 2020)

The confirmation of human-to-human transmission by Zhong Nanshan on 20 January 2020 marks the beginning of Stage 2 of the outbreak. From 20 January to the end of February, the epidemic quickly spread across the country, and all provinces reported cases by end of February. The number of confirmed cases during this stage was 80,251. On 20 January, President Xi Jinping, gave instructions on the work related to the epidemic, emphasized that party committees, governments, and relevant departments at all levels must put people's lives and health first. The NHC started making daily reports of the new cases in each province. The next day (21 January), the WHO announced that it would set up an emergency committee to monitor the outbreak of the epidemic.

Figure 3.3 shows the distribution of the first batch of reported cases across China. Numerous provinces reported their first confirmed cases during the week of 19–25 January, highlighting the rapid spread of the epidemic.

---

2   Fieldwork, Shenzhen, January 2020.

Figure 3.3 Distribution of the first confirmed cases in 31 provinces in Mainland China

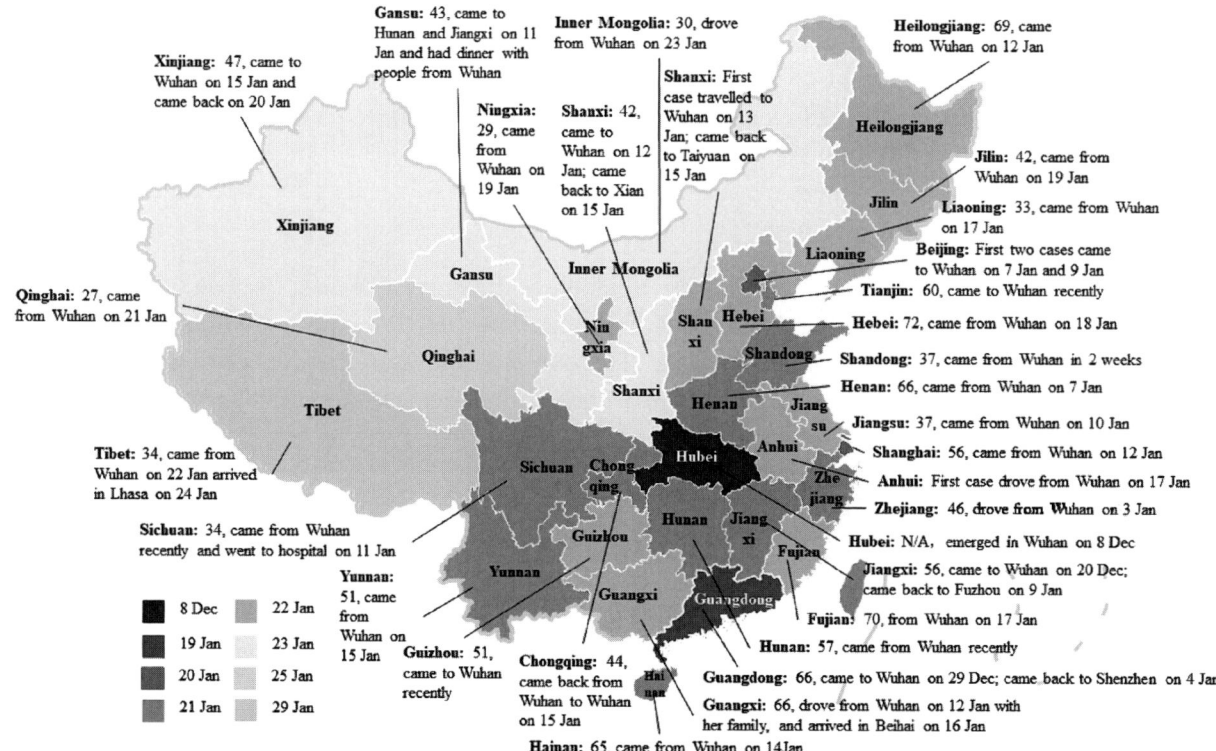

The first batch of areas reporting confirmed cases included the more economically developed cities, such as Shenzhen, Beijing, and Shanghai. On 19 January, Shenzhen City announced its first confirmed case, a traveler from Wuhan. On 20 January, Beijing and Shanghai announced their first confirmed cases. On 21 January, Tianjin, Zhejiang, Hainan, and several provinces adjacent to Wuhan, including Henan, Shandong, Chongqing, Sichuan, Yunnan, Hunan, and Jiangxi, announced their first cases. On 22 January, the remaining areas in eastern and central inland areas announced their first cases, including Liaoning, Jilin, Heilongjiang, Hebei, Shanxi, Jiangsu, Anhui, Fujian, Guizhou, Guangxi, and Ningxia. On 23 January, infections were reported in the western provinces of Shanxi, Gansu, and Xinjiang, as well as Inner Mongolia. On 25 January, Qinghai announced its first case, and four days later, on 29 January, Tibet made a similar announcement. By then, the virus had spread to all provinces of Mainland China. All of these first cases were either from, or had recently been, to Wuhan, the epicenter.

While the virus spread, the situation in Wuhan worsened. In the early morning of 22 January, Hubei Province announced the implementation of a Second-Level response to the public health emergency. On the same day, the National Healthcare Security Administration and the Ministry of Finance issued a notice that coronavirus treatment costs would be covered by medical insurance. The NHC also issued the "New Coronavirus Infection Pneumonia Diagnosis and Treatment Plan (Trial Version 3)" and advised citizens not to travel to Wuhan and for Wuhan citizens not to leave the city.

From 10 a.m. local time on 23 January, Wuhan, a city with more than 10 million people, shut down its public transport as it tried to halt further spread of the virus. All flights and passenger train services out of Wuhan were stopped. Bus, subway, and ferry services were also terminated. However, in the interval of several hours between the announcement of the city-wide shutdown and the actual closure of roads and facilities, about three million Wuhan citizens reportedly left Wuhan.

The news of a city-wide lockdown in Wuhan alerted the rest of the country to the serverity of the epidemic. Many netizens criticized Wuhan and Hubei authorities for concealing the information about the virus and failing to contain the outbreak in its early stages in Wuhan. Faced with serious public criticism, the Wuhan governor emphasized that they had dealt with the situation in strict compliance with national laws and regulations.

On the same day of the Wuhan lockdown, the provincial governments of Zhejiang and Guangdong launched a First-Level response to the public health emergency. The Central Government also urgently allocated 1 billion yuan in financial prevention and control subsidies to Wuhan. Following these actions, other provinces also launched First-Level responses. Many inter-provincial roads set up body temperature monitoring points to identify possible patients. In some cities, public transportation was reduced or suspended. Roadblocks were also set up between the villages to prohibit outsiders from entering. Urban residential communities used access passes or electronic "health codes"[3] to control the movements of residents.

In Wuhan, hospitals and clinics were flooded with patients, while many were turned away due to a shortage of doctors, nurses, and medical resources. Medical teams from other parts of China arrived to assist. In order to solve the problem, learning from the "Xiaotangshan" hospital model during the 2003 SARS outbreak, which was built in Beijing in six days, the Wuhan Urban Construction Bureau urgently held a special meeting on 23 January and decided to build two emergency hospitals, "Huoshenshan" and "Leishenshan", to provide the necessary isolation beds for infected patients, with intensive care units, general wards, and auxiliary departments (such as infection control, inspection, special diagnosis, and radiological diagnosis). Construction of Huoshenshan started two days later, on 25 January.

Multiple issues emerged in the local emergency epidemic prevention measures in the weeks after the commencement of the lockdown, however. The livelihood resources which were donated to Wuhan from various parts of China, intended to help Wuhan residents, were slow to arrive to front-line medical staff and citizens, and the Red Cross and local government units were found to be grossly inefficient and ineffective in their coordination role. The local medical sector was overwhelmed by the escalating number of cases. Images of exhausted front-line medical workers in overcrowded wards flooded social media. Many patients were not isolated and treated in time, resulting in the rapid spread of the virus among family members and the community.

Social anxiety and criticism reached a high point in February. Capturing the social atmosphere, the online *Wuhan diaries* by Wuhan writer Fangfang registered the difficult lives of ordinary people in Wuhan during the lockdown. The *"diaries"* quickly gained currency among netizens and became an important source of information about the epidemic for people outside Wuhan. As the *"diaries"* attracted nationwide attention, different views emerged over its possible repercussions, from both a positive and a negative perspective. Some people criticized the *"diaries"* for exaggerating the situation. In March, the

---

3   The "health code" is based on real data, by the public or rework personnel through their own online declaration, which can generate a personal QR code after the background audit. The QR code, as an electronic certificate, can achieve a declaration of universal access to all parts of the local region. On 11 February 2020, Hangzhou City, Zhejiang Province, took the lead in launching the health code model. The local government implemented the dynamic management of residents and people who planned to enter Hangzhou under the three-color system of "green code, red code, and yellow code". Members of the public and prospective visitors to Hangzhou can make their own online declaration through APPs such as Alipay; after filling in information such as health condition, whether they have come into contact with a newly diagnosed patient or a suspected patient within 14 days, a color code will be generated after verification. The persons with a green code can pass through by code, while persons with a red code or yellow code should be isolated and do daily health report online; only when the conditions are met, the color of their code will be converted to green. Since then, the "health code" management information system enabled in Zhejiang Province has quickly spread throughout the country.

news that Fangfang's diary would be published overseas in several foreign languages added fuel to the criticism, and Fangfang was fiercely denounced for amplifying the dark side of the city's response to the epidemic, and for causing damage to China's international image.

On 2 February, the Central Government enlisted relevant units from the People's Liberation Army to assist in Wuhan's anti-epidemic work, including the management of the newly built Huoshenshan hospital and vaccine research. In addition, 16 mobile field hospitals, or "Fangcang" (literally a "cabin") hospitals, with over 200,000 beds were set up in Wuhan through conversion of existing facilities, such as stadiums and exhibition halls, to provide community care and quarantine facilities for patients with mild symptoms.

In addition to the worries over public health, the health of the economy was also at risk. By the end of January, in order to prevent people from gathering, all workplaces and social facilities were closed down, with the exception of factories that produced virus prevention materials. The government also centralized the allocation of anti-epidemic protective materials, given the emerging shortage, to ensure adequate supply to the medical sector. It was difficult for people to buy face masks in the market at the time, for example. Seeing the large demand, some firms started to modify their production lines to produce face masks and protective clothing.

Economic hardship was increasingly felt because of the closure of businesses. In mid-to-late February, two manufacturing powerhouses in the country, Zhejiang and Guangdong, took the lead in restarting economic activities. In Zhejiang, special buses were hired to take workers who had returned home for the Chinese New Year in January back to work in the factories. Other provinces quickly followed suit and by the end of February, all provinces had re-opened their workplaces except Hubei.

As China's neighbors, North Korea and Russia moved first and closed their borders with China on 22 and 30 January, respectively. On 17 January, the United States imposed entry screening on passengers from China. At the end of January, Xi Jinping met WHO Director-General Tedros Adhanom in Beijing to discuss the response to the epidemic. At the meeting, Adhanom showered praise on China for its quick response. However, as the epidemic soon worsened, there were allegations that the Chinese government concealed information during the early stages. By the end of January, the United Kingdom had suspended flights to and from China. The United States, Japan, and Australia also successively imposed restrictions on entry from China. International criticisms over the lack of transparency of the Chinese government in the epidemic intensified. By the end of February, more countries turned their attention to developing COVID-19 vaccines.

Stage 3: The Disruption of Imported Cases (March to April 2020)

Domestic transmission of the epidemic was mostly under control by early March, with case numbers dropping significantly across the country. In the meantime, many Chinese students in overseas universities returned to China as the outbreak spread in Europe and North America. The anti-epidemic focus of the Chinese government turned to containment of imported cases. Beijing and Guangdong faced a relatively high risk due to their large overseas communities, as well as the fact that many returning students flew into these cities before heading to other Chinese cities. Starting from 1 April, all incoming passengers were required to undergo a nucleic acid test upon arrival and were put in centralized quarantine for 14 days.

As the outbreak in Europe and the United States deepened during March and April, complaints from other countries against China surged. The Chinese government sought to help and shipped face masks and other medical supplies to Italy, the first European country suffering an outbreak, followed by other countries. These actions had mixed results. Despite an initial welcome by segments of the population, China was quickly criticized for using "mask diplomacy" to win the hearts and minds of people around the world.

Wuhan ended its lockdown on 8 April. On 10 April, the number of critically ill patients with COVID-19 in Hubei Province fell to double digits for the first time. On 26 April, all confirmed cases in hospitals in Wuhan were cured. In this stage, the number of confirmed cases dropped to 2,712.

Stage 4: Normalization of Epidemic Prevention (since May 2020)

Since May 2020, anti-epidemic measures have focused on controlling the number of imported cases and preventing a rebound of cases in the community. There were 3,123 confirmed cases during this stage (1 May – 31 October). On 7 May, the State Council proposed to (1) prioritize prevention; (2) strengthen infection control measures in public places, such as entertainment venues, medical institutions, campuses and communities, and susceptible populations; (3) expand the scope of nucleic acid tests, optimize the health code by leveraging big data, and strengthen scientific research and international cooperation; and (4) dynamically adjust the risk level and emergency response level in different areas.[4] These measures subsequently proved effective, as no major outbreak has happened since, including during the high risk periods of "Golden Week" or during the annual sessions of the People's Congress and Political Consultative Conference in May.

When new clusters of cases re-emerged in Beijing, Xinjiang, and the North-East, these four measures were ruthlessly adopted to contain the epidemic. On 7 May, Shulan district in Jilin City in North-East China reported its first locally confirmed case. As the number of confirmed cases increased, four districts in Jilin City were defined as high or medium-risk areas. On 13 May, Jilin closed the city's borders. The lockdown lasted until 6 June, 14 days after no new local cases were recorded. This local outbreak registered a total of 48 locally confirmed cases and one death.

On 11 June, a cluster of cases broke out in a wet market (Xinfadi Market) in southern Beijing. The similarity with the Huanan Market outbreak in Wuhan caused alarm, especially in the context of Beijing as the nation's capital. In order to curb the spread of the epidemic, local areas were classified into high-, medium-, or low-risk levels according to their distance from Xinfadi Market, and residents in the high-risk areas were required to have a nucleic acid test. At the same time, Beijing upgraded its control measures in many districts. The government of Fengtai District, where Xinfadi Market is situated, implemented a "wartime" control strategy, closing the Xinfadi Market immediately and adopting isolation measures in several of the neighboring communities. At midnight on 30 July, a total of 335 confirmed cases had been reported, with 326 recoveries and no deaths. By 6 August, there were no longer any confirmed cases.

On 22 July, Dalian city in Liaoning province, reported a new confirmed local case. The infected person was an employee of an imported aquatic product processing enterprise, Kai Yang Seafood Company. Dalian immediately implemented its control plan. It started an epidemiological investigation and began enforcing personnel quarantine and nucleic acid testing. However, the infection chain of the epidemic in Dalian had expanded to six cities in Heilongjing, Jilin, and Liaoning provinces by 24 July. Dalian City restricted the movement of people in medium- and high-risk areas and also advised people in low-risk areas not to leave Dalian unless necessary. By 30 July, Dalian had a total of 68 confirmed

---

4   Guiding Opinions of the State Council on the Normalization of Prevention and Control of the Covid-19 Epidemic (Guo Fa Dian [2020] No. 14) [EB/OL], www.gov.cn/zhengce/content/2020-05/08/content_5509896.htm, 2020-08-08.]

cases, of which 34 were employees of Kai Yang Seafood Company and another 11 were related parties. By 30 August 2020, all patients had recovered.

There was a similar outbreak of cases in Xinjiang on 15 July. On 19 July, some places in Xinjiang were categorized as high- and medium-risk, and adopted corresponding control measures. In contrast to the outbreaks in Beijing and Dalian, where the number of confirmed cases dropped within 14 days, the number of newly confirmed cases in Xinjiang kept on an upward trend. At the same time, two rounds of nucleic acid tests were completed in Urumqi, the capital of Xinjiang. On 30 July, the communities in Urumqi were blocked off. On 31 July, the number of newly confirmed cases dropped to 31 from 111 of the previous day, marking the turning point of the Xinjiang outbreak. With the alleviation of the epidemic, the high- and medium-risk areas were adjusted to low-risk on 30 August. By 7 September, the number of confirmed cases was reduced to zero.

However, in a comment about these local clusters, Zeng Guang, the former chief epidemiologist of the CDC in China, stated that there was no need to feel so apprehensive, even though the clusters meant that the epidemic was rebounding. As people understand more about the disease and become more skilled at implementing the anti-epidemic measures, the risk of a national epidemic is decreasing.[5]

In May, over 120 WHO member nations, led by Australia, the United States, and others, called for an independent probe into the origins of COVID-19 in China. This initially drew an angry response from the Chinese government, but the Chinese President Xi Jinping later endorsed a WHO-led inquiry. On 10 July, a two-person WHO team arrived in Wuhan for a three-week trip to identify the origins of COVID-19. In August, it was reported that the WHO team was merely laying the groundwork in advance of a full international mission to investigate the virus but it was also vague on whether this larger task force would visit Wuhan. This report sparked international concerns over the credibility of the inquiry.[6]

The Response to COVID-19 in Mainland China

Comprehensive Management and Control: Centralized Decision-making and Command System

On 7 January, President Xi Jinping convened a meeting of the Politburo Standing Committee of the Chinese Communist Party (hereafter referred to as PSCCCP), which laid the parameters for the prevention and control of a "pneumonia epidemic with unknown cause".[7] On 20 January, in a directive on anti-epidemic work, President Xi stressed that "we must attach great importance to the epidemic and do our best to prevent and control it". On 25 January, the first day of the Chinese Lunar New Year, President Xi presided over another meeting of the PSCCCP to discuss the growing epidemic. Reportedly this was the first time a formal PSCCCP meeting was ever held on Chinese Lunar New Year's Day, showing the urgency of the anti-epidemic work.[8] At the meeting, the Committee decided to set up a new Central Leading Group to lead the work on the epidemic and dispatch a Central Steering Group to

---

5　*Xinlang News.* http://finance.sina.com.cn/wm/2020-07-29/doc-iivhvpwx8140089.shtml

6　"Failure by WHO team to visit Wuhan sparks concerns over virus probe". *Financial Times.* www.ft.com/content/f9dea077-66fb-4734-9d1d-076dc93568e1.

7　The State Council Information Office of the People's Republic of China, "Fighting Covid-19 China in Action" [EB/OL]. www.scio.gov.cn/ztk/dtzt/42313/43142/index.htm.

8　Xinhuanet, www.xinhuanet.com/politics/xxjxs/2020-02/17/c_1125587543.htm.

Wuhan to strengthen national oversight. The State Council would play a coordinating role through its Joint Prevention and Control Mechanism program.

President Xi presided over a series of special sessions to fine-tune prevention and control strategies. In the initial outbreak stage of the epidemic, the Central Committee of the CCP (hereafter referred to as CCCCP) formulated a policy stressing the containment of infections in the community and across borders, whether inward or outward. On 25 January, the CCCCP instructed Hubei Province to make the anti-epidemic work its top priority, to take more stringent measures, and resolutely prevent the spread of the epidemic.[9] On 10 February, it was noted that Beijing, as the national capital, had a major responsibility for the prevention and control of the epidemic, and a policy stressing the containment of infections in the community and across borders was formulated.[10] On 23 February, the different emphases on work by different localities were further clarified: Hubei Province would focus on containment, while other large cities and provinces with large population flow, cities in Hubei, and provinces neighboring Hubei, were to take measures to prevent infections. Together, the goal was to minimize the number of imported cases from other regions and the number of exported cases to other regions.

During March, the second phase of anti-epidemic work, the virus was largely contained domestically, while the risk of importing cases from Europe and North America was on the rise. The strategy was refocused to minimize importation risks and the subsequent rebound of local community cases. On 23 March, Premier Li Keqiang said at a meeting of the Central Leading Group that while the spread of the epidemic across the country had basically halted, the risk of sporadic cases and local outbreaks still existed, and the global pandemic situation was still complex and severe. He called for continuous application of vigilance to guard against a rebound of cases.[11] On 8 April, President Xi noted during a meeting of the PSCCCP that "in the face of a severe and complex international epidemic and economic situation, we should always think about worst-case scenarios and make ideological and work preparations to cope with future changes in the external environment".[12]

The Joint Prevention and Control Mechanism of the State Council played a key coordinating role. Regular meetings were held to monitor and analyze the epidemic, allocate human and material resources across provinces, and adjust work strategies and measures. In mid-to-late February, the State Council initiated a plan to steer the economy back to normal operations after the earlier lockdown and partial closures. All provinces, cities, and counties had set up emergency command mechanisms to coordinate the work of not only government departments, but also party units, enterprises, social organizations, and resident associations in local neighborhoods.

Rapid Societal Mobilization

The response of communities across Mainland China is best described by the Chinese saying 一方有難，八方支援 ("When trouble occurs at one spot, help comes from all quarters"). The national anti-epidemic response was characterized by centralized and unified deployment from the top and the mobilization of a broad range of organizations, corporations, and residents, down to the community and household levels. This mechanism played a critical role in the defensive battle of Wuhan as well as in the successful control of epidemics in other areas.

---

9 *The People's Daily*, http://paper.people.com.cn/rmrb/html/2020-01/26/nw.D110000renmrb_20200126_2-01.htm.

10 *The People's Daily*, http://paper.people.com.cn/rmrb/html/2020-02/11/nw.D110000renmrb_20200211_2-01.htm.

11 *The People's Daily*, http://paper.people.com.cn/rmrbhwb/html/2020-03/24/content_1977844.htm.

12 *The People's Daily*, http://paper.people.com.cn/rmrb/html/2020-04/09/nw.D110000renmrb_20200409_2-01.htm

Take the case of Wuhan. First, it organized the largest medical support operation since the founding of the People's Republic of China. On 24 January, medical teams from various provinces and from the army set out overnight and rushed to Wuhan. According to official statistics, more than 330 medical teams and more than 41,600 medical personnel from 29 provinces, autonomous regions, and municipalities, as well as the Xinjiang Production and Construction Corps and the military, provided assistance to Wuhan over the course of the outbreak. Sixteen mobile cabin hospitals with more than 14,000 beds were built within 10 days. Meanwhile, for other cities in Hubei Province (except for Wuhan), 19 provinces sent medical teams to assist, based on arrangements by the Central Government.[13]

Second, priority was given to the medical and food supply in Hubei Province. Although many workers in medical enterprises had been away during the Spring Festival holiday, many enterprises cut the holiday short and resumed production early. At the same time, other industries also quickly modified their production lines to produce masks, protective clothing, disinfectants, thermometers, and other anti-epidemic materials. At the beginning of February, the daily production of N95 and other medical-grade masks were only130,000 and 5.86 million, respectively. However, these numbers were increased to 5 million and 200 million by the end of April. These materials were delivered continuously to key areas through unified distribution networks. At the same time, the Central Government made arrangements to provide living materials to people in Hubei Province, where a lot of cities had been shut down since late January and the economy was at a standstill. Altogether nine provinces and 500 companies were engaged in providing emergency supplies and transportation. The products included, for example, frozen pork, originally in the central reserve stock, and vegetables.

Shortages still posed a lot of challenges, however. Some localities found it necessary to scramble for resources to meet local needs even at the risk of defying central command. For example, in February, officials in Dali City, Yunnan Province, once intercepted the anti-epidemic materials on transit in its jurisdiction but which were scheduled for Chongqing City and other places. The officials in Qingdao City and Shenyang City also detained each other's supplies.[14]

Strict Measures and Community Participation

Soon after Wuhan started its lockdown on 23 January, many regions launched their first-level emergency responses to the public health emergency and entered states of "emergency during wartime". The most comprehensive, strict, and thorough anti-epidemic measures were soon launched across the nation.

Although it was the Lunar New Year holiday, the Central Government urged people to stay at home and not to visit relatives or friends. The state-run media repeatedly broadcast basic knowledge of epidemic prevention, such as proper washing hands procedures, and advocated wearing masks. In order to reduce the size of crowds, some parks and public facilities were closed and large-scale performances were cancelled. For those few who did not immediately wear masks, the staff at community venues, subways, shopping malls, and other places warned them or prevented them from entering the premises. The Spring Festival holiday, which usually lasts for two weeks, was also extended to keep people home.

Since the beginning of February, some provinces have introduced the "health code", an electronic device to track infected patients, and many local communities also strengthened the control over the

---

13 *The People's Daily*, http://paper.people.com.cn/rmrb/html/2020-02/24/nw.D110000renmrb_20200224_1-02.htm

14 Netease News. http://news.163.com/20/0206/19/F4NNRS960001899O.html

flow of people. For example, some local communities required that only one person in a family could go out once a day with a pass. In-city public transport services was also drastically reduced, with some areas even going out of service. Roadblocks were erected on inter-provincial and inter-city highways. Most people simply stayed home. Many cities looked like ghost towns, with only a lone car or two on the streets.

Strict measures and tiers of interlocking deployments pressed the "pause button" on social operation. With the goal of "missing no one (patient)", grass-roots party organizations, as well as neighborhood and village committees, worked hard on the anti-epidemic front-lines to find suspected cases, measured everyone's body temperature, implemented closed-off community management procedures, and tracked the travel paths of confirmed cases. Government departments and relevant units at all levels invested a large number of personnel during the period, which was a part of the huge social costs incurred by these measures.[15]

Social forces had a limited role in this grid-based, grass-roots governance system. At the beginning of the outbreak, official non-governmental organizations, such as the Red Cross, were responsible for distributing all kinds of donations to Wuhan and other cities in Hubei Province. The authorities stressed the need for order in disaster relief work, and rules concerning the role and participation of civil society in this circumstance were not yet in place. They did not exist and there was no precedent of good practices to give any guidance. Many problems soon emerged, such as a lack of manpower, low administrative efficiency, and insufficient use of information technology, which turned the Wuhan Red Cross into a target for complaints. The agency was criticized for monopolizing its role in disaster relief and its failure to deliver.[16] In response to the failure of the Red Cross, CCP members and cadres were organized to work in the communities. In addition, local residents were encouraged to participate in community work on infection control. Some residents also joined bottom-up neighborhood mutual assistance activities, such as guarding and disinfecting the local area, logistics support to fellow residents (e.g., buying food or medicine), or taking body temperatures at community gates.

A high degree of social cooperation with the government was a key factor in the effective control of the epidemic. Mainland people basically understood the necessity of closed-off management of communities and villages, registration and control of personnel movement, temperature measurement, quarantine, and wearing masks, and thus, obeyed the rules. Many families gave up the traditional habit of family reunions during the Spring Festival, and many businesses and workers suffered huge economic losses because of the infection-control measures, but they still cooperated with the government. Meanwhile, workers in industries that support social operation kept working regardless of the risk of infection. A large number of enterprises, organizations, individuals, and overseas Chinese citizens donated money and materials, demonstrating the spirit of solidarity and a high sense of social responsibility.

However, it is clear that the strict prevention and control measures carry very high costs which are difficult to sustain. The severe lockdown of Wuhan City and Hubei Province, and the nationwide suspension of production and the practice of "not giving up anyone", have resulted in a high recovery rate of 94.3%. The estimated economic cost of this recovery rate was 3 trillion yuan in the first quarter of 2020 alone.[17] With an effective, well-tested vaccine still a long way from use, finding a sustainable strategy to contain the uncertain trend of infection is a question that require more thought.

---

15 Xinhuanet, www.xinhuanet.com/politics/2020-02/10/c_1125553920.htm

16 IFeng.com, http://finance.ifeng.com/c/7tmzqD8ZRDc

17 Wechat. https://mp.weixin.qq.com/s/UZeF5sHImWGBGsbEaicvQQ

Evolving Measures

A comprehensive understanding of a new virus is an outcome of research and evolves over time. In the beginning, knowledge about this strain of COVID-19 coronavirus was limited. Expert opinions on the matter of human-to-human transmission shifted over time. After an initial judgment of no human-to-human transmission, a team of six experts, including Professor Zhong Nanshan, concluded the existence of human-to-human transmission on 20 January. Based on this information, epidemiology expert Professor Li Lanjuan of Chinese Academy of Engineering proposed the closure of Wuhan to stop the spread out of the city. Next came the suggestion of using the Spring Festival holiday to implement a nation/community-wide self-quarantine at home, by Professor Zhong Nanshan and other experts, which reduced social contact, and thus the spread of infection, during what is otherwise an intensive social festival. Professor Wang Chen of the Chinese Academy of Medical Science proposed establishing temporary mobile field hospitals to achieve the objective that "all suspected and confirmed patients should be admitted to the hospital". These proposals were quickly adopted by the Central Leading Group on the epidemic.

Experts in virology, epidemiology, clinical medicine, and other related fields have played a prominent role in anti-epidemic control in China. The scientific research explores the source of infection and transmission routes, and tracks virus mutations. The resultant deepening of knowledge of the disease enables the government to adjust and optimize its infection-control measures in a timely manner. The NHC has revised and issued six editions of plans for the prevention and control of COVID-19, and an additional 15 types of plans for infection-control and 6 plans for psychological counseling for key population groups, places, and units. A total of 50 technical guidelines are provided in these plans, greatly improving the accuracy of epidemic prevention and control. The NHC also revised eight editions of the diagnosis and treatment plan for COVID-19, three of which were for severe and critical cases, two for the management standards for light and ordinary cases, two for convalescent plasma therapy, and one for rehabilitation therapy for primary dysfunction of discharged patients.[18] Chinese experts were the first team to publish the entire genome of the virus in January, facilitating further research on the virus, including the development of diagnostic kits, therapeutic drugs, and vaccines. At present, there are six COVID-19 vaccines in Phase III clinical trials worldwide, three of which are from China.[19] Medical experts, such as Dr Zhang Wenhong of Shanghai Medical College of Fudan University, have been active in popularizing the practical knowledge of daily prevention and control tips to the public.

At times, questions have been asked about the infection control approach that has been taken in China. Some scholars have pointed out that China has basically controlled the epidemic through tight control and isolation, but has not formed the herd immunity. With a high risk of imported cases, the epidemic is likely to re-emerge. Chinese society cannot remain in such a tight state of control.[20] Another controversy is over the efficiency of traditional Chinese medicine in the treatment of COVID-19. The official reports suggest that 92 percent of the newly diagnosed cases have been treated with Chinese medicine, and the utilization rate and total effective rate of Chinese medicine in Hubei Province are all above 90 percent, showing the unique advantages of Chinese medicine as a treatment.[21] Indeed, Professor Zhong Nanshan and another famous academician, Zhang Boli, were among the advocates of the Lian Hua Qing Wen capsule, a specific form of

---

18 The State Council Information Office of the People's Republic of China, "Fighting Covid-19 China in Action" [EB/OL]. www.scio.gov.cn/ztk/dtzt/42313/43142/index.htm

19 Xinhuanet. https://baijiahao.baidu.com/s?id=1674319891157566904&wfr=spider&for=pc

20 Caixin, http://opinion.caixin.com/2020-03-14/101528385.html

21 The State Council Information Office of the People's Republic of China, "Fighting Covid-19 China in Action" [EB/OL]. www.scio.gov.cn/ztk/dtzt/42313/43142/index.htm

concentrated Chinese medicine, as a cure for COVID-19 symptoms. However, the medical communities at home and abroad have remained critical and unconvinced.[22]

Big data technology features conspicuously in China's response to COVID-19. The personal "health code" has become the residents' credential for daily travel, a de facto permit to go back and forth to work or school, and regain access to public places. The process has seen a number of internet companies taking a lead, by launching instruments such as the epidemic map, a platform to refute rumors and online medical services, which provide great convenience to everyday life in the context of an epidemic. Despite these benefits, criticism of this tech boom falls into two areas. The first is an equity issue. Vulnerable groups have been left out of this frenzied pursuit of technology and their lives marginalized. For example, most elderly do not have a smart phone or cannot apply independently for a health code. Thus, their ability to travel independently has been negatively affected. Moreover, although many citizens have agreed to give up their private information now to meet the urgent need to control the epidemic, they are always alert to the risk of abuse. In May 2020, when the city government of Hangzhou tried to normalize the use of the health code by collecting health data of Hangzhou residents after the primary outbreak there had subsided, it caused a strong backlash. Netizens ferociously criticized the attempt, saying it was beyond the boundaries of epidemic prevention and that it violated individuals' rights to privacy. The Hangzhou Health Commission was forced to back down, stating that the health code "is only a concept, there is no plan to go online now".[23]

Anti-epidemic Diplomacy and International Tension

In March 2020, as the domestic epidemic came under control, the developing spread in other countries started to change the global environment and led to a period of heightening international tension, which remains unabated at the time of writing in September 2020.

The official stance has emphasized multi-lateral cooperation. The Central Government took the initiative to cooperate and exchange information with the WHO starting from the initial outbreak phase in January 2020. The specific measures taken include: (1) regularly informing the WHO and other countries about the epidemic situation in China; (2) sharing the whole genome sequence of COVID-19 and information about nucleic acid detection primers for COVID-19 with other countries; (3) exchanging experiences with epidemic prevention and control with international organizations and countries, such as Korea, Japan, Russia, the United States, and Germany; and (4) compiling the guidelines for diagnosis, treatment, and prevention of COVID-19 and translating them into three languages. In addition, the Chinese government sent professional medical teams abroad to render assistance with anti-infection measures and donated medical protective equipment to 150 countries. In fact, by the end of May, 29 teams of medical experts had been sent from China to 27 countries, including Serbia, Cambodia, and Pakistan. Two hundreds countries and regions have bought medical supplies, such as masks, protective clothing, goggles, breathing machines, test kits, and infrared thermometers, from Chinese companies. A moratorium on debt repayment was arranged for 77 developing countries, and assistance was expanded for more than 50 African countries.[24]

---

22 Sohu, www.sohu.com/a/393684665_114835. Separately, another patented Chinese medicine, Shuanghuanglian, an oral liquid that had once been described by the Shanghai Institute of Medicine of the Chinese Academy of Sciences and the Wuhan Institute of Virology as an effective cure, caused a crash toward the medicine in the market. Medical opinions on its efficacy for COVID-19 remain divided amongst Chinese medical experts, however.

23 Sohu, www.sohu.com/a/398263993_223323.

24 The State Council Information Office of the People's Republic of China, "Fighting Covid-19 China in Action" [EB/OL]. www.scio.gov.cn/ztk/dtzt/42313/43142/index.htm.

However, Western countries, in particular the United States, are wary of the possibility that China could expand its geopolitical influence through medical aid. China's aid has been criticized as "mask diplomacy" to seek benefits from the epidemic and highlights "a struggle for influence". U.S. President Donald Trump described COVID-19 as the "China virus" in a tweet message, sparking a heated wrangle between the United States and China.[25]

In May, President Xi Jinping endorsed a WHO-led inquiry by inviting a WHO team to investigate the origins of COVID-19. However, the news that the two-person WHO team had not visited Wuhan during its three-week trip in July again aroused concerns over the credibility of the inquiry.[26]

China claims that the U.S.-led criticism of its public diplomacy in fighting the epidemic is primarily based on the desire to make China a scapegoat for the United States' failure in anti-epidemic control. In addition, China accused some Western media of using the pandemic to alienate China's relations with African countries. For several months now, China and the United States have repeatedly scolded the other for "dumping the blame", and the atmosphere is getting increasingly tense.

Socio-economic Measures

The suspension of socio-economic operations in late January and February had an unprecedented and significant impact on China's economy. Restrictions on the movement of people and on assembly activities led to a significant decline in consumer demand. Retail sales of consumer goods in China fell 20.5 percent in February compared with that a year earlier. Business profits, government taxes, and household income fell, while the risks of bank and local debt increased. The urban unemployment rate rose to 6.2 percent in February, with unemployment increasing by nearly 4 million people. The electricity consumption of society as a whole dropped by 8.2 percent compared with that a year earlier.[27]

In mid-February, with the exception of Hubei Province, the number of newly confirmed cases nationwide was declining. In order to minimize the economic losses caused by the epidemic, the Central Government decided on 16 February that all government departments except those in Hubei Province would restart work, and economic production would resume. Four measures were adopted to facilitate the recovery: (1) offering special preferential interest rates and loans to enterprises that produce essential products, and those that have suffered huge losses because of the epidemic; (2) kick-starting a number of major construction projects to stimulate the economy; (3) maintaining the previous consumption level; (4) organizing the return of migrant workers in key industries.[28]

After March, the economy began to recover quickly as the domestic epidemic was largely contained. The Central Government issued a series of circulars calling for the cancelation of all obstacles that impeded the movement of people or goods, and the "resumption of work according to the risk classification". At

---

25　The Chinese official accounts of the origin of COVID-19 have undergone several changes. In early March, a foreign ministry spokesman told a news conference that the outbreak first appeared in China, but did not necessarily originate there. On the evening of 12 March, Foreign Ministry spokesman Zhao Lijian tweeted that COVID-19 may have been brought to Wuhan by the U.S. military. After triggering an international outcry and backlash from the United States, China softened its stance. On the 13th, Foreign Ministry spokesperson Geng Shuang said at a press conference that "[t]he international community has different views on the source of the virus. The Chinese side always believes that this is a scientific issue and we need to listen to scientific and professional opinions." Source: Sohu, www.sohu.com/a/379900773_655796.

26　*The Financial Times*, www.ft.com/content/f9dea077-66fb-4734-9d1d-076dc93568e1.

27　Hu Angang. "China's epidemic prevention and control and expansion of domestic demand against the background of the new global pandemic". *Journal of the Xinjiang Normal University*, 2020(6) : 7-19.

28　Qstheory.com, www.qstheory.cn/yaowen/2020-01/25/c_1125502099.htm.

the same time, the government adopted some supportive policies, such as tax relief, suspension of the collection of old-age pensions, reduction of or exemption from highway fees, provision of loan interest subsidies to alleviate some people's financial burdens.

From April to May, various economic indicators changed from negative to positive, indicating the recovery of the domestic economy. In the face of the global economic recession caused by the spread of the virus, the Chinese government put forward the strategy of expanding domestic demand. On 22 May, Premier Li Keqiang, in his report on the work of the government at the third meeting of the 13th National People's Congress, called for greater efforts to strengthen the "six stability and six guarantee" issues[29] and to provide a package of economic recovery plans to expand domestic demand. By this point, the following four economic stimulus policies had been adopted to hedge the negative impact of COVID-19 and push society and the economy back on the track for normal growth.

The first economic stimulus policy involves a number of *proactive fiscal measures*. For instance, special anti-epidemic bonds totaling one trillion yuan were issued at the end of July. The proceeds from these bonds were allocated to local governments to cover their expenditures toward infection control and the construction of public health infrastructure, and financial difficulties at the grassroots levels. These measures also involve the expansion of special local debts. According to the 2020 government work report, the new debt limit for local governments will be 3.08 trillion yuan this year, of which 2.15 trillion yuan will be earmarked for special debt, an increase of 800 billion yuan over last year. In order to promote the expansion of consumption and effective investment, the government will pool funds in a targeted way, support the construction of major projects under construction (such as railways supported by the state, national highways and local highways, and power and gas supply projects that support the advancement of the state's major strategy), and strengthening the weak links. Another proactive fiscal mesure is the implementation of reduced taxes and fees. The government will continue to reduce the value-added tax rate and the enterprise pension insurance premium rate this year, with a scale of about 500 billion yuan. The expiration of tax and fee reduction policies[30] has also been extended to the end of 2020. The income tax payment of small and micro enterprises and individual businesses will be postponed to 2021. It is estimated that taxes and fees for enterprises will be reduced by more than 2.5 trillion yuan over the whole year. In addition, to lower production and operating costs, industrial and commercial electricity prices have been reduced by five percent, and the average tariff for broadband and private lines will be reduced by 15 percent by the end of 2020. The government report went on to state: "We must firmly persist in implementing the policy of reducing taxes and fees, and win the future."[31]

The second economic stimulus policy is the *relaxation of the pre-existing "prudent monetary policy"*. The measures under this policy include lowering the reserve requirement, increasing the amount of refinance by 1.8 trillion yuan, and launching the small-scale enterprise credit loan support program. The financial sector will support enterprises by: lowering interest rates, adopting direct monetary policy tools, and reducing bank fees. These measures are expected to help enterprises save 1.5 trillion yuan

---

29 "Six stability" refers to stable employment, stable finance, stable foreign trade, stable foreign investment, stable investment, stable expectations; "Six guarantees" refers to the protection of employment, the basic livelihood of the people, the main market, food and energy security, industrial chain stability, and grass-roots operation.

30 These tax reduction and fee reduction policies specifically include exempting small and medium-sized and micro-sized enterprises from the payment of old-age, unemployment, and industrial injury insurance units; reducing or exempting small-scale taxpayers from value-added tax; exempting value-added tax on public transport, catering and accommodation, tourism and entertainment, cultural and sports services; and reducing or exempting civil aviation development fund and port construction fees.

31 State Council Research Office. *The third session of the National People's Congress*, Beijing: People's Publishing House, 2020.

in 2020. By the end of May 2020, the M2 balance of broad money had increased by 11.1 percent and the stock of social financing had increased by 12.5 percent. The above-mentioned monetary and credit support policies will make the national loan balance in 2020 exceed 175 trillion yuan.[32] Through the above measures, key medical goods and living materials enterprises can get some support, and this financial support will become an important driver of economic growth.

The next economic stimulus policy involves adopting measures to save jobs. This includes: (1) maintaining the existing employment rate; (2) creating new jobs; (3) promoting the employment of college graduates; and (4) helping the unemployed get back to work. To reduce the cost of hiring workers, the policy of exempting small and medium-sized enterprises from paying premiums for old-age pension, unemployment insurance, and industrial injury insurance has been extended until the end of 2020. The value-added tax for small-scale taxpayers has also been reduced or exempted. The unemployment insurance premiums will also be returned to small and medium-sized enterprises that do not lay off employees or reduce the number of employees. Banks, especially small and medium-sized banks, have been encouraged to reduce the financing costs of small and micro enterprises, to defer their loan repayments, to stabilize the cash flow of enterprises, and to enhance the ability of enterprises to operate normally and stabilize employment. Significant effort has been made to help the nearly 200 million self-employed people in urban and rural areas, such as small businesses, hourly workers, and temporary workers, to tide them over through the difficulties of the epidemic. Job creation will be increased by expanding effective investment. Indeed, the government has vigorously supported the "three new" economies (platform economy, sharing economy, and digital economy) that have achieved rapid development in the midst of the epidemic, and has advocated for the acceleration of the construction of key national projects to increase the rate of resuming work and promote employment growth. Similarly, to promote the employment of college graduates in 2020 and 2021, many vacancies in public institutions nationwide will be earmarked for their special recruitment. College graduates are also encouraged to work in grassroots public institutions in remote areas and start up business by themselves. While these effort focus on students new to the job market, significant effort will also be made to help the unemployed get back to work. A unified national service platform for unemployment registration was launched on 31 March to provide those affected with job transfer or re-employment services. A number of temporary public welfare posts have also been developed in various regions to provide job-hunting opportunities for the unemployed. Large-scale vocational skills training has been organized, especially job-transfer training specifically geared toward those that have lost their jobs because of the virus.[33]

The last economic stimulus policy is the implementation and acceleration of *a new economic development pattern*, which pays more attention and energy on the domestic market and considers the global market as complementary. The Chinese government believes that economic development must be adjusted against the expected decline in world trade post-COVID-19. On 21 July, President Xi Jinping hosted a symposium for entrepreneurs and said that China must take advantages of the super-large-scale domestic market, and "gradually form a new pattern of development with the domestic market as the main body, and the domestic and international market develop together (逐步形成以國內大循環為主體、國內國際雙循環相互促進的新發展格局)".[34] On 30 July, the PSCCCP re-emphasized that China should accelerate the formation of a new development landscape. They suggest that this can be accomplished by first building a strong domestic consumer market by increasing government expenditure on public services (such as the development of the life service industry, the old-age and child

---

32 Xinhuanet, www.xinhuanet.com/finance/2020-06/18/c_1126128464.htm.

33 *The People's Daily*, http://paper.people.com.cn/rmrb/html/2020-06/22/nw.D110000renmrb_20200622_1-18.htm.

34 Xinhuanet, www.xinhuanet.com/politics/leaders/2020-07/21/c_1126267575.htm.

care industries, and the supply of community life services). This is intended to drive the consumption expenditure of residents, especially the consumption demand for services. Another measure to help achieve this goal is to build a strong domestic investment market. This includes investment in new-type infrastructure construction (such as the new-generation 5G information network) to achieve nationwide coverage at the prefecture, city, and county levels; investment in new-type urbanization to improve the public infrastructure and service capacity of county-level cities and speed up the transformation of old urban areas; and investment in transportation, water conservancy, and other major projects to enhance agricultural and rural infrastructure. This policy also includes measures aimed at stabilizing foreign trade, which is suffering from the double impacts of the epidemic and the sharp contraction of international market demand. These measures include increasing the export tax rebate rate, simplifying the export tax rebate procedures, and reducing taxes and other financial policies. At the same time, the opening of air, sea, and land logistics networks to facilitate the import and export of goods and the cross-border movement of business people is being promoted under the precondition of effective prevention and control of the epidemic. In addition, the government actively supports export enterprises, takes advantage of the domestic super-large-scale market, promotes turning export products into domestic sales, and advocates opening parallel industrial supply chains in the domestic and foreign markets.

The government has stressed that holding China's domestic economy in a primary position does not mean closing its doors to other countries. The so-called "new development pattern" is essentially a way to achieve stronger and more sustainable development by giving full play to the potential of domestic demand, enhancing connections between the domestic and international markets, and making better use of international and domestic resources. Professor Liu Yuanchun, vice-president of Renmin University of China, said: "In the future, China will not build a simple and unconditional open system, but rather seek a more diversified, balanced, safe and efficient open system. Such a new system must be built on a solid foundation. That is the efficient domestic cycle."[35]

Conclusion

In January 2020, after the sudden outbreak of COVID-19, the epidemic spread rapidly to all provinces and regions of China in a few weeks. Adopting a mode of comprehensive management and control, the government soon adopted drastic measures, including city-wide lockdowns which cut off each city from the rest of the country and the world, closures of most business activities, severe restrictions of resident movements, and strict home quarantine measures. Social and economic activities were halted. In the early days of the outbreak, officials in Wuhan City were guilty of withholding information and malfeasance in disease prevention and control. In addition, the ineffective administrative systems, over-formalism, and bureaucratism of many officials in patient care and supply management came under public criticism. The tsunami of online tributes to Dr. Li Wenliang after his death from COVID-19 and the attention drawn to the online "Wuhan Diaries" are the tip of the iceberg of societal anger that stemmed from how the early months of the epidemic were handled.

Since then, a "comprehensive, whole country management approach" to epidemic prevention and control was put in place. Through a strict grid-based grassroots governance system and high-tech support by experts, the epidemic situation was basically under control in just over a month. Public psychology also dramatically reversed, from the initial heavy grief and anger to one of pride for Chinese citizens,

---

35   Youth.cn, http://pinglun.youth.cn/ll/202007/t20200707_12399585.htm.

although international diplomacy suffered (and still suffers) as other countries have dealt with their own epidemics.

The outbreak of COVID-19 in China and the process of fighting the disease have exposed many deficiencies in China's state governance system and modern governance capabilities. For China, the epidemic is both a threat and an opportunity. Despite the huge social and economic costs, the comprehensive, all-society management approach to epidemic control has worked for China. This has won back a good deal of trust among the Chinese population towards the government. In July 2020, Edelman, a well-known public relations corporation in the United States, released trust survey which reports that the Chinese people's trust in their government reached 95 percent, up 5 percentage points from the beginning of the COVID-19 outbreak in January 2020.[36] China was ranked number one among the countries surveyed. In contrast, the global average trust in government stood at 65 percent, up only 11 percentage points from January. Some Chinese scholars even believe that the epidemic will "provide a good opportunity to launch further reforms".[37] The threat comes from the changes in the international environment. The disputes concerning the source of the epidemic, and the conspicuous differences in the approaches and performances between the West and China in fighting the epidemic, as well as other geopolitical issues such as Hong Kong and the South China Sea, have triggered a new wave of conflicts.[38] Relations between China and the West, particularly the United States, have continued to deteriorate, with an accelerating "decoupling" and a *de facto* "new Cold War" taking shape. Domestically this has triggered a new economic policy stressing domestic consumption and "in-country circulation". How to manage sustainable growth amid the escalating international tension is the greatest challenge.[39] Against this, achieving successful containment of the COVID-19 will be an important prerequisite. The question is: how does China (and the rest of the world) sustain the current approach of control in view of the immense social costs involved?

---

36 Xinhuanet, www.xinhuanet. COM/MRDX/2020-07/27/C_139243339.HTM, 2020-08-18.

37 Zhao Dingxin." New Crown Disease and China Reform". *Beijing Cultural Review,* 2020(8) : 69–77.

38 *Lianhe Zaobao*, www.zaobao.com/forum/expert/zheng-yong-nian/story20200505-1050797.

39 Clifford, Zheng Tao. "The crisis of epidemic situation and the task of Chinese ideological circle". *Beijing Cultural Review*, 2020(8) : 36-41.

Mainland China

Dingyi You, City University of Hong Kong, Hong Kong, China
Guilan Zhu, Tsinghua University, Beijing, China

17–23.11.2019–31.10.2020 Total 85,997 cases / 4,634 deaths

AIDS = acquired immunodeficiency syndrome
CAA = Civil Aviation Administration
CAS = Chinese Academy of Sciences
CCP = Chinese Communist Party
CDC = Center for Disease Control
CFA = China Film Administration
GAC = General Administration of Customs
GASC = General Administration of Sport of China
MARA = Ministry of Agriculture and Rural Affairs
MC = Ministry of Commerce
MCA = Ministry of Civil Affairs
MCT = Ministry of Culture and Tourism
ME = Ministry of Education
MERS = Middle-East respiratory syndrome
MF = Ministry of Finance
MFA = Ministry of Foreign Affairs
MHC = Wuhan Municipal Health Commission
MHRSS = Ministry of Human Resources and Social Security
MHURD = Ministry of Housing and Urban-Rural Development
MIIT = Ministry of Industry and Information Technology
MJ = Ministry of Justice
MPS = Ministry of Public Security
MST = Ministry of Science and Technology
MT = Ministry of Transport
MVA = Ministry of Veterans Affairs

NATCM = National Administration of Traditional Chinese Medicine
NBS = National Bureau of Statistics
NDRC = National Development and Reform Commission
NFDA = National Forestry and Grassland Administration
NHC = National Health Commission
NHSA = National Healthcare Security Administration
NIA = National Immigration Administration
NIH = National Institutes of Health
NIPA = National Intellectual Property Administration
NMPA = National Medical Products Administration
NPR = National Public Radio
PCR = polymerase chain reaction
PSB = Public Security Bureau
SAMR = State Administration for Market Regulation
SARS = severe acute respiratory syndrome
SASAC = State-owned Assets Supervision and Administration Commission
SME = small and medium sized enterprises
SPC = Supreme People's Court
SPP = Supreme People's Procuratorate
SSC = State Supervisory Commission
STA = State Taxation Administration
WHO = World Health Organization
WIV = Wuhan Institute of Virology

The majority of the contents in this timeline are drawn from the official websites of the Chinese Government, Hubei Provincial Government, and Wuhan City Government. Other sources are listed individually when referenced.

Key and Abbreviations:

(*P) = Policy of Chinese Central Government:
    www.gov.cn/zhengce/index.htm

(*C)= News of Chinese Central Government
    www.gov.cn/xinwen/index.htm

(*N) = National Health Commission of the People's Republic of China (PRC)
    www.nhc.gov.cn/xcs/xxgzbd/gzbd_index.shtml

(*H) = Hubei Provincial Government
    wjw.hubei.gov.cn/bmdt/ztzl/fkxxgzbdgrfyyq/index.shtml

(*W) = Wuhan City Government
    wjw.wuhan.gov.cn/ztzl_28/fk/tzgg/

(*O) = Timeline from the World Health Organization (WHO)
    www.who.int/zh/news-room/detail/29-06-2020-covidtimeline

(#) = Numbers and text in brackets denote possible cases and developments as demonstrated in retrospective studies. However, at the time, these had not yet been reported in any of the official Chinese Government sources. This is the case for much of the information for November and December 2019.

*   values reported by Prof Cao Bin's team in The Lancet on 24 January 2020;

**   values reported by the Center for Disease Control (CDC) team directed by Gao Fu in *The New England Journal of Medicine* on 29 January 2020. Notably, the data reported in these two papers were not consistent. As Gao Fu's work provides more details concerning the daily confirmed cases, we mostly refer to his work.

17–23.11.2019

Major Development

17.11 There is a report of a patient who manifests symptoms of a previously unknown virus in Wuhan.[1]

01–07.12.2019 (1)**

Major Development

01.12 Confirmation of the first patient to manifest symptoms in Wuhan.[2]

08–14.12.2019 (3)**

Major Development

08.12 Another "first" confirmed case.[3]

15–21.12.2019 (17)**

Major Development

15.12 A 65-year-old delivery man in the South China Seafood Market in Wuhan runs a fever and antibiotic treatment is ineffective.[4]

22–28.12.2019 (34)**

Major Development

24.12 The Guangzhou Vision Medicals Company receives clinical

specimens from Wuhan's pneumonia patients for investigation.[5]

26.12 Dr. Zhang Jixian of the Wuhan Xinhua hospital reports four suspicious cases to the local CDC via the hospital management system.[6]

BGI Genomics receives clinical specimens from Wuhan's pneumonia patients taken on 24 Dec.[7]

The Shanghai Public Health Clinical Center receives clinical specimens from Wuhan's pneumonia patients.[8]

27.12 The Guangzhou Vision Medicals Company tells the Wuhan Centre Hospital that the 24 Dec clinical specimens sample indicates a new strain of coronavirus.[9]

Clinical specimens from the 41-year-old man who sought hospital treatment in Wuhan are sent to CapticalBio Medlab for testing.[10]

29.12.2019 – 04.01.2020

44 cases of unknown origin in Wuhan; (74) by 3 Jan; and (87) by 4 Jan**

Public Health Policies

30.12 The Wuhan CDC issues an emergency directive regarding a stream of patients with symptoms of pneumonia of unknown origin and requires all medical institutions to closely monitor and report similar cases. (*W)

31.12 Large-scale disinfection is carried out at the South China Seafood Market in Wuhan. A number of suspicious cases are connected to the market.[11]

Wuhan Union Hospital establishes an isolation zone for infectious respiratory disease patients.

01.01 The South China Seafood Market closes.[12]

The NHC establishes the Central Leading Group to help mediate the response to the epidemic. (*C)

Major Development

29.12 BGI Genomics says that the test results on the 26 Dec clinical specimen indicate that the genes of the virus are similar to, but not the same as, SARS. It is a new coronavirus.[13]

The WIV and CAS receive clinical specimens from Jin Yin-tan Hospital.[14]

One hospital in Wuhan reports cases to the CDCs at provincial, city, and district levels in Hubei Province, as well as province-wide. The Wuhan MHC asks the Wuhan CDC, district CDC, and another hospital to begin an epidemical investigation into the new virus.[15]

30.12 CapitalBio Medlab reports a SARS-like coronavirus found in the

---

1 According to the *South China Morning Post* on 13 March: www.scmp.com/news/china/society/article/3074991/coronavirus-chinas-first-confirmed-covid-19-case-traced-back

2 Study by Prof Cao Bin (China-Japan Friendship Hospital), Huang Chaolin (Jin Yin-tan Hospital), Li Xinwang (Beijing Ditan Hospital), and Ren Lili (Chinese Academy of Medical Sciences) published on 24 January in The Lancet: www.thelancet.com/journals/lancet/article/PIIS0140-6736(20)30183-5/fulltext

3 Reported by the Wuhan MHC on 11 January. (*W)

4 https://user.guancha.cn/main/content?id=250814

5 https://user.guancha.cn/main/content?id=250814

6 https://health.huanqiu.com/article/3wwgMTxps6b

7 www.dxy.cn/bbs/newweb/pc/post/42862108

8 www.21jingji.com/2020/2-4/xOMDEzNzlfMTUzMDYxOA.html

9 www.dxy.cn/bbs/newweb/pc/post/42862108

10 www.dxy.cn/bbs/newweb/pc/post/42862108

11 www.lifeweek.com.cn/2020/0212/53254.shtml

12 https://finance.sina.cn/china/gncj/2020-01-01/detail-iihnzhfz9652655.d.html

13 www.dxy.cn/bbs/newweb/pc/post/42862108

14 www.dxy.cn/bbs/newweb/pc/post/42862108

15 www.lifeweek.com.cn/2020/0212/53254.shtml

27 Dec clinical specimens. It raises the alarm within the medical team.[16]

Doctors, among them Li Wenliang issue a report for "seven confirmed SARS cases from the South China Seafood Market", causing concern in a WeChat group.[17]

31.12 An NHC team of experts arrives at Wuhan to conduct testing and verification. (*H)

The Wuhan MHC states that there are "no obvious human-to-human cases and no infections among medical staff". (*W)

02.01 The whole-genome sequence of the new coronavirus is first discovered by WIV and CAS (archived, but not published).[18]

The Wuhan PSB files a case against eight persons who "spread rumors."[19]

03.01 The Wuhan City Government launches a city-wide investigation into unknown pneumonia cases and begins to collect environmental and animal specimens from the South China Seafood Market. (*W)

The NHC issues a directive that the samples from unknown pneumonia cases from Wuhan should be sent to designated pathogen testing agencies; specimens and related information should not be released to other non-designated agencies or individuals.[20]

The Wuhan MHC reports a total of 44 cases of "unknown pneumonia" and again states there is no "obvious human-to-human transmission" or "infections among medical staff". (*W)

China begins to regularly report to the WHO and relevant countries and regions, including the United States, Hong Kong, Macao, and Taiwan.[21]

04.01 The National CDC develops a PCR detection reagent with a high specificity for the new coronavirus.[22]

05–11.01 (41/1)2 recoveries[23] (295)**

Public Health Policies

07.01 President Xi Jinping presides over a meeting where he puts forward requirements for the prevention and control of the epidemic. (*C)

11.01 The National CDC provides PCR detection reagents to Wuhan hospitals and institutions for the detection and diagnosis of suspected cases.[24]

Major Development

06.01 The WHO reports recent cases of unknown pneumonia in Wuhan, and states that they do not recommend any travel or trade restrictions on China.[25]

07.01 The National CDC successfully isolates the virus from clinical specimens.[26]

08.01 The NHC task force confirms the new coronavirus as the cause of the outbreak. (*N)

09.01 The first death due to the new coronavirus is reported in Wuhan. (*W)

11.01 The Wuhan MHC traces the first confirmed case to 8 Dec 2019. (*W)

The Wuhan MHC again says that there are no infections among medical staff and no clear evidence of human-to-human transmission. (*W)

The gene sequence of the new coronavirus is first shared by Zhang Yongzhen's team at the Shanghai Public Health Clinical Centre.[27]

12–18.01 (45/2)15 recoveries[28] (418)**

Public Health Policies

14.01 The NHC holds a national video conference on the deployment of anti-epidemic measures. (*N)

15.01 The NHC releases the first version of the treatment plan. (*N)

18.01 The NHC releases the second version of the treatment plan. (*N)

---

16 www.dxy.cn/bbs/newweb/pc/post/42862108

17 https://app.bjtitle.com/8816/newshow.php?newsid=5533898&typeid=26&uid=1&did=&mood=

18 http://hb.people.com.cn/BIG5/n2/2020/0219/c192237-33811169.html

19 www.xinhuanet.com/2020-01/01/c_1125412773.htm

20 http://wsjkw.hlj.gov.cn/index.php/Home/News/show/newsid/8045/id/navid/37

21 http://news.cri.cn/wifihezuo/20200510/915bb6e4-3e7d-1419-fa2f-ae454813959c.html#

22 http://m.chinacdc.cn/xwzx/zxyw/202003/t20200312_214348.html

23 Reported by the Wuhan MHC

24 www.cbnweek.com/articles/theme/24378

25 www.who.int/csr/don/05-january-2020-pneumonia-of-unkown-cause-china/zh/

26 http://m.chinacdc.cn/xwzx/zxyw/202003/t20200312_214348.html

27 www.dxy.cn/bbs/newweb/pc/post/42862108

28 Reported by the Wuhan MHC

Major Development

12.01 The laboratory at the Shanghai Public Health Clinical Centre, which first shared the coronavirus genome, is ordered to close for "rectification".[29]

The NHC shares the new coronavirus gene sequence with the WHO. (*C)

The name "new coronavirus" is adopted to replace "unknown pneumonia" in Wuhan. (*O)

Wuhan begins a daily notification system for the epidemic. (*W)

13.01 Hong Kong, Macao, and Taiwan task forces visit Wuhan for investigative purposes.[30]

14.01 The Wuhan MHC states that the existing findings show that there is no clear evidence of human-to-human transmission, but that the possibility of limited human-to-human transmission cannot be ruled out. However, the risk of sustained human-to-human transmission is low. (*W)

17.01 In a report, Yuen Kwok-yung (an expert from Hong Kong and a member of the NHC task force) alerts Gao Fu (Director of the National CDC and the Guangdong CDC) to the risk of human-to-human transmission and asymptomatic infection.[31]

The U.S. CDC announces it will screen Chinese tourists at ports of entry.[32]

19–25.01 (1748/50)20 recoveries; 291 confirmed cases by 20 Jan[33]

Public Health Policies

19.01 The NHC starts to release test kits. (*N)

20.01 The NHC publishes a directive to classify the new coronavirus-induced pneumonia as a Class B infectious disease and to adopt preventive and control measures required for Class A infectious diseases. (*N)

President Xi Jinping emphasizes that people's lives and health are the main priority and that the country must take prevention and control measures seriously. (*C)

22.01 The Hubei Provincial Government initiates a "Second-Level Response" to the public health emergency. (*H)

The NHSA and the MF issue a directive that patient medical expenses related to COVID-19 will be covered by state-owned medical insurance and other financial subsidies. (*P)

The NHC releases the third version of the treatment plan. (*N)

The NHC advises travelers not to visit Wuhan and that Wuhan citizens should remain there. (*C)

23.01 At 2:39 a.m., an official announcement is made online in Wuhan stating that the airport and railway station departures from Wuhan will be temporarily closed starting at 10 a.m. that day. About five million people leave Wuhan for the Spring Festival and to flee the epidemic. Within the 10 hours before the official close of the border, around 300,000 people leave Wuhan.[34] The highway is finally closed around 2 p.m.[35][36]

The construction of a new emergency hospital, Huoshen Hospital, begins. (*C)

Zhejiang and Guangdong initiate a "First-Level Response" to the public health emergency. (*C)

The MF allocates a one billion-yuan subsidy to Hubei Province for the prevention and control of COVID-19. (*C)

The MHRSS, MF, and NHC release a directive stating that illness, death, or injury of medical staff while carrying out anti-COVID-19 work will be treated as occupational injuries. (*P)

24.01 The State Council Joint Prevention and Control Mechanism Network begins to hold daily press conferences to report nation-wide COVID-19 cases. (*N)

The State Council encourages the public to post suggestions and criticism on the work of local governments and departments in the prevention and control of COVID-19 on the government e-platform. (*P)

The MT issues a directive to exempt vehicles with emergency supplies, doctors, and patients from road tolls. (*P)

The Hubei Provincial Government initiates a "First-Level Response" to the public health emergency. (*H)

---

29 www.scmp.com/news/china/society/article/3052966/chinese-laboratory-first-shared-coronavirus-genome-world-ordered
30 www.nhc.gov.cn/gjhzs/s7952/202001/83b5d0f29dfd48e580fe8d940f125f9d.shtml
31 www.cbnweek.com/articles/theme/24378
32 www.bjnews.com.cn/news/2020/01/22/677703.html
33 Reported at the national level for the first time
34 www.thepaper.cn/newsDetail_forward_5654383
35 https://card.weibo.com/article/m/show/id/2309404463724621594742?_wb_client_=1
36 www.bbc.com/zhongwen/simp/chinese-news-52197004

Shanghai and Guangdong sends a team of medical professionals to Wuhan. (*N)

25.01 The CCP Central Committee establishes a task force to deal with the epidemic. (*C)

The MF and the NHC issue a directive to implement the subsidy policy for patient treatment and provide temporary work subsidies to medical staff and epidemic prevention workers. (*P)

Wuhan decides to build another emergency hospital: Wuhan Leishen Hospital. (*W)

The NDRC issues a 300 million-yuan special subsidy to finance the building and equipment procurement for the Wuhan Huoshen Hospital and Leishen Hospital. (*N)

Major Development

19.01 The first case in Guangdong is diagnosed and confirmed by the NHC. (*N)

The Wuhan MHC issues a report stating that some cases had no history of exposure to the South China Seafood Market. (*W)

20.01 The first cases are diagnosed in Beijing and Shanghai, respectively. (*N)

Academician Zhong Nanshan confirms that the new coronavirus could be transmitted from human to human. (*N)

The number of new cases is to be reported every day at the national level. (*C)

21.01 The first cases are diagnosed in Tianjin, Zhejiang, Jiangxi, Shandong, Henan, Hunan, Chongqing, Sichuan, Yunnan, and Taiwan. (*N)

A task force on pandemic emergency research in China is launched and led by Zhong Nanshan.[37]

The WHO says that there is evidence of limited human-to-human transmission, but there is no clear evidence of sustained human-to-human transmission.[38]

22.01 The first cases are diagnosed in Anhui, Fujian, Guangxi, Guizhou, Hebei, Heilongjiang, Jilin, Jiangsu, Liaoning, Ningxia, Shanxi, Hainan, Hong Kong, and Macau. (*N)

The WHO warns that the new coronavirus pneumonia might carry a human-to-human risk.[39]

22.01 The National CDC says that the virus originated in wild animals in the South China Seafood Market, with 33 environmental samples positive out of 585 taken.[40]

23.01 first cases are diagnosed in Gansu, Inner Mongolia, Shanxi, and Xinjiang. (*N)

From midnight on 24 Jan, all ticket holders for trains, buses, ferries, and flights can receive a refund for their tickets and be exempt from the refund fee.[41]

24.01 A study by Cao Bin (China-Japan Friendship Hospital),Huang Chaolin (Jin Yin-tan Hospital), Li Xinwang (Beijing Ditan Hospital), and Ren Lili (Chinese Academy of Medical Sciences) et al. is published in *The Lancet* and traces the first confirmed case to 1 Dec 2019. The patient had no history of contact with the South China Seafood Market.[42]

25.01 The first case is diagnosed in Qinghai. (*N)

The U.S. announces the closure of the Consulate General Office in Wuhan and evacuates its personnel.[43]

26.01–01.02 (14,380/304) 328 recoveries

Public Health Policies

26.01 By 8 a.m., 30 provinces have launched a "First-Level Response" to the health crisis. (*C)

Local governments are required to establish task forces for infection control. (*C)

27.01 Premier Li Keqiang visits Wuhan to inspect and guide the prevention and control activities for the epidemic. (*C)

The NHC sends supervision teams to seven provinces to oversee the prevention and control activities for the epidemic. (*N)

A total of 959 medical staff from seven provinces are sent to Wuhan to support the medical sector there. The establishment of a follow-up medical team continues. (*C)

The MF allocates 4.4 billion yuan for the prevention and control of the epidemic, including an additional 500 million yuan for Hubei Province. (*C)

The NHSA, MF, and NHC order treatment fees for suspected cases (as well

---

37 http://m.xinhuanet.com/2020-01/24/c_1125499305.htm

38 www.bjnews.com.cn/news/2020/01/21/677244.html

39 www.who.int/zh/news-room/detail/27-04-2020-who-timeline---covid-19

40 http://m.chinacdc.cn/xwzx/zxyw/202003/t20200312_214348.html; www.chinacdc.cn/yw_9324/202001/t20200127_211469.html

41 www.xinhuanet.com/politics/2020-01/24/c_1125498514.htm

42 www.thelancet.com/journals/lancet/article/PIIS0140-6736(20)30183-5/fulltext

43 www.sohu.com/a/368938386_120044982

as those of confirmed cases) to be covered by insurance, local governments, and the Central Government. (*P)

The State Council publishes a directive to strengthen control over wildlife sales and consumption; coordinate all nationwide activities; minimize travel; and reducing public gatherings and group dining during the Spring Festival. (*P)

The GAC publishes a directive to reduce or exempt the customs duties on imported epidemic prevention materials and set up a green channel for imported epidemic prevention materials and donated materials. (*P)

The NHC and NATCM release the fourth version of their treatment plan. (*P)

28.01 The MCA issues an emergency directive to strengthen infection control in nursing institutions for the aged, as well as carefully managing the mental health of the elderly and employees there. (*P)

The NHC publishes a directive which requires mild cases and asymptomatic infections be re-ported; the close contacts of confirmed, suspected, and asymptomatic cases to go into quarantine and observation; and screenings and tests to be performed on those who came from Wuhan and who exhibit symptoms of respiratory diseases. (*N)

29.01 The State Council issues an emergency directive to organize the re-opening of businesses that produce materials for epidemic prevention and control at the provincial and city levels, and unify the management and allocation of these materials. (*P)

Socio-Economic Policy Packages

30.01 The MARA, MT, and MPS issue an emergency directive to secure the supply chain of agricultural products and agricultural production materials. (*P)

Hubei organizes the resumption of businesses that produce epidemic prevention materials. (*H)

01.02 The State Council says that there will be no tariffs on materials for the epidemic imported from the US. (*C)

Major Development

26.01 The NHC says that the virus is different from that of SARS and that the spread of the epidemic is only in the early stage. (*N)

27.01 The State Council announces that the 2020 Chinese Spring Festival holiday will be extended to 2 February. (*C)

The WHO changes the global risk of the new coronavirus pneumonia outbreak from medium to high, indicating that the outbreak poses a very high risk to China and the Asia-Pacific region in general.[44]

28.01 President Xi Jinping meets with Dr. Tedros Adhanom Ghebreyesus, Director-General of the WHO. (*C)

The WHO announces a plan to dispatch an international team of experts to China to gain a deeper understanding of the epidemic and provide guidance to global prevention efforts. (*O)

The Chinese Academy of Medical Sciences identifies bats as the origin of the virus, but the intermediate host remains unknown.[45]

A research and development project between Tongli University and the pharmaceutical industry to find a new coronavirus mRNA vaccine is officially established.[46]

29.01 The first case is diagnosed in Tibet. (*N)

The WIV screens and identifies several drugs that may inhibit the effects of the novel coronavirus.[47]

The Shenzhen Municipal Health Commission launches a clinical study on the feasibility of using AIDS drugs to combat the epidemic.[48]

British Airways announces the suspension of all direct flights to China.[49]

The White House announces that it would not, for the time being, suspend flights between China and the U.S.[50]

Questions are raised online about the deployment of donated materials by the Red Cross Society of Hubei.[51]

30.01 Beijing and Shandong launch a data portal for local outbreaks on their open platforms.[52]

The Lancet publishes a paper by the China CDC

---

44   http://news.cctv.com/2020/01/28/ARTIv0wjlHZrLo4GJ5wDWCwW200128.shtml
45   http://m.cyol.com/content/2020-01-28/content_18343288.htm
46   http://sh.xinhuanet.com/2020-01-28/c_138739276.htm
47   www.xinhuanet.com/politics/2020-01-29/c_1125511036.htm
48   www.chinanews.com/sh/2020/01-29/9072792.shtml
49   www.bbc.com/zhongwen/simp/chinese-news-51296646
50   www.voachinese.com/a/china-flight-airline-virus-20200128/5264686.html
51   www.bbc.com/zhongwen/simp/chinese-news-51338241
52   www.echinagov.com/info/273325

research team stating that the new virus is comparable to that of SARS and MERS, and confirms that bats might be the origin of the virus.[53]

31.01 The WHO announces that the epidemic constitutes a public health emergency of international concern, but emphasizes that travel and trade restrictions are not recommended. (*N)

The Central Government decides to bring back Hubei citizens stranded overseas.[54]

The MPS issues an emergency directive calling for a severe crackdown on illegal and criminal activities related to wildlife. (*N)

02.02–08.02 (37,198/811) 2,649 recoveries

Public Health Policies

02.02 Huoshen Hospital is formally turned over to the Medical Team of the People's Liberation Army. (*C)

03.02 Wuhan decides to build "mobile cabin hospitals" to treat patients. (*C)

05.02 The NHC and the NATCM release the fifth version of the treatment

plan, which now includes CT results in the criteria for clinical diagnostics within Hubei Province. (*P)

06.02 Wuhan's first three "mobile cabin hospitals" open, with approximately 4,400 beds for treating patients with mild symptoms.[55]

08.02 Wuhan Leishen Hospital is officially opened.[56]

Socio-Economic Policy Packages

03.02 The CAA requires domestic airlines to ensure the operation of international flights as 46 foreign airline companies suspend flights to Mainland China.[57]

04.02 The MARA issues an emergency directive to ensure the supply of meat, eggs, and milk.[58]

The ME requires universities to implement online teaching. (*P)

Major Development

03.02 The MFA spokesperson, Hua Chunying, says that on 30 occasions, China has notified the U.S. of its epidemic information and defense measures, adding a call

for rational and prudent responses worldwide.[59]

06.02 Dr. Zhang Dingyu (the then- president of Jin Yin Tan hospital), and Dr. Zhang Jixian (Director of the Department of Respiratory Medicine, Hubei Hospital of Integrated Traditional Chinese and Western Medicine) receive awards from the Hubei Provincial Government for outstanding performance in epidemic prevention and control. (*H)

07.02 Dr. Li Wenliang dies. In response to public outrage over his death and his earlier reprimand, the SSC sets up a team to investigate related issues.[60]

08.02 Mohammed Bandi, Chairman of the 74th Unite Nations General Assembly, says the information provided by China is timely, transparent, and helpful.[61]

09.02–15.02 (68,500/1,665) 9,419 recoveries

Public Health Policies

10.02 The Hubei Bureau of Housing and Urban-Rural Development issues a directive that residential

areas should be closed-off/isolated and people entering and leaving must register and have their temperatures taken. (*H)

Socio-Economic Policy Packages

09.02 The State Council issues a directive to promote the resumption of enterprises and production by backing the resumption of work in an orderly manner and as soon as possible; ensuring the safety of transportation; improving screening and testing capabilities; and strengthening the quarantine and treatment of key populations. (*P)

12.02 The ME requires students in primary and secondary schools to learn at home and avoid taking a "one-size-fits-all" approach.

15.02 The SAMR, NMPA, and NIPA issues "Ten Supporting Measures for Resumption". These include online handling of registrations; implementing notice pledges; establishing emergency green channels for administrative permits; extending the period of administrative permits; accelerating

53 www.thelancet.com/journals/lancet/article/PIIS0140-6736(20)30251-8/fulltext
54 www.xinhuanet.com/politics/2020-01/31/c_1125515234.htm
55 www.hb.xinhuanet.com/2020-02/06/c_1125537724.htm
56 http://tv.cctv.com/2020/02/08/VIDEhxC7g6OVcKW7xV79l0Gn200208.shtml
57 www.xinhuanet.com/politics/2020-02/04/c_1125529780.htm
58 www.moa.gov.cn/gk/tzgg_1/tfw/202002/t20200204_6336566.htm
59 www.xinhuanet.com/2020-02/03/c_1125527184.htm
60 www.ccdi.gov.cn/toutiao/202003/t20200319_213880.html
61 www.xinhuanet.com/world/2020-02/09/c_1125549126.htm

standard conversion and application; cautiously administering the catalogue of enterprises with irregular operations; strict investigation of arbitrary fees and price increases; strengthening quality and technical service support; reducing or waiving technological service fees; and encouraging businesses to participate in the "three guarantees" action. (*P)

Major Development

13.02 Ying Yong is appointed Party Secretary of Hubei Province and Wang Zhonglin is appointed Party Secretary of Wuhan.[62]

14.02 Larry Kudlow, the Director of the U.S. White House National Economic Committee, says that the Chinese Government lacks transparency in its response to the epidemic. In response, Michael Ryan, the WHO's health emergency project leader, points out that Kudlow's remarks are falsehoods, stating that the Chinese Government has actively cooperated with the WHO and shown a high level of transparency.[63]

16.02–22.02 (64,084/2,346) 15,299 recoveries

Public Health Policies

17.02 Wuhan starts a three-day "net-pull" survey of 100 percent coverage of treatment, tests, quarantine, and community isolation. All local communities, urban and rural, are to be covered by the survey. All movement of persons within Wuhan is banned. (*W)

The State Council issues a guideline on the classification of epidemic risk levels and the employment of different measures in areas with different risk levels. The adoption of strict measures in Hubei and Wuhan will continue to secure the safety of the capital, Beijing. (*P)

The Wuhan government issues a directive establishing a system to reward outstanding individuals in anti-epidemic work. (*W)

The Guangxi Provincial Government issues a directive establishing a system for rewarding people who report information regarding the prevention and control of COVID-19. This is in response to the anti-epidemic deployment by the Central Government.[64]

18.02 Hubei strengthens policy incentives for frontline medical staff, such as granting their children an additional 10 points to their total marks in high school entrance examinations. (*H)

The NHC and the NATCM release the sixth version of the treatment plan, excluding CT results from the criteria of clinical diagnostics. (*N)

19.02 COVID-19 patients who donate convalescent plasma will enjoy the honor and status of voluntary blood donors. (*N)

20.02 Communities in some cities begin to use "smart seals" to prevent people in quarantine from leaving their homes.[65]

22.02 The Justice Department of Sichuan Province orders prisons and drug addiction treatment centers to be strictly managed to prevent the spread of the virus.[66]

The "Wuhan Health Code" is launched to facilitate more efficient community management. (*W)

Socio-Economic Policy Packages

18.02 After a meeting, Premier Li Keqiang decides to reduce corporate social insurance premiums and postpone their housing accumulation fund. (*C)

20.02 The MHRSS, MF, and STA issue a directive to exempt SMEs from paying pensions, unemployment, and work-related injury insurance; reducing pension and insurance fees of other enterprises by 50 percent; and allowing businesses to apply for deferred payments. (*P)

Major Development

19.02 Twenty-seven internationally renowned medical experts from eight different countries issue a joint report in *The Lancet*, stating that the virus comes from wild animals.[67]

22.02 A joint study by the CAS found that the South China Seafood Market was not the birthplace of the new coronavirus. Two expanded spreads on 8 December and 6 January were found prior to 12 February.[68]

62   www.xinhuanet.com/renshi/2020-02/13/c_1125568253.htm
63   www.xinhuanet.com/politics/2020-04/06/c_1125819214.htm
64   http://wsjkw.gxzf.gov.cn/zhuantiqu/ncov/ncovzcwj/2020/0217/68955.html
65   http://m.mp.oeeee.com/a/BAAFRD000020200220267589.html
66   www.sc.gov.cn/10462/10464/10797/2020/2/24/08de2d11f7ce4fa49815f11bed6a0664.shtml
67   www.thelancet.com/journals/lancet/article/PIIS0140-6736(20)30418-9/fulltext
68   http://eprint.las.ac.cn/abs/202002.00033

23.02–29.02
(66,907/2,761)
31,187 recoveries

Public Health Policies

23.02 The Central Government orders increases in the remuneration of prevention and treatment personnel, as well as an increase in the scope of subsidies covered. (*P)

24.02 From 21 to 24 February, Gansu, Liaoning, Guizhou, and Yunnan successively adjust the emergency response level to the public health emergency from the First-Level to the Third-Level, while Shanxi and Guangdong adjust it from the First-Level to the Second-Level. (*N)

Socio-Economic Policy Packages

28.02 The ME requests classes start at different times based on the local situation.[69]

Major Development

28.02 The WHO says that more than 20 new coronavirus pneumonia vaccines are in the research and development phase and some are undergoing clinical trials.[70]

The WHO announces a rise in the global risk level of the new coronavirus epidemic from "high" to "very high".[71]

29.02 A medical team from the Red Cross Society of China arrives in Iran.[72]

The "China-WHO COVID-19 Joint Investigation Report" is released. It states that the new coronavirus is animal-derived, with bats appearing to be its original host. However, the intermediate host has not been identified.[73]

01.03–07.03
(67,707/2,986)
45,011 recoveries

Public Health Policies

01.03 The State Council holds a press conference to introduce measures on prevention and control of imported cases from overseas. (*C)

03.03 The Guangdong Provincial Government declares that persons who have come from or have traveled to countries with severe epidemic conditions should quarantine for 14 days after entering Guangdong.[74]

The NHC and the NATCM publish the seventh version of the treatment plan. (*N)

Socio-Economic Policy Packages

02.03 The MARA issues a directive to promote the employment of rural labor forces by providing job information and carefully managing incoming populations to prevent disease; creating jobs for the local community; and promoting the resumption of rural businesses.[75]

03.03 The All-China Federation of Trade Unions requests enterprises pay the same wages they would normally receive to employees who work flexible hours or from home. (*C)

04.03 The State Council issues a directive to accelerate the resumption of work and production by simplifying approval procedures and promoting online government services. (*P)

So far, 110.48 billion yuan of funding has been allocated to anti-epidemic work; of that amount, 71.43 billion yuan has been used.[76]

07.03 The Central Government issues a directive to ensure the welfare of people in difficult circumstances, including those now at the poverty level as a result of the epidemic. This includes the distribution of relief funds, social welfare subsidies, and temporary subsidies for price increases in full and on time for those enrolled in the relief and assistance system and families with members who have COVID-19. (*P)

Major Development

02.03 Public security agencies have investigated 948 criminal cases and 2,147 administrative cases involving wild animals, confiscating 92,000 wild animals and more than 5,300 kg of wild animal products.[77]

03.03 A senior adviser to the WHO Director-General says that China has not concealed any data.[78]

05.03 The Standing Committee of Hubei Provincial People's Congress prohibits the consumption of wild animals. (*H)

69   www.moe.gov.cn/srcsite/A17/s7059/202002/t20200228_425499.html

70   www.who.int/zh/dg/speeches/detail/who-director-general-s-opening-remarks-at-the-media-briefing-on-covid-19---28-february-2020

71   www.who.int/zh/dg/speeches/detail/who-director-general-s-opening-remarks-at-the-media-briefing-on-covid-19---28-february-2020

72   www.xinhuanet.com/politics/2020-04/06/c_1125819214.htm

73   www.xinhuanet.com/politics/2020-04/06/c_1125819214.htm

74   www.gd.gov.cn/gdywdt/bmdt/content/post_2913089.html

75   www.moa.gov.cn/gk/tzgg_1/tfw/202003/t20200304_6338197.htm

76   www.xinhuanet.com/2020-03/06/c_1125669615.htm

77   www.bj.xinhuanet.com/jzzg/2020-03/02/c_1125651242.htm

78   www.vox.com/2020/3/2/21161067/coronavirus-covid19-china

06.03 An MFA spokesperson emphasizes that the epidemic first appeared in China but did not necessarily originate in China, stressing a need to fight against "information viruses" and "political viruses".[79]

07.03 China announces a donation of US$20 million to the WHO to support international cooperation to combat COVID-19.[80]

A Chinese medical team and a supply of epidemic prevention equipment arrives in Iraq.[81]

**08.03–14.03
(67,794/3,085)
54,278 recoveries**

Public Health Policies

10.03 All mobile cabin hospitals in Wuhan are closed. Sixteen square cabin hospitals in Wuhan allowed more than 12,000 patients with mild cases of the new pneumonia to fully recover. (*C)

Hubei Province decides to distribute the Hubei Health Code to achieve hierarchical management of people. (*H)

13.03 As of midnight on 12 March, there are 63 low-risk cities and counties in Hubei and 12 medium-risk ones. Wuhan is the only city categorized as high-risk. (*H)

Socio-Economic Policy Packages

11.03 The Organization Department of the CCP and the MHRSS issue a directive requiring public institutions to expand public recruitment of college graduates, especially those in Hubei. (*P)

Major Development

12.03 The first group of Chinese anti-epidemic medical experts arrives in Italy with medical supplies.[82]

13.03 The *South China Morning Post* publishes a report that traces the first confirmed case of the virus to 17 Nov 2019, stating that "Government records suggest the first person infected with the new disease may have been a Hubei resident aged 55, but 'patient zero' has yet to be confirmed."[83]

**15.03–21.03
(81,054/3,261)
72,244 recoveries**

Public Health Policies

16.03 The SPC, SPP, MPS, MJ, and GAC issue guidelines to strengthen frontline health and quarantine work and punish those who violate the law by concealing infections or forging health documents. (*C)

Beijing opens Xiaotangshan Hospital to test and treat personnel returning to Beijing from overseas, providing over 1,000 beds.[84]

17.03 The Wuhan City Government announces that from midnight on 17 March, people who enter Wuhan from other areas must quarantine for 14 days. (*W)

Socio-Economic Policy Packages

15.03 The Chengdu City Government announces the "Five Permits, One Standard" program to promote economic development by allowing temporary stalls that pose no safety hazards. (As of 28 May, these measures enabled about 100,000 persons to obtain employment at temporary stalls or as floating vendors.)

20.03 The MHRSS initiates a 100-day online recruitment campaign.[85]

Major Development

16.03 A recombinant COVID-19 vaccine is successfully developed by a team from the Academy of Military Sciences, led by Academy Fellow Chen Wei.

17.03 Five well-known scholars from the U.S., the UK, and Australia publish a paper in *Nature Medicine*, stating that there is no evidence that the virus was manufactured in a laboratory or designed in other ways.[86]

18.03 The second group of medical experts from China arrives in Milan, Italy.[87]

The *New England Journal of Medicine* publishes a paper from researchers in the China-Japan Friendship Hospital and Wuhan Jin Yin-tan Hospital, stating that the "Lopinavir/ritonavir combined standard treatment" was not effective for treating critical adult COVID-19 patients.[88]

19.03 The investigation team of the SSC publishes a directive regarding the investigation related to Dr. Li Wenliang and requests the public security

79   www.xinhuanet.com/politics/2020-04/06/c_1125819214.htm

80   www.xinhuanet.com/politics/2020-04/06/c_1125819214.htm

81   www.xinhuanet.com/politics/2020-04/06/c_1125819214.htm

82   www.xinhuanet.com/politics/2020-04/06/c_1125819214.htm

83   www.scmp.com/news/china/society/article/3074991/coronavirus-chinas-first-confirmed-covid-19-case-traced-back

84   www.xinhuanet.com/photo/2020-03/17/c_1125724935.htm

85   www.mohrss.gov.cn/SYrlzyhshbzb/dongtaixinwen/buneiyaowen/202003/t20200320_363047.html

86   www.nature.com/articles/s41591-020-0820-9

87   www.xinhuanet.com/politics/2020-04/06/c_1125819214.htm

88   www.nejm.org/doi/full/10.1056/NEJMoa2001282

agencies to withdraw the reprimand and prosecute those responsible for it.[89]

Wuhan police withdraw the reprimand of Li Wenliang, apologize, and take disciplinary actions against the deputy director and a police officer.[90]

20.03 The journal *Pharmacological Research* publishes a paper from Chinese researchers (Zhong Nanshan included) stating that Lianhua Qingwen can significantly inhibit the replication of the new coronavirus (SARS-CoV-2) in cells.[91]

22.03–28.03 (67,801/3,182) 62,565 recoveries

Public Health Policies

24.03 Restrictions on leaving Hubei will be lifted from midnight on 25 March, and restrictions on leaving Wuhan will be lifted from midnight on 8 April. People who left Hubei must use a Health Code to travel in other provinces. (*H)

26.03 The MFA and the NIA issue an announcement that from midnight on 28 March, the entry of foreigners holding

valid Chinese visas and residence permits will be suspended.[92]

Socio-Economic Policy Packages

25.03 The Sichuan Provincial Government announces that mahjong parlors, tea houses, and Internet cafes will be allowed to re-open.[93]

Major Development

26.03 The G20 Leaders' Special Summit on COVID-19 is conducted via video conference. (*C)

Francis Collins, President of the NIH, says in a blog post that the virus naturally exists in humans and was not artificially created in a lab.[94]

28.03 The MARA, ME, MST, NHC, GAC, NFGA, and CAS issue a directive to strengthen the supervision of laboratories and research projects for pathogenic animal microbes. (*P)

29.03–04.04 (81,669/3,329) 76,964 recoveries

Public Health Policies

31.03 The NHC indicates that it will begin reporting cases of asympto-

matic infections on 1 April. Close contacts with asymptomatic patients should also quarantine for 14 days. (*C)

01.04 Customs agencies and local governments stress that they will work together to implement nucleic acid testing for all passengers entering Mainland China. (*C)

02.04 The CAA announces that the first batch of 310,000 health kits will be distributed to overseas students.[95]

Socio-Economic Policy Packages

31.03 The National Unified College Entrance Examination for 2020 is postponed for one month.[96]

Major Development

31.03 The central task force says that the spread of the epidemic in Wuhan, the main battlefield in China, has been stopped, attaining a progressive achievement. (*C)

The Standing Committee of Guangdong National People's Congress issues a regulation that prohibits eating wild animals

beginning 1 May.[97]

02.04 The Hubei Provincial Government designates 14 staff members on the frontline of prevention and control of COVID-19 as martyrs, including Dr. Li Wenliang. (*H)

03.04 The State Council announces a National Day of Mourning will be held on 4 April. (*C)

05.04–11.04 (82,052/3,339) 77,575 recoveries

Public Health Policies

06.04 The State Council advises that there is a risk of transmission from asymptomatic patients, and that cases of asymptomatic infections should quarantine for 14 days and strictly regulated. (*P)

07.04 China and Russia agree to temporarily close the Suifenhe-Pogranici Port Travel Inspection Channel.[98]

10.04 The State Council issues a directive requiring improved pre-examination and triage management of outpatient and emergency cases and promoting the practice of scheduled appointments

89   www.ccdi.gov.cn/toutiao/202003/t20200319_213880.html
90   https://xw.qq.com/cmsid/TWF202003190142861G
91   www.sciencedirect.com/science/article/pii/S104366182030743X
92   https://s.nia.gov.cn/mps/tztg/202003/t20200327_1194.html
93   www.sc.gov.cn/zcwj/xxgk/NewT.aspx?i=20200325080646-342864-00-000
94   https://directorsblog.nih.gov/2020/03/26/genomic-research-points-to-natural-origin-of-covid-19/
95   www.moe.gov.cn/jyb_xwfb/s5147/202004/t20200401_437133.html
96   www.moe.gov.cn/jyb_xxgk/s5743/s5744/202003/t20200331_436662.html
97   www.gd.gov.cn/gdywdt/zwzt/fkyq/pfzl/content/post_2962738.html
98   www.suifenhe.gov.cn/contents/1962/80412.html

and Internet consultations. (*C)

Socio-Economic Policy Packages

07.04 The State Council announces a plan to guide the hierarchical management of the resumption of business, requiring that persons with normal temperatures and from low-risk areas can start work immediately. (*P)

08.04 The State Council orders low-risk areas to gradually open for work and resume normal activities, while restrictions for medium- and high-risk areas will remain in place. (*P)

The NDRC, MCA, MF, MHRSS, MVA, and NBS publish a directive to double the amount of the monthly temporary price subsidy and pay it on time; and expand the number of people receiving the price subsidy, reflecting a total of 8 million additional recipients. (*P)

09.04 The Central Government issues guidelines to promote the resumption of enterprises, requiring that businesses ensure the orderly and smooth flow of personnel; guard against falsification of data regarding resumption ; and reducing reporting processes and inspections. (*P)

Major Development

07.04 *Nature* publishes three editorials in April apologizing for associating the novel coronavirus with Wuhan and China. Admitting its error, it calls for an immediate end to associating the virus with specific locations.[99]

08.04 Northeastern University research shows that New York state's first confirmed coronavirus strain did not originate in China.[100]

The New York Times quotes research from American experts that confirms the main source of the New York outbreak was not from Asia.[101]

09.04 The ME has suspended the pilot program for Mainland students to study in the Taiwan Region in 2020.[102]

12.04–18.04 (82,735/4,632) 77,062 recoveries

Public Health Policies

14.04 The MCA and NHC issue guidelines on prevention and control of the epidemic in the community, highlighting four aspects: community infection control, community service, mass participation, and information dissemination. (*P)

16.04 The Army medical team sent to Hubei has completed its task and returns to base.[103]

Socio-Economic Policy Packages

13.04 The MCT and the NHC order scenic areas popular with tourists to only open outdoor areas and that the number of tourists should not exceed 30 percent of the maximum capacity. (*P)

Major Development

13.04 U.S. NPR says on its website that according to analysis reports from many top virus researchers in the U.S., it was virtually impossible for the new coronavirus to be caused by a laboratory accident in China or anywhere else. The virus spreads to humans in the same way as other coronaviruses.[104]

15.04 The seroepidemiological investigation of asymptomatic patients is carried out in nine provinces in China. (*C)

The MFA announces that China has donated US$20 million to the WHO.[105]

17.04 The Office of the French President states that there is no evidence to suggest a relationship between the P4 laboratory in Wuhan and COVID-19.[106]

Wuhan revises the number of confirmed cases and deaths (325 confirmed cases and 1290 deaths were added). (*W)

19.04–25.04 (82,827/4,632) 77,394 recoveries

Public Health Policies

21.04 Guangzhou decides to conduct nucleic acid testing on nearly 30,000 faculty members and 167,000 junior and senior students who are the first to return to school.[107]

---

99 www.nature.com/articles/d41586-020-01009-0

100 www.nytimes.com/2020/04/08/us/coronavirus-live-updates.html?searchResultPosition=93

101 www.nytimes.com/2020/04/08/us/coronavirus-live-updates.html?searchResultPosition=93

102 www.moe.gov.cn/jyb_xwfb/xw_zt/moe_357/jyzt_2020n/2020_zt03/yw/202004/t20200409_441791.html

103 www.mod.gov.cn/shouye/2020-04/16/content_4863672.htm

104 www.npr.org/sections/goatsandsoda/2020/04/23/841729646/virus-researchers-cast-doubt-on-theory-of-coronavirus-lab-accident

105 www.fmprc.gov.cn/web/fyrbt_673021/t1770018.shtml

106 www.reuters.com/article/us-health-coronavirus-france-lab/france-says-no-evidence-covid-19-linked-to-wuhan-research-lab-idUSKBN21Z2ME

107 www.gz.gov.cn/zfjg/gzswsjkwyh/zwlb/content/post_5799751.html

Socio-Economic Policy Packages

20.04 The MHRSS and MHURD issue a directive allowing construction companies that have not been in arrears of wages within a certain period to suspend the deposit of migrant workers' wages. (*P)

24.04 A spokesperson for the MCA says that 3.71 billion yuan in temporary price subsidies has been issued to 81.689 million people in need so far this year.[108]

Major Development

20.04 A total of 33 people, including Dr. Li Wenliang, were awarded for their sacrifices in anti-epidemic work.[109]

U.S. independent news website The Greyzone publishes an article alleging that U.S. conservative and right-wing news outlets are cooperating with the Trump administration by disseminating false information about the virus to attack China.[110]

21.04 A WHO spokesperson says that all available evidence indicates that the new coronavirus has its origin in animals and was not artificially created in a laboratory. The virus' likely host is bats, but how it spreads from bats to humans is unknown.[111]

23.04 An MFA spokesperson announces that China will add an additional US$30 million to support the WHO's international coalition to fight COVID-19. China previously donated US$20 million to the WHO coalition.[112]

24.04 The U.S. NIH announces the end of a cooperative research project between a non-profit organization and WIV, and withdraws all funding. The move reflects the position of the Trump Administration. This latest move sparks widespread doubt and criticism from the American scientific community.[113]

The U.S. news outlet Politico reports that the National Republican Senatorial Committee sent a detailed, 57-page memo advising Republican candidates to address the coronavirus crisis by aggressively attacking China.[114]

26.04–02.05 (82,877/4,633) 77,713 recoveries

Public Health Policies

29.04 At midnight on 30 April, the emergency response level in Beijing will be lowered to the Second-Level. (*C)

30.04 The Central Government sets up a liaison group to coordinate the anti-epidemic work in Hubei Province and Wuhan City, and dispatches a supervision team to direct and guide the work in Heilongjiang Province. (*C)

01.05 The Central Government issues a directive to strengthen infection control measures in medical institutions. (*P)

The Harbin City Government issues an emergency directive suspending dining in catering units from midnight on 2 May.[115]

At midnight on 2 May, the First-Level Response to the public health emergency in Hubei Province is adjusted to the Second-Level. (*H)

Socio-Economic Policy Packages

30.04 The MIIT orders the publication of 94 big data products and solutions to support epidemic prevention and control as well as the resumption of production and school attendance. (*P)

Major Development

26.04 Dr. Peter Daszak, President of the Eco-Health Alliance and an expert on disease ecology who has been working with the WIV for 15 years, says that WIV did not create the virus. Two days later, Donald Trump orders the NIH to terminate EcoHealth's grant to study bat viruses.[116]

27.04 Richard Horton, editor-in-chief of The Lancet, praises China's prompt notification of the virus to the WHO and its attempts to warn the international community.[117]

28.04 Economists Chistoffer Koch and Ken Okamura publish a paper

108 http://m.xinhuanet.com/2020-04/24/c_1125902187.htm

109 http://qnzz.youth.cn/qckc/202004/t20200420_12294143.htm

110 https://thegrayzone.com/2020/04/20/trump-media-chinese-lab-coronavirus-conspiracy/amp/?__twitter_impression=true

111 https://edition.cnn.com/us/live-news/us-coronavirus-update-04-21-20/h_802e1e857336975e196e3c25c647b02e

112 www.xinhuanet.com/2020-04/23/c_1125897152.htm

113 https://sports.yahoo.com/m/c1d3ceb1-df40-373a-b28c-7b058a223310/%E7%BE%8E%E5%9C%8B%E4%B8%AD%E6%AD%A2%E8%B3%87%E5%8A%A9%E5%86%A0%E7%8B%80%E7%97%85%E6%AF%92%E7%A0%94%E7%A9%B6-%E9%A0%85%E7%9B%AE%E6%9B%BE%E8%88%87%E6%AD%A6%E6%BC%A2%E7%97%85%E6%AF%92%E7%A0%94%E7%A9%B6%E6%89%80%E5%90%88%E4%BD%9C.html

114 www.politico.com/news/2020/04/24/gop-memo-anti-china-coronavirus-207244

115 http://news.cctv.com/2020/05/02/ARTIUPnLbWKvmrNjQ2p5H2j1200502.shtml

116 https:/edition.cnn.com/videos/tv/2020/04/26/exp-gps-0426-daszak-int.cnn

117 http://m.haiwainet.cn/middle/3544276/2020/0507/content_31784482_1.html

that says the distribution of cases reported by China is the same as those in the U.S. and Italy. The paper says no manipulation of the data is corroborated by Benford's law, an observation about the frequency distribution of leading digits in real life sets of numerical data.[118]

29.04 An MFA spokesperson announces that China and South Korea will establish a green channel for the flow of important business, logistics, production, and technical services between the two countries.[119]

Dr. Nicholas A. Christakis from Yale University co-authors a paper published in *Nature*, stating that the number of cases reported in China is accurate based on studies of population movements.[120]

The finding of clinical trials which showed no significant clinical benefit of Remdesivir are published in *The Lancet*, by Professor Cao Bin (China-Japan Friendship Hospital) and Academician Wang Chen (Chinese Academy of Medical Sciences).[121]

03.05–09.05
(82,901/4,633)
78,120 recoveries

Public Health Policies

08.05 The NHC and the ME issue guidelines for infection control in primary and secondary schools. (*N)

The Central Government issues guidelines on anti-epidemic measures that include limited gatherings; maintaining safe distances and wearing masks; the implementation of "early detection, early reporting, early quarantine, and early treatment" measures; the opening of public places in an orderly manner; strengthening anti-epidemic measures in medical institutions, schools, pension, and welfare institutions; expanding the scope of nucleic acid testing; and promoting mutual recognition of "health codes" in different areas. (*C)

09.05 At 9 a.m., the emergency response level in Guangdong is adjusted from the Second-Level to the Third-Level.[122]

Jilin Province announces a local confirmed case of

COVID-19. According to the national COVID-19 classification standards, the risk level of Shulan City is adjusted from low to medium.[123]

Socio-Economic Policy Packages

06.05 At the executive meeting of the State Council, relevant departments report on measures to support businesses. These include expanding the reduction of added-value tax for SMEs and individual businesses; reducing and remitting 600 billion yuan in social insurance premiums paid by businesses; securing over 84 million jobs by reinstating unemployment insurance; waiving more than 140 billion yuan in road tolls; lowering electricity and gas prices, saving 67 billion yuan for businesses; calibrating interest rates to release 1.75 trillion yuan in funds; providing 2.85 trillion yuan in low-cost loans to enterprises, especially SMEs and individual businesses; extending the deadline for repayment of SME and individual business loans, affecting more than 1.1

million businesses and over 1 trillion yuan in loans; and increasing support for spring farming production and animal husbandry development.[124]

08.05 The NDRC, MHURD, MF, MC, People's Bank of China, SASAC, STA, and SAMR publish guidelines to exempt three-months of housing rents for SMEs in the service sector and for individuals that rent state-owned houses for business operations, while encouraging other landlords to waive or defer rents. (*P)

Major Development

03.05 A paper published in *the International Journal of Antimicrobial Agents* by French scholars found that a 42-year-old man without any connection to China or foreign travel came down with COVID-19 before 16 January, suggesting the spread of COVID-19 in France may have occurred at the end of December 2019.[125]

04.05 *National Geographic* magazine publishes an interview with Dr. Anthony Fauci, Director of the U.S. National Institute

---

118 https://chinaminutes.com/News/News-Article/benfords-law-and-covid-19-reporting

119 www.xinhuanet.com/world/2020-04/30/c_1125930854.htm

120 https://twitter.com/NAChristakis/status/1255466011672879109

121 www.thelancet.com/journals/lancet/article/PIIS0140-6736(20)31022-9/fulltext

122 http://wsjkw.gd.gov.cn/xxgzbdfk/content/post_2989765.html

123 www.xinhuanet.com/politics/2020-05/09/c_1125961491.htm

124 www.gov.cn/guowuyuan/2020-05/07/content_5509476.htm

125 www.sciencedirect.com/science/article/pii/S0924857920301643

of Allergy and Infectious Diseases, in which he says that the best evidence shows that the virus behind the pandemic was not made in a lab in China.[126]

Nature publishes a paper by research teams from China, the UK, and the U.S. that concludes that the major non-pharmaceutical interventions used in China — intercity travel restrictions, early identification and quarantine, exposure restrictions, and social distancing — were effective. Without these interventions, the number of cases in China might have increased 67-fold, to more than 7 million people.[127]

05.05 Dr. Jeffrey Sachs, Director of the Center for Sustainability at Columbia University, criticizes the U.S. government's groundless and unreasonable placing of blame on China for the epidemic.[128]

Dr. Gao Li, the WHO representative in China, says that since 3 January,

the WHO and China have kept communication open and reported to the world in detail.[129]

06.05 *USA Today* reports that 171 people in Florida were infected in January and February, two months before officials announced confirmed cases.[130]

The British Health Minister, Matthew Hancock, says in an interview with British Sky TV that there is no evidence that the new coronavirus has been artificially created, nor is there any connection between it and the WIV.[131]

Swedish authorities test the Chinese herbal medicine Lianhua Qingwen Jiaonang. The results indicate that the drug only contains menthol and would have no effect on the virus. The medicine has been embargoed by Swedish Customs.[132]

07.05 Mayor Michael Melham of Belleville, New Jersey, says he has tested positive for coronavirus antibodies, and thinks

he may have been sick with the virus back in November 2019. The U.S. reported the first case on 20 January 2020.[133]

08.05 Peter Embarek of the WHO says that the new coronavirus had its origins in wild bats and the reason why so few cases went undetected at the beginning was because most cases were mild or asymptomatic.[134]

10.05–16.05 (82,947/4,634) 78,227 recoveries

Public Health Policies

10.05 Eleven new confirmed COVID-19 cases are reported in Shulan City, Jilin Province. The risk level of Shulan city is adjusted from medium to high.[135]

12.05 Beijing implements normalized prevention and control measures. Measures to help the elderly include using mobile devices and the Internet to make hospital appointments. (*C)

13.05 The Jilin City government begins to implement strict prevention and control measures.[136]

14.05 To discover and clear all asymptomatic cases, Wuhan begins to carry out nucleic acid testing on all citizens. (*W)

16.05 From midnight on 17 May, all stand-alone clinics in Jilin city will be temporarily closed. People should seek medical treatment in relevant medical institutions when needed. Patients with fever should go to the special fever clinic.[137]

Socio-Economic Policy Packages

13.05 The MF and the CFA announce that the special film funding fee will be waived by location: Hubei is exempt for all of 2020, while other provinces will be exempt for the first eight months of 2020. (*P)

15.05 The MF and the STA announce that the tax and fee policies to

126 www.yicai.com/news/100617851.html

127 www.nature.com/articles/s41586-020-2293-x

128 www.jeffsachs.org/blog/m222zmwdpm83mc32ntfbgr38hml4mj

129 www.gov.cn/xinwen/2020-05/06/content_5508977.htm

130 www.usatoday.com/story/news/nation/2020/05/05/patients-florida-had-symptoms-covid-19-early-january/3083949001/

131 www.sky.com/new-search/ask-the-health-secretary-06-05-20-ccc49a95-e2ca-47af-ad14-aa31d75ab92b?q=Matt%20Hancock

132 https://baijiahao.baidu.com/s?id=1666123581352009560&wfr=spider&for=pc

133 https://news.cgtn.com/news/3149444e79514464776c6d636a4e6e62684a4856/index.html

134 http://m.news.cctv.com/2020/05/08/ARTI1j8TOpWps7sD9JRrTeQD200508.shtml

135 www.jl.xinhuanet.com/2020-05/10/c_1125964669.htm

136 http://wjw.jlcity.gov.cn/gsgg/202005/t20200513_777836.html

137 http://wjw.jlcity.gov.cn/gsgg/202005/t20200516_778658.html

support epidemic prevention and enterprises will be valid through 31 December 2020. (*P)

Major Development

10.05 A research report is published in *Science* by experts from China, the UK, and the .US., stating that the national emergency response imposed by China delayed the spread of the COVID-19 epidemic.[138]

The New York Times reports that the FBI and the U.S. Department of Homeland Security are preparing to issue a warning that "China's most skilled hackers and spies are working to steal American research in the crash effort to develop vaccines and treatment for the coronavirus." [139]

17.05–23.05 (82,974/4,634) 78,261 recoveries

Public Health Policies

17.05 Jilin Province announces three new confirmed COVID-19 cases in Fengman District, Jilin City. The risk level of Fengman District is adjusted from medium to high.[140]

Major Development

18.05 President Xi Jinping delivers a speech at the opening ceremony of the 73rd World Health Assembly video conference, announcing that China would provide US$2 billion in international assistance over two years to support anti-epidemic work and the recovery of economies and society. Additionally, China will cooperate with the United Nation to set up global humanitarian emergency warehouses and hubs in Africa, establish cooperation arrangements with 30 countries in Africa and construct an African CDC. He also promised that when a Chinese vaccine was completed it would be available globally. He also assured that China would work with G20 members to implement the "Debt Repayment Suspension Initiative for the Poorest Countries".(*C)

When asked about an "independent inquiry" into COVID-19, an MFA spokesperson said that WHO members, including China, agreed that there would be a fair, independent, and comprehensive assessment to review the lessons from the anti-epidemic work and tracing of the virus. It was not an inquiry.[141]

22.05 *The Lancet* publishes a study authored by Academician Chen Wei and his team, stating that the first Phase 1 clinical trial of a COVID-19 vaccine was safe and generated an immune response in humans. However further tests are needed to see whether the immune response was effective in preventing SARS-COV-2 infection.[142]

24.05–30.05 (83,001/4,634) 78,304 recoveries

Public Health Policies

29.05 Several districts in Guangzhou issue directives indicating that while on campus, students and teachers do not need to wear masks, while service staff should wear masks. (*C)

Socio-Economic Policy Packages

27.05 The Central Civilization Office says that roadside stall businesses, street markets, and traders will not be involved in this year's national civilized city evaluation index.[143]

29.05 The GASC issues guidelines on the resumption of sporting events. These include the orderly re-opening of sports venues, with appointment systems and reduced capacity; and holding non-contact individual sporting events. However, international and national comprehensive sporting events are still temporarily on hold. (*C)

Major Development

29.05 The WHO launches a "COVID-19 Technology Access Pool" to accelerate research and development of vaccines, tests, treatments, and other technologies for COVID-19.[144]

31.05–06.06 (83,036/4,634) 78,332 recoveries

Public Health Policies

02.06 A total of 9,899,828 persons have undergone nucleic acid testing in Wuhan, with a total of 300 asymptomatic cases and no confirmed symptomatic cases.[145]

---

138 https://science.sciencemag.org/content/368/6491/638

139 www.nytimes.com/2020/05/10/us/politics/coronavirus-china-cyber-hacking.html?searchResultPosition=1

140 http://wjw.jlcity.gov.cn/gsgg/202005/t20200517_778720.html

141 www.fmprc.gov.cn/web/fyrbt_673021/t1780224.shtml

142 www.thelancet.com/journals/lancet/article/PIIS0140-6736(20)31208-3/fulltext

143 www.wenming.cn/bwzx/jj/202005/t20200527_5623955.shtml

144 www.who.int/zh/news-room/detail/29-05-2020-international-community-rallies-to-support-open-research-and-science-to-fight-covid-19

145 www.xinhuanet.com//mrdx/2020-06/03/c_139110161.htm

04.06 The CAA says that from 8 June, incentives will be given to inbound flights if no positive cases are found onboard. However, if there are more than five positive cases on a flight, the airline company must suspend their flights for a week.[146]

06.06 As of midnight on 6 June, the emergency response level in Beijing is lowered to the Third-Level.[147]

Socio-Economic Policy Packages

01.06 Premier Li Keqiang visits an old residential area in Yantai, Shandong Province, to support the development of the small shop and street vendor economy.

Major Development

03.06 At the regular MFA press conference, a journalist says that the Associated Press has obtained a recording of a January internal WHO meeting that indicated that the WHO was dissatisfied with China's transparency. The MFA spokesperson questions the source of the information and says it was seriously inconsistent with the facts: China shared the information

with the world openly and in a timely manner.[148]

07.06–13.06
(83,132/4,634)
78,369 recoveries

Public Health Policies

08.06 The Central Government issues an advisory to expand nucleic acid testing that includes mandatory testing for key groups and voluntary testing for others, as well as strengthening public monitoring, early warnings, and conducting sampling tests among populations. (*C)

12.06 Beijing will conduct nucleic acid tests on all people in the Xinfadi wholesale market.[149]

13.06 Beijing plans to conduct nucleic acid tests on those who had close contact with the Xinfadi wholesale market as early as 30 May.[150]

At 3 a.m., the Xinfadi wholesale market is temporarily closed for cleaning and disinfection.[151]

Epidemiological investigation and community isolation are deployed in Beijing's Fengtai District, where five confirmed cases were reported on 12 June.[152]

Socio-Economic Policy Packages

09.06 Premier Li Keqiang announces the establishment of a special transfer payment that will add 2 trillion yuan to the government deficit, and sale of special government bonds to fight COVID-19. The monies will be released to cities and counties as soon as possible. (*C)

Major Development

07.06 The State Council publishes a white paper on China's efforts to fight COVID-19. The paper lists 346 state-run medical teams, 42,600 medical staff, and 960 public health personnel that aided Hubei Province. By 2 June, the national cure rate of COVID-19 was 94.3 percent, exceeding the worldwide average rate. Four inactivated vaccines and one adenovirus vector vaccine have been approved for clinical trials. By 31 May, China had sent 29 medical teams to 27 countries, and aided 150 countries and four international organizations. (*P)

09.06 When asked about a report that said COV-

ID-19 might have begun spreading in Wuhan as early as the end of August 2019, based on analysis on data of traffic flow and related Baidu searches, the MFA spokesperson says that it was absurd to draw such a conclusion from superficial phenomena such as traffic flow.[153]

14.06–20.06
(83,378/4,634)
78,413 recoveries

Public Health Policies

15.06 The Beijing City Government announces Third-Level emergency response, Second-Level anti-epidemic measures, and First-Level working status. Resume taking temperatures and performing sterilization in public areas; indoor entertainment venues will close; community residents should use access cards, and non-residents must register and check the health code before entering the community. Those returning to Beijing must check their itinerary and fill in their personal information online.[154]

16.06 The level of emergency response in Beijing is upgraded to the Second-Level. Measures

146 www.caac.gov.cn/XXGK/XXGK/TZTG/202006/t20200604_202928.html

147 www.beijing.gov.cn/shipin/szfxwfbh/19765.html

148 www.fmprc.gov.cn/web/fyrbt_673021/t1785499.shtml

149 www.beijing.gov.cn/gongkai/ldhd/202006/t20200613_1924417.html

150 http://wjw.beijing.gov.cn/wjwh/ztzl/xxgzbd/gzbdjkts/202006/t20200613_1924480.html

151 www.beijing.gov.cn/ywdt/yaowen/202006/t20200613_1924428.html

152 www.beijing.gov.cn/ywdt/gzdt/202006/t20200613_1924472.html

153 www.fmprc.gov.cn/web/fyrbt_673021/t1787296.shtml

154 www.beijing.gov.cn/ywdt/gzdt/202006/t20200615_1925204.html

include the restoration of community isolation; those who have gone to Xinfadi, Yuquan East, Tiantao Honglian markets, and other key areas (and people in close contact with them) in the past 14 days should undergo nucleic acid testing; online teaching will resume and college students will not be allowed to return to campus. Unnecessary travel from Beijing is prohibited, while those who must leave Beijing will undergo a nucleic acid test and show a negative test report within seven days.[155]

18.06 All inter-provincial passenger transport operating in Beijing will be suspended from 19 June. Passengers who have already bought tickets will receive full refunds.[156]

People at risk of infection are strictly prohibited from leaving Beijing, including all those previously diagnosed and their close contacts; persons who went to Xinfadi market since 30 May and their close contacts; and persons who live in the area at medium and high risk of infection. (*C)

19.06 The NHSA issues a directive requiring local governments to include nucleic acid testing in state-owned health insurance.[157]

Socio-Economic Policy Packages

19.06 The MF issues regulations to simplify the accounting for rent concessions related to COVID-19. (*P)

Major Development

16.06 The Phase I/II clinical study of an inactivated vaccine by the Wuhan Institute of Biological Products reveals the vaccine to be safe and effective.[158]

17.06 President Xi Jinping hosts a special summit on China-Africa Solidarity against COVID-19 in Beijing. The summit issues a joint statement of fighting against the diseases together and appealing to the international community to strengthen cooperation. (*C)

18.06 The CDC officially shares globally the genome sequence data of the novel coronavirus that caused the epidemic in Xinfadi via a national platform, GISAID, and the WHO. (*C)

21.06–27.06 (83,500/4,634) 78,451 recoveries

Public Health Policies

23.06 The Beijing City Government now requires that the number of tourists at indoor public venues shall not exceed 30 percent of the maximum capacity, while civil aviation, railways, and highway checkpoints must strengthen checks.[159]

25.06 The NHC issues a directive correcting unreasonable measures of restriction on the movement of people beyond regular infection control measures. (*C)

28.06–04.07 (83,553/4,634) 78,516 recoveries

Public Health Policies

28.06 The NHC issues a directive further normalizing epidemic prevention and control measures with the support of information systems. (*P)

03.07 The State Council's Joint Prevention and Control Mechanism mandates stronger prevention and control measures in farmers' markets. (*C)

Socio-Economic Policy Packages

01.07 The MF issues a directive requiring local governments to allocate discounted interest funds directly to businesses as soon as possible. The Central Government allocates 2.92885 trillion yuan in discounted interest funds. (*P)

04.07 Employers in Shenzhen are allowed to use 80 percent of their housing provident fund to pay for housing rents (up from 65 percent), and the estimated addition of 2.5 billion yuan will be paid by the fund to reduce the pressure on employers. (*C)

Major Development

30.06 The European Union announces it will reopen entry permits for travelers from China only if China declares its borders open to them.[160]

05.07–11.07 (83,594/4,634) 78,634 recoveries

Socio-Economic Policy Packages

08.07 The MC, MPS, and NHC publish guidelines for exhibitions. (*P)

---

155 www.beijing.gov.cn/ywdt/gzdt/202006/t20200616_1926324.html

156 www.beijing.gov.cn/fuwu/bmfw/bmzt/yqzt/jt/202002/t20200228_1855700.html

157 www.nhsa.gov.cn/art/2020/6/19/art_37_3265.html

158 www.xinhuanet.com/health/2020-06/17/c_1126124573.htm

159 www.beijing.gov.cn/gongkai/ldhd/202006/t20200624_1931441.html

160 www.consilium.europa.eu/en/press/press-releases/2020/06/30/council-agrees-to-start-lifting-travel-restrictions-for-residents-of-some-third-countries/

Major Development

06.07 The China-Arab States Cooperation Forum is held via video and issues a joint statement on solidarity between China and Arab countries in the fight against COVID-19. (*C)

12.07–18.07

Public Health Policies

17.07 Starting from 10 a.m. on 17 July, anyone entering Mainland China through the Shenzhen-Hong Kong port must have a negative nucleic acid testing report within 72 hours and take 14 days of centralized quarantine for medical observation.[161]

The Urumchi Government expands nucleic acid testing to all who have reason to be tested and to those who would like to be tested.[162]

18.07 The NHC issues a directive requiring medical institutions to establish a green channel for critically ill patients, emphasizing that no delay or avoidance of treatment should exist in the name of epidemic prevention and control. (*C)

Socio-Economic Policy Packages

15.07 The MCT issues a directive and guidelines for conditionally restarting cultural and tourism activities. Air flights, ticketing, and hotels can resume with strict preventive measures, with the usable capacity of services adjusted from 30 percent to 50 percent. Middle- and high-risk regions are excluded from the new measures. (*C)

16.07 The CFA issues a directive to re-open cinemas in low-risk areas from 20 July. (*P)

Major Development

16.07 *The New York Times* reports that the employees of state-owned enterprises were among the first in China to receive a coronavirus vaccine, raising ethical concerns.[163] It was later reported on 26 September that thousands in China, such as government officials and vaccine company staff, were also injected with the unproven vaccines whose Phase 3 trials are not yet completed with risks unknown.[164] A later report by Nikkei Asia on

29 September said that at least 350,000 people were inoculated with the unproven vaccines.[165]

19.07–25.07
(83,830/4,634)
78,908 recoveries

Public Health Policies

19.07 At midnight on 20 July, the emergency response level in Beijing is lowered to the Third-Level. (*C)

23.07 Dalian City, Liaoning province, begins nucleic acid testing for 190,000 people.[166]

The Central Government issues a directive strengthening anti-epidemic measures in meat processing plants. (*C)

Socio-Economic Policy Packages

21.07 The MT issues a directive in alignment with that issued by the MCT on 15 July, allowing cross-provincial tourist transport and cross-provincial group travel to resume. (*P)

According to a report by SASAC, thanks to the lowering of electricity prices, gas prices, transportation fees, and rents, business operating costs in China

were reduced by more than 120 billion yuan in the first half of 2020. (*C)

Major Development

20.07 *The Lancet* publishes a paper by Academician Chen Wei's team that says the Phase 2 clinical trials of a novel coronavirus vaccine proved it to be effective.[167]

22.07 Director of the NHC announces in an interview with state broadcaster CCTV that the Central Government authorizes the "emergency use" of a vaccine.[168]

23.07 The foreign ministers of China and Latin American and Caribbean countries hold a special video conference on COVID-19, later issuing a joint statement of strengthening cooperation between China and Latin American and Caribbean countries in fighting COVID-19 and resuming economic and social development. (*C)

26.07–01.08
(84,385/4,634)
79,003 recoveries

Public Health Policies

26.07 Dalian City Government issues a directive that the nucleic

---

161 www.sz.gov.cn/szzt2010/yqfk2020/szzxd/content/post_7899512.html
162 www.xinjiang.gov.cn/xinjiang/xjyw/202007/0a8dfcff60884bb7a283187cbb12d356.shtml
163 www.nytimes.com/2020/07/16/business/china-vaccine-coronavirus.html
164 www.nytimes.com/2020/09/26/business/china-coronavirus-vaccine.html?referringSource=articleShare
165 https://asia.nikkei.com/Spotlight/Coronavirus/China-inoculates-350-000-while-coronavirus-vaccine-still-in-trials
166 http://dl.gov.cn/yqfk2020/info/1052136_1114143.vm
167 http://news.cctv.com/2020/07/21/ARTIHIkyDoT0KJViJiyAvqPa200721.shtml
168 https://tech.sina.com.cn/roll/2020-08-22/doc-iivhuipp0127950.shtml

testing for all citizens will be financed with public funds.[169]

28.07 Dalian bans gatherings such as wedding and birthday banquets.[170]

The director of the NHSA reports that by 19 July, 135,500 confirmed and suspected COVID-19 patients in China had been covered by medical insurance, with 1.232 billion yuan paid by national medical insurance. The total medical cost was 1.847 billion yuan. (*C)

Socio-Economic Policy Packages

27.07 In Urumqi, relief subsidy funds for July are released, and the August relief subsidy funds will be released by the end of July. (*C)

Major Development

01.08 The NHC plans to send support teams for nucleic acid testing and mobile cabin hospitals to Hong Kong soon. (*N)

***02.08–08.08
(84,619/4,634)
79,168 recoveries***

Public Health Policies

03.08 The NHSA will include the cost of drugs to test COVID-19 in the list of medical insurance procedures. (*C)

Socio-Economic Policy Packages

03.08 The Urumqi City Government adopts a social security payment policy stating: "The lower limit shall not be increased, and individuals can hold off payment." (*C)

05.08 Beijing allocates 20 million yuan from a special film fund to give subsidies to 232 cinemas in Beijing. (*C)

Major Development

07.08 NBC News becomes the first foreign news organization to be granted access to the WIV. It met with senior scientists there and ran a report.[171]

08.08 A spokesperson for the U.S. State Department, Morgan Ortagus, criticizes NBC's 7 August report, stating that "they just regurgitated CCP propaganda and didn't press for facts."[172]

09.08–15.08

Public Health Policies

12.08 The NHC issues guidelines for control of COVID-19 in farmers' markets. (*N)

Socio-Economic Policy Packages

09.08 The Urumqi City Government releases a series of corporate subsidy policies to businesses, including subsidies, subsidized loans, and lower interest rates. (*C)

10.08 The MCT issues guidelines for opening entertainment venues, that the number of spectators must not exceed 50% of the seats in the theatre. (*C)

13.08 The China Securities Regulatory Commission will solicit public opinion until 6 September regarding the rules to remove mandatory credit ratings for companies that will make it easier for them to issue debt and raise funds on the country's stock exchanges.[173]

Major Development

11.08 In response to Morgan Ortagus's comments on 8 August, an MFA spokesperson says that the U.S. Government always has a way to define the "facts". The spokesperson further commented that "In their [the U.S.] eyes, as long as they can attack and discredit China, lies are facts."[174]

***16.08–22.08
(84,951/4,634)
79,895 recoveries***

Public Health Policies

19.08 The NHC and the NATCM publish the eighth version of the treatment plan. (*N)

Socio-Economic Policy Packages

17.08 The MF issues a directive regarding the refund of education fees during the epidemic period by the end of August. (*C)

20.08 The ME publishes a directive to comprehensively resume normal education and adopt effective anti-epidemic measures in schools. (*C)

Major Development

20.08 The China National Biotec Group (CNBG) is given the green light to begin the third phase of testing for one of its vaccine candidates in Peru, Morocco, and Argentina. Yang Xiaoming, the Chairman of CNBG, said in an interview with state broadcaster CCTV that 20,000 people had taken part in the overseas trials and the preliminary results were positive.[175]

***20.09–26.09
(85,351/4,634)
80,541 recoveries***

Major Development

24.09 At the 13th China Bioindustry Convention held in Wuhan, Zhong Nanshan claims that

169 http://dl.gov.cn/yqfk2020/info/1052156_1114741.vm

170 http://dl.gov.cn/yqfk2020/info/1052156_1120456.vm

171 www.nbcnews.com/news/world/inside-wuhan-lab-center-coronavirus-storm-n1236254

172 http://news.sina.com.cn/c/2020-08-12/doc-iivhuipn8285667.shtml

173 Ren, D. Mandatory Credit Ratings to be Scrapped. *South China Morning Post*, 13 August 2020, B1.

174 www.fmprc.gov.cn/web/fyrbt_673021/t1805487.shtml

175 https://tech.sina.com.cn/roll/2020-08-22/doc-iivhuipp0127950.shtml

in one to two years, all people in China will be vaccinated for the virus.[176]

04.10–10.10 (85,557/4,634) 80,705 recoveries

Major Development

09.10 China joined the COVID-19 Vaccines Global Access (COVAX) Facility, bringing the total number of countries and economies that are part of the global initiative for vaccine access to 171. According to WHO Director-General, countries and economies that are part of COVAX can distribute vaccines simultaneously to priority populations, including health workers, older people and those with underlying conditions. The aim of COVAX is to ensure that 2 billion doses are manufactured and distributed equitably by the end of 2021.[177]

11.10–17.10 (85,672/4,634) 80,786 recoveries

Public Health Policies

13.10 As a response to the emergency of 3 asymptomatic carriers on 11 Oct, Qingdao organized large-scale nucleic acid testing. By 8:00 am, 13 Oct, 3,078,528 samples were taken, and 1,107,883 of them were tested. 9 people tested positive.[178, 179]

14.10 Sui Zhenhua, director of Qingdao Health Commission, and Deng Kai, deputy secretary of the Party Committee and Dean of Qingdao Chest Hospital, were suspended for investigation.[180]

17.10 Live COVID-19 virus is tested and isolated in the outer packaging of cold chain food.[181]

The 22nd meeting of the 13th NPC Standing Committee voted to pass the Biosafety Law. It will come into effect on April 15, 2021.[182]

18.10–24.10 (85,790/4,634) 80,891 recoveries

Public Health Policies

19.10 Jiaxing City Center for Disease Control released the instruction of new vaccination. The vaccine has not yet been officially registered for marketing, and it is only approved for emergency vaccination.[183]

Major Development

24.10 Wu Zunyou, chief epidemiologist of China CDC told China Newsweek that (1) Due to the serious situation in European and American countries, China can only afford "gradual and stable opening based on its handling capacity" to ensure safety. (2) There is still a risk from contaminated frozen food packing. (3) It is not science-based or cost efficient to carry out citywide nucleic acid testing, but it reassures residents and officials.[184]

---

176 www.cjrbapp.cjn.cn/toutiao/p/204062.html

177 www.who.int/dg/speeches/detail/who-director-general-s-opening-remarks-at-the-media-briefing-on-covid-19---9-october-2020

178 wsjsw.qingdao.gov.cn/n28356065/n32563060/n32563061/201012134807954745.html

179 wsjsw.qingdao.gov.cn/n28356065/n32563060/n32563061/201013084424642633.html

180 www.bjnews.com.cn/news/2020/10/16/778091.html

181 www.chinacdc.cn/yw_9324/202010/t20201017_222144.html

182 http://legal.people.com.cn/gb/n1/2020/1017/c42510-31895822.html

183 www.jiaxing.gov.cn/art/2020/10/19/art_1228921205_59000977.html

184 www.guancha.cn/politics/2020_10_24_569115.shtml

COVID-19 in Germany:
Learning to Dance with the Virus

H. Christoph Steinhardt

Germany's fairly successful management of the first eight months of the COVID-19 pandemic proceeded through three phases of government response: (1) being caught off-guard, (2) taking decisive actions and (3) searching for a "new normal". An elite consensus regarding the severity of the threat to public health and the necessity for counter-measures was supported by a large majority. Although noisy opposition emerged on the fringes, political polarisation over the pandemic remained limited.

In contrast to Asian societies such as Taiwan, Hong Kong or Vietnam,[1] Germany did not succeed in preventing sustained community transmission of SARS-CoV-2 in the early phases of the pandemic. Nonetheless, its comparatively mild lock-down—the "hammer" [2]—succeeded in suppressing the virus better than other large European countries. Since then the country has managed the "dance"[3] of controlling the spread of the disease fairly successfully. Yet as decision-makers decided against an elimination strategy, the pandemic continued to simmer over summer. By the time of writing in August 2020 Germany had avoided a second wave of fast-paced community transmission.

In spite of intense discussions on the most appropriate measures, the political, media and scientific elites were relatively united in their assessment of the threat and the necessity for decisive counter-measures. Overall popular support for government policy was strong. Nonetheless, Germany became a victim of its own success as a noisy minority of dissenters used the absence of a public health crisis to cast doubts on the rationale for anti-pandemic policies. In contrast to other large democracies such as the US or Brazil, however, the dissenting camp did not find effective brokers among the elites. Thus, so far political polarization over the pandemic has remained limited.

This report begins by tracing the development of the pandemic in Germany from January to August 2020, based on publicly available data. It then reviews the three phases of government counter-measures before it analyses public debates and selected indicators of public opinion. It concludes with a summary of findings and an outlook on the months ahead.

---

1   Viet-Phuong La et al., "Policy Response, Social Media and Science Journalism for the Sustainability of the Public Health System Amid the COVID-19 Outbreak: The Vietnam Lessons," *Sustainability* 12, no. 7 (January 2020): 2931, https://doi.org/10.3390/su12072931; C. Jason Wang, Chun Y. Ng, and Robert H. Brook, "Response to COVID-19 in Taiwan: Big Data Analytics, New Technology, and Proactive Testing," *JAMA* 323, no. 14 (April 14, 2020): 1341–42, https://doi.org/10.1001/jama.2020.3151; Kin-Man Wan et al., "Fighting COVID-19 in Hong Kong: The Effects of Community and Social Mobilization," *World Development* 134 (October 1, 2020): 105055, https://doi.org/10.1016/j.worlddev.2020.105055.

2   Tomas Pueyo, "Coronavirus: The Hammer and the Dance," Medium (blog), May 28, 2020, https://medium.com/@tomaspueyo/coronavirus-the-hammer-and-the-dance-be9337092b56.

3   Pueyo.

The Spread of the Virus from January to August

Germany's first infections with of SARS-CoV-2 were detected on 28 January 2020 in a subsequently contained cluster at car component supplier, Webasto, near Munich. The Chinese employee, who brought the virus in, developed symptoms upon returning to China, got tested, and warned her German colleagues.[4] Community transmission began on 24 February at the latest, when the first cases without a traceable origin were detected among participants of a carnival party in Heinsberg county in western Germany.[5] Heinsberg subsequently turned into Germany's first COVID-19 hotspot.[6] In the following days, more infections were diagnosed from holiday returnees and business travellers. By early March, a growing number of infections could not be traced back to travel history and community transmission was established in multiple locations. On 9 March, the first two COVID-19 deaths occurred in the state of North-Rhine Westphalia.[7]

Figure 4.1 COVID-19 infections and deaths in Germany (January–August 2020)

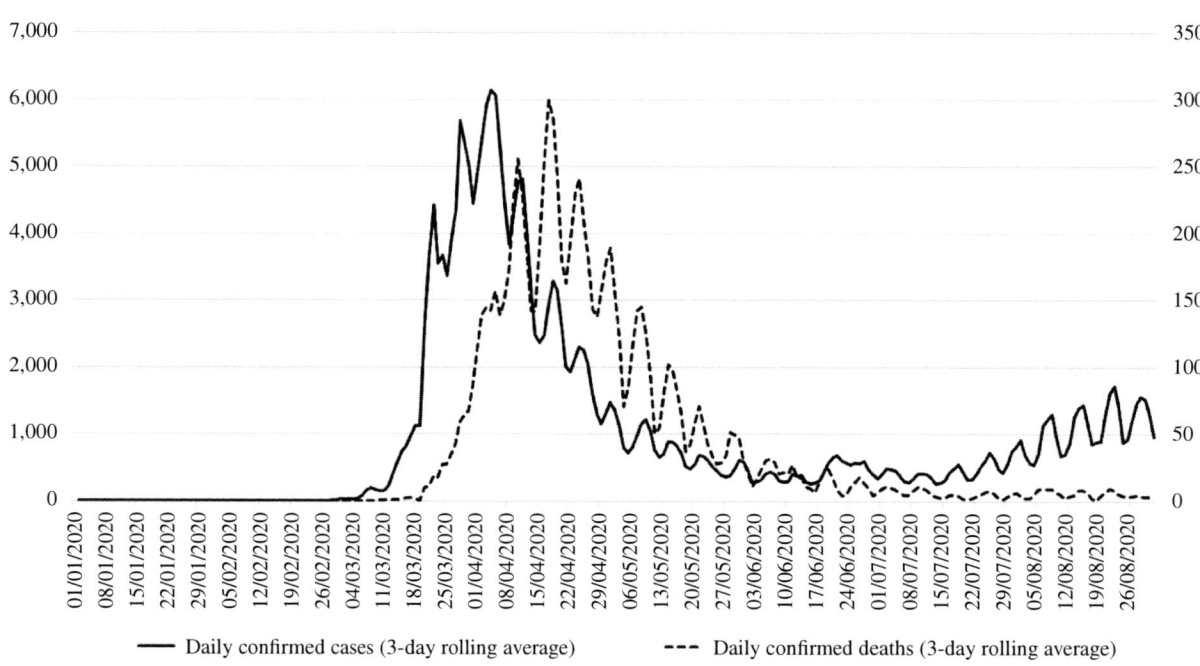

— Daily confirmed cases (3-day rolling average)   - - - Daily confirmed deaths (3-day rolling average)

Note: Daily cases are displayed on the left axis, daily deaths on the right axis. Source: Our World in Data[8]

Figure 4.1 illustrates how the number of confirmed cases shot up in early March. After the authorities mandated social distancing measures from 16 March (see below), the reproduction rate R estimated by the Robert Koch Institute (RKI, the German central agency for disease control) dropped below 1 a few days later. New infections peaked on 29 March. The number of deaths peaked on 16 April.

---

4   Camilla Rothe et al., "Transmission of 2019-NCoV Infection from an Asymptomatic Contact in Germany," *New England Journal of Medicine* 382, no. 10 (March 5, 2020): 970–71, https://doi.org/10.1056/NEJMc2001468.

5   Andreas Walker et al., "Genetic Structure of SARS-CoV-2 Reflects Clonal Superspreading and Multiple Independent Introduction Events, North-Rhine Westphalia, Germany, February and March 2020," *Eurosurveillance* 25, no. 22 (June 4, 2020): 2000746, https://doi.org/10.2807/1560-7917.ES.2020.25.22.2000746.

6   www1.wdr.de/nachrichten/rheinland/corona-virus-zusammenfassung-donnerstag-100.html, accessed August 31, 2020.

7   www.dw.com/de/erste-corona-todesf%C3%A4lle-in-deutschland/a-52597027, accessed September 10, 2020.

8   https://ourworldindata.org/coronavirus/country/germany?country=~DEU, accessed August 31, 2020.

After a sustained decline of new infections over April and May, cases remained at a low level and the estimated reproduction number R hovered around 1. Local outbreaks in June and July occurred but were brought under control through localised measures. In August, case numbers picked up again gradually on a broader geographic scale with a significant share of them among holiday returnees and younger age groups. However, R rose only somewhat above 1. The total number of registered COVID-19 deaths in Germany, at almost 9,300 on 31 August 2020,[9] has remained far below that of all other large European countries.

Figure 4.2 Estimate of the COVID-19 reproduction number (March–August 2020)

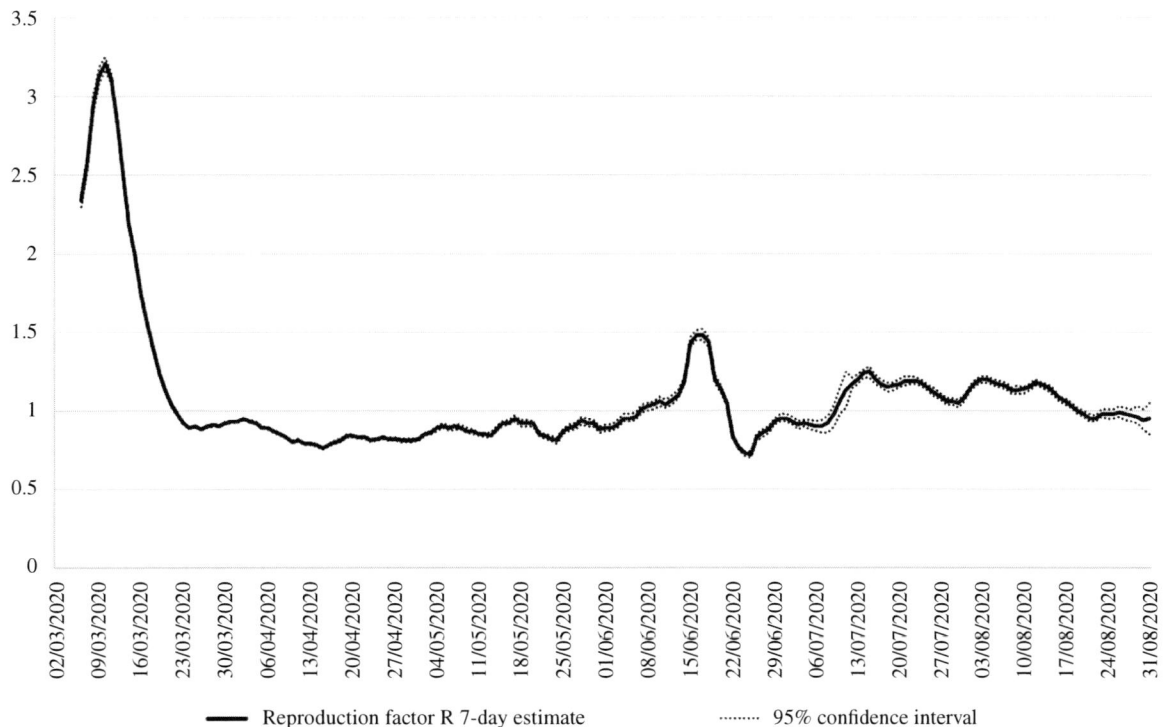

Source: Robert Koch Institute[10]

Phase I: The Government Caught off-guard (13 January–25 February 25)

On 13 January 2020, the first case of COVID-19 was confirmed outside of China in Thailand.[11] Germany's leading healthcare officials' early assessment of the threat posed by the disease can, in hindsight, only be characterised as a misjudgement. On 22 January, a day before the Chinese government decided to lock down the province of Hubei, German Health Minister, Jens Spahn, declared that the virus posed "a very minor" risk to public health in Germany, that there was "no reason for alarm."[12] A few days later Spahn

---

9 www.rki.de/DE/Content/InfAZ/N/Neuartiges_Coronavirus/Situationsberichte/2020-08-31-en.pdf?__blob=publicationFile, accessed August 31, 2020.

10 www.rki.de/DE/Content/InfAZ/N/Neuartiges_Coronavirus/Projekte_RKI/Nowcasting.html, accessed August 31, 2020.

11 www.who.int/emergencies/diseases/novel-coronavirus-2019/events-as-they-happen, accessed September 10, 2020.

12 https://rp-online.de/panorama/ausland/bundesregierung-coronavirus-nur-geringes-gesundheitsrisiko-in-deutschland_aid-48488333, accessed September 10, 2020.

stated that the country was "well prepared" for COVID-19.[13] On 22 January the director of the RKI, Lothar Wieler, professed the expectation that the virus "will not spread very widely." His assessment was publicly challenged by virologist and epidemiologist, Alexander Kekulé, whose more pessimistic assessment turned out to be more realistic.[14]

The initial miscalculation contributed to a lack of decisive measures to prevent community spread in February. Two missed opportunities stand out here. First, February is the season of carnival that is celebrated widely in southern and western Germany. These large public gatherings went ahead largely unhindered and served as accelerators for community transmission. Second, many federal states have school holidays in late February and early March, during which tourists frequently travel to southern Europe and the Alpine regions. Although the outbreak in Northern Italy and COVID-19 hotspots in Austrian ski resorts were known by then, returnees from these regions were not comprehensively tested and quarantined. Thus, Germany did not succeed in preventing sustained community transmission of SARS-CoV-2 in the early phases of the pandemic.

However, after the government swung into action in late February, Germany eventually managed to contain the spread of the virus and control the number of deaths significantly better than all other large European countries. Aside from the dramatic pictures emerging from Northern Italy since late February, which convinced the political elite and the public of the need for action, two factors possibly contributed to this outcome: first, one of the leading authorities on coronaviruses, Christian Drosten, and his team at Charité Hospital, Berlin, developed the first diagnostic test for the novel coronavirus on 16 January 2020.[15] The researchers subsequently distributed the test protocol to a wide and decentralised network of government and private labs which were authorized to conduct SARS-CoV-2 tests.[16] Germany, partly for that reason, had a very high capacity to test early on and was able to detect significant local outbreaks.[17] Second, the first contained and extensively documented outbreak at car component supplier, Webasto, near Munich served as a warning shot for decision makers on COVID-19's ease of transmission, and provided a rich case study for virologists, epidemiologists and clinicians to learn about the disease under controlled conditions.[18]

Phase II: Decisive Counter-measures (26 February–14 April)

The Federal Government initiated a first set of anti-epidemic measures after the initial cases of local transmission had been detected. On 26 February, Health Minister Spahn declared that Germany was at the beginning of an epidemic.[19] One day later, the Ministries of Health and Interior Affairs formed a

---

13 www.welt.de/regionales/bayern/article205400853/Spahn-nach-Coronavirus-Fall-in-Bayern-Sind-gut-vorbereitet.html, accessed September 10, 2020.

14 www.merkur.de/welt/corona-rki-robert-koch-institut-hopkins-zahlen-infektionen-statistik-kritik-wieler-deutschland-zr-13602916.html, accessed September 10, 2020.

15 www.charite.de/en/service/press_reports/artikel/detail/researchers_develop_first_diagnostic_test_for_novel_coronavirus_in_china, accessed September 10, 2020.

16 www.bbc.com/news/health-5223406, accessed September 10, 2020.

17 Ned Stafford, "Covid-19: Why Germany's Case Fatality Rate Seems so Low," *BMJ* 369 (April 7, 2020), https://doi.org/10.1136/bmj.m1395.

18 For instance, the cluster was the first one where scientist noted and systematically researched asymptomatic transmission of Covid-19. www.nytimes.com/2020/06/27/world/europe/coronavirus-spread-asymptomatic.html; Camilla Rothe et al., "Transmission of 2019-NCoV Infection from an Asymptomatic Contact in Germany," *New England Journal of Medicine* 382, no. 10 (March 5, 2020): 970–71, https://doi.org/10.1056/NEJMc2001468.

19 www.welt.de/vermischtes/article206136215/Coronavirus-Spahn-sieht-Deutschland-am-Beginn-einer-Epidemie.html, accessed July 18, 2020.

crisis group.[20] Travelers from COVID-19 hotspot countries had to fill in registration forms upon arrival. However, a travel ban, similar to measures adopted elsewhere, was explicitly rejected.[21] On 28 February, the RKI recommended cancelling large events. However, it took until 8 March for Health Minister Spahn to recommend cancelling events above 1,000 participants.[22] The federal states, which are in charge of these matters, followed suit over the following days.

Between 12 and 23 March, the authorities swung into action and enacted a series of sweeping anti-epidemic measures. On 12 March, Chancellor Merkel appealed to the public to stay home, to reduce social contact wherever possible and to cancel all non-essential events.[23] Between 12 and 18 March, all federal states closed schools, kindergartens and universities.[24] On 16 March, Bavaria declared a state of emergency.[25] On 22 March, an internal Federal Government document, which estimated over 1 million deaths if no counter-measures were taken, was leaked to the public.[26] On that day, the Federal Government and the states agreed on nationwide social distancing measures. These included maintaining a minimum distance of 1.5 m between individuals from different households in public areas, a temporary ban on public gatherings, a closure of restaurants except for take-aways, additional hygiene measures in all workplaces, etc. The measures explicitly permitted going to work, exercising or walking outside. Mandatory mask wearing was not included at the time.[27] Some local governments, however, enacted mask requirements of their own,[28] while certain states, such as Bavaria, mandated stricter stay-at-home orders.

In terms of travel restrictions, the government changed its earlier position and closed the borders to most neighbouring countries on 16 March.[29] A day later, the Ministry of Foreign Affairs issued a worldwide travel warning.[30] On the same day, EU member countries closed their external borders for non-essential travel.[31] Germany issued a full travel ban for Iran on 31 March.[32] On 10 April, it was mandated that incoming travellers, with only a few exceptions, were required to go into 14 days quarantine.[33]

20 www.spiegel.de/politik/deutschland/coronavirus-in-deutschland-bundesregierung-fuehrt-registrierung-von-reisenden-aus-betroffenen-laendern-ein-a-d718ed8d-6d3c-4acd-9cf7-98fdba4bce68, accessed July 18, 2020.

21 www.spiegel.de/politik/deutschland/coronavirus-in-deutschland-bundesregierung-fuehrt-registrierung-von-reisenden-aus-betroffenen-laendern-ein-a-d718ed8d-6d3c-4acd-9cf7-98fdba4bce68, accessed July 18, 2020. www.tagesschau.de/ausland/eu-coronavirus-101.html, accessed July 18, 2020.

22 www.n-tv.de/panorama/Spahn-Alle-Grossveranstaltungen-absagen-article21627196.html, accessed July 18, 2020.

23 www.bundeskanzlerin.de/bkin-de/aktuelles/pressekonferenz-von-bundeskanzlerin-merkel-ministerpraesident-soeder-und-dem-ersten-buergermeister-tschentscher-1730300, accessed July 20, 2020.

24 www.mz-web.de/halle-saale/wegen-corona-halle-schliesst-als-erste-deutsche-grossstadt-alle-schulen-und-kitas-36404152; www.spiegel.de/panorama/coronavirus-wo-schulen-und-kitas-geschlossen-werden-a-30dc65e6-b6bc-4787-9113-f8a4945005bb, accessed July 15, 2020.

25 www.merkur.de/bayern/coronavirus-soeder-bayern-katastrophenfall-tote-massnahmen-schliessung-geschaefte-news-sars-cov-2-zr-13599530.html, accessed July 20, 2020.

26 https://fragdenstaat.de/dokumente/4123-wie-wir-covid-19-unter-kontrolle-bekommen/, accessed September 10, 2020.

27 www.bundesregierung.de/breg-de/themen/coronavirus/besprechung-der-bundeskanzlerin-mit-den-regierungschefinnen-und-regierungschefs-der-laender-1733248, accessed July 20, 2020.

28 According to recent research, the city of Jena, which was the first to adopt a mandatory mask policy in Germany, achieved a significant reduction of local transmission through that measure. Timo Mitze et al., "Face Masks Considerably Reduce COVID-19 Cases in Germany: A Synthetic Control Method Approach," IZA Discussion Papers, IZA Discussion Papers (Institute of Labor Economics (IZA), June 2020), https://ideas.repec.org/p/iza/izadps/dp13319.html.

29 www.tagesschau.de/inland/corona-grenzschliessung-deutschland-101.html, accessed July 20, 2020.

30 www.spiegel.de/panorama/gesellschaft/coronavirus-bundesregierung-spricht-weltweite-reisewarnung-aus-a-9209a1d9-ec60-4619-84e1-c25318d676a5, accessed July 20, 2020.

31 https://home.kpmg/xx/en/home/insights/2020/07/flash-alert-2020-305.html, accessed July 18, 2020.

32 www.bundesgesundheitsministerium.de/fileadmin/Dateien/3_Downloads/C/Coronavirus/Anordnung_BMG_31._Maerz_2020.pdf, accessed July 20, 2020.

33 www.tagesschau.de/inland/corona-reisende-quarantaene-101.html, accessed July 20, 2020.

On the economic front, the Federal Government announced a EUR 40 billion rescue package for self-employed individuals and small businesses on 19 March.[34] A second, much larger crisis relief package of over EUR 122 billion was announced on 23 March.[35] It covered EUR 50 billion for small companies and self-employed persons, including direct subsidies,[36] a further expansion of the state-subsidised short-time work programme,[37] support measures for hospitals and clinics, EUR 55 billion for anti-pandemic measures, EUR 3.5 billion for protective equipment procurement, vaccination research, support for families with children, etc. Simultaneously, the parliament cleared a temporary increase of the debt ceiling by EUR 100 billion for 2020.[38] On 31 March, the Federal Government introduced an additional economic stabilisation package of EUR 600 billion in loans and guarantees for larger companies.[39]

Phase III: Towards a "New Normal" (since 15 April)

As new infections experienced a sustained decline and hospitals were never overwhelmed, even in the hardest hit regions in western and southern Germany, calls for an exit from the social distancing measures and a restart of the economy began to emerge in April. Advice by some epidemiologists, however, recommended to suppress the spread of the virus more thoroughly before reopening public life.[40] Ultimately, however, the authorities gave in to pressure for reopening.

On 15 April, the Federal Government and the states agreed on a gradual relaxation of social distancing measures.[41] Shops of up to 800 m2 sales area, all book shops, bike shops, and car sellers were allowed to reopen from 20 April. A gradual reopening of schools began from 4 May. Large events remained banned until 31 August. Some states announced additional loosening or restricting measures. On 15 April, the Federal Government began to "strongly recommend" mask wearing in public transport and in shops. In the following days, most federal states issued mandatory mask-wearing rules.[42] This was followed by a further relaxation of distancing measures on 30 April (covering religious gatherings, play grounds, museums, exhibitions, zoos, etc.)[43] and on 6 May (including an extension of social distancing under relaxed rules until 5 June, the reopening of all shops, restricted permission for sports and a further broadening of emergency child care in schools and kindergartens). The 6 May agreement also included an "emergency break" of 50 new infections per 100,000 individuals at the city/county level, above which renewed local anti-epidemic measures become necessary.[44]

On 3 June, the parliament passed a record-breaking economic growth programme (Konjunkturprogramm) of EUR 130 billion, aimed at strengthening economic demand, supporting

---

34 www.spiegel.de/wirtschaft/soziales/corona-krise-bundesregierung-will-40-milliarden-euro-fuer-kleinstunternehmen-bereitstellen-a-ca1f6b3f-8156-4258-a31b-ff335095c9f2, accessed July 20, 2020.

35 www.bundesfinanzministerium.de/Content/DE/Standardartikel/Themen/Schlaglichter/Corona-Schutzschild/2020-03-13-Milliarden-Schutzschild-fuer-Deutschland.html, accessed July 20, 2020.

36 www.bundesregierung.de/breg-de/themen/coronavirus/soforthilfen-beschlossen-1733604, accessed July 19, 2020.

37 www.bundesregierung.de/breg-de/themen/coronavirus/kurzarbeitergeld-1729626, accessed July 19, 2020.

38 www.faz.net/aktuell/wirtschaft/wegen-des-coronavirus-die-schuldenbremse-faellt-16688082.html, accessed July 19, 2020.

39 www.bundesregierung.de/breg-de/themen/coronavirus/wirtschaftsstabilisierung-1733458, accessed July 15, 2020.

40 www.helmholtz.de/fileadmin/user_upload/01_forschung/Helmholtz-COVID-19-Papier_02.pdf, accessed July 19, 2020.

41 www.spiegel.de/politik/deutschland/corona-krise-bund-und-laender-einigen-sich-auf-erste-schritte-aus-dem-lockdown-a-42d774df-b457-4cf4-9b2e-6d3baf164c20, accessed July 16, 2020.

42 www.mdr.de/brisant/maskenpflicht-bayern-sachsen-100.html, accessed July 16, 2020.

43 www.bundesregierung.de/resource/blob/975226/1749804/353e4b4c77a4d9a724347ccb688d3558/2020-04-30-beschluss-bund-laender-data.pdf?download=1, accessed September 10, 2020.

44 www.tagesschau.de/inland/lockerungen-bund-laender-101.html, accessed September 10, 2020

local government investments as well as investments in strategic areas of modernisation (environmental sustainability, digitalisation, pandemic protection, education and research).[45]

Since June the government also began to gradually reopen the borders. On June 5, the EU interior ministers agreed to reopen borders within the Schengen area until the end of the month. The federal government further announced the cancellation of its travel warning for all EU member states plus the UK, Switzerland, Liechtenstein, Norway and Iceland from June 15.[46] On July 1, Germany opened its borders for a first batch of 11 non-EU countries.[47] In order to mitigate the introduction of infections from incoming and returning travelers, on 24 July federal and state health ministers announced to offer free Sars-Cov-2 tests at entry points.[48]

Societal Responses: Mainstream Consensus and Minority Dissent

The COVID-19 pandemic took the German public by surprise. Arguably, it was only when the first pieces of dramatic visual footage from Northern Italy emerged in late February that a significant section of the public began to take the issue seriously. According to the COVID-19 Snapshot Monitoring (COSMO) Internet panel study, by 3 March, 50% of respondents reported that they "almost never/rarely" thought of the novel coronavirus and 39% reported that they were "(rather) not afraid" of it. By 24 March, after the government anti-pandemic measures were initiated, 54% reported that they "constantly/rather often" thought of the virus, while 60% were "(rather) afraid" of it. Subsequently, concern and fear gradually declined, but as of July both indicators remained at a higher level than in early March.[49]

Figure 4.3 Satisfaction with federal government crisis management

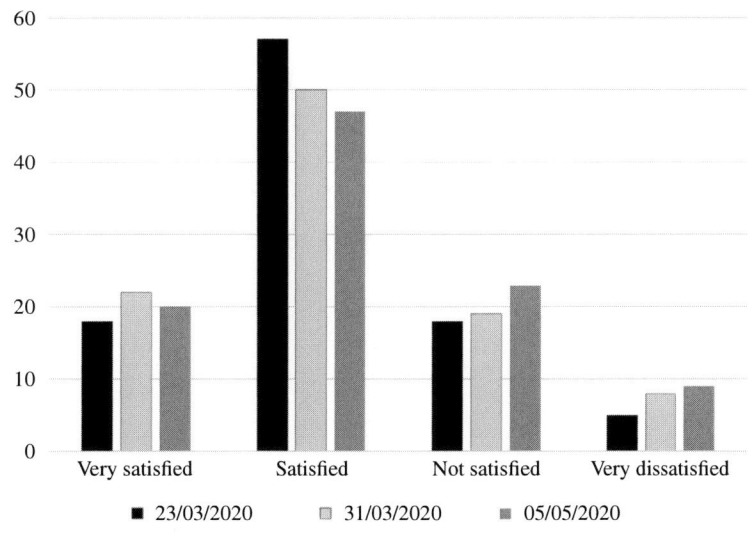

Source: Infratest-Dimap[50]

---

45 www.bundesfinanzministerium.de/Content/DE/Standardartikel/Themen/Schlaglichter/Konjunkturpaket/2020-06-03-eckpunktepapier.pdf?__blob=publicationFile, accessed September 11, 2020

46 www.tagesschau.de/inland/kabinett-reisewarnung-aufhebung-101.html, accessed September 11, 2020.

47 www.tagesschau.de/inland/einreise-deutschland-kabinett-101.html, accessed September 11, 2020.

48 www.gmkonline.de/documents/final_gmk-beschluss-nach-tsk-2407_reinschrift_1595838561.pdf, accessed September 11, 2020.

49 https://projekte.uni-erfurt.de/cosmo2020/cosmo-analysis.html#3_psychologische_lage, accessed August 20, 2020.

50 www.infratest-dimap.de/umfragen-analysen/bundesweit/ard-deutschlandtrend, accessed July 24, 2020.

The government's anti-pandemic measures enjoyed broad public support. Shortly after social distancing measures had been initiated, a telephone survey from 23 March found that 95% of respondents supported contact restrictions in public spaces.[51] Support somewhat decreased over the course of April and May but remained substantial. In mid-May, 66% believed the present measures were "just right", 15% found them "too weak", while 17% believed they were "exaggerated". After a brief public debate over masks and relevant mandatory mask-wearing policies in mid-April, mask wearing became widely publicly accepted. By early July, 90% of respondents to the COSMO Internet panel study thought it was a "useful measure". 90% also reported to have worn a mask over the preceding week.[52] Confidence in state and government increased to record levels in April.[53] Overall satisfaction with government crisis management stood at 75%, 72% and 67% in March, April and May respectively (Figure 3).[54]

Figure 4.4 Voting intention from January to July

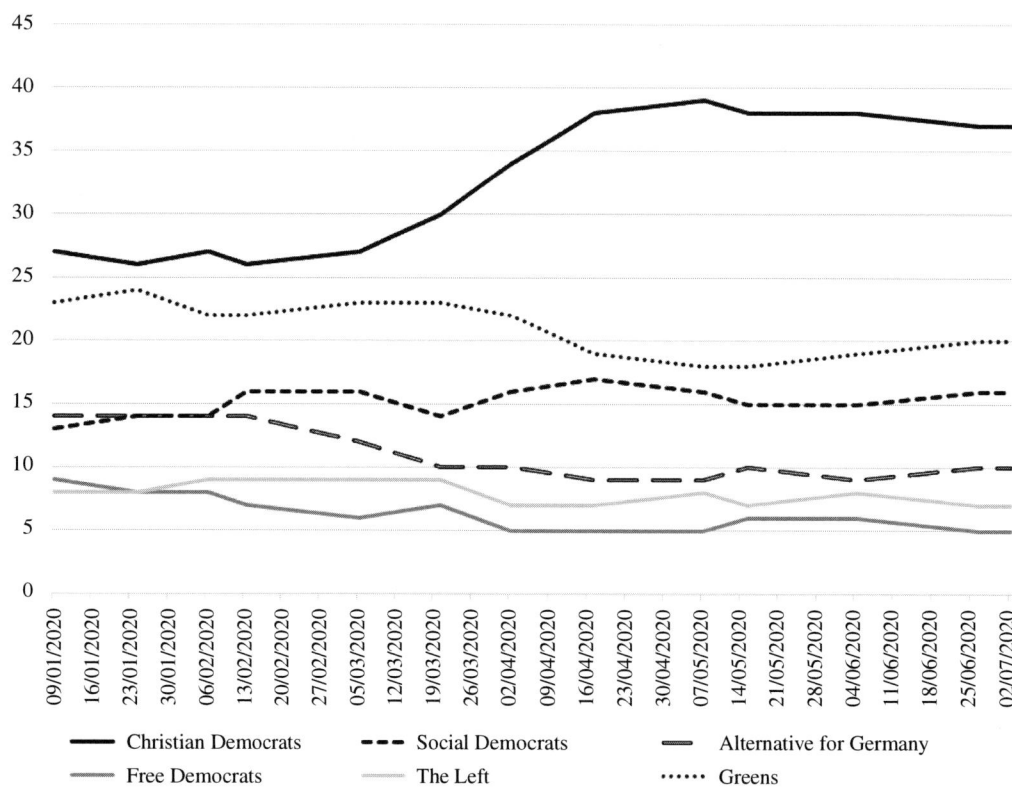

Source: Infratest-Dimap[55]

51 www.infratest-dimap.de/umfragen-analysen/bundesweit/ard-deutschlandtrend/2020/maerz-extra/, accessed July 24, 2020.

52 https://projekte.uni-erfurt.de/cosmo2020/cosmo-analysis.html#11_tragen_einer_maske_in_der_%C3%B6ffentlichkeit, accessed August 20, 2020.

53 www.tagesspiegel.de/politik/rekordwert-in-der-pandemie-vertrauen-in-regierung-erreicht-in-corona-krise-hoechstwert/25819304.html, accessed July 24, 2020.

54 www.infratest-dimap.de/umfragen-analysen/bundesweit/ard-deutschlandtrend/2020/maerz-extra/, accessed July 24, 2020.; www.infratest-dimap.de/umfragen-analysen/bundesweit/ard-deutschlandtrend/2020/april/, accessed July 24, 2020.; www.infratest-dimap.de/umfragen-analysen/bundesweit/ard-deutschlandtrend/2020/mai/; accessed July 24, 2020; www.politico.eu/europe-poll-of-polls/germany/, accessed July 24, 2020.

55 www.infratest-dimap.de/umfragen-analysen/bundesweit/sonntagsfrage/, accessed July 24, 2020.

In terms of party support (Figure 4), Angela Merkel's right-centre Christian Democrats have received a major popularity boost since March, as the public apparently honoured her crisis management. The Christian Democrats' junior coalition partner, the left-centre Social Democrats, have also made modest gains. All opposition parties have lost support. The Greens and the Alternative for Germany (AfD) have lost most. The Greens' strong environmental agenda was possibly eclipsed by rising popular concerns over public health and the economy. The AfD, a right-wing populist outfit that rose to prominence in the aftermath of the European sovereign debt and refugee crises, had difficulties in positioning itself on the pandemic. For one, the issue distracts from identity and immigration, the AfD's trademark issues. For another, although a majority of its support base is drawn towards resistance against the government's anti-pandemic policies, a sizable minority of its comparatively old, and at-risk, voters supports the measures.[56]

Another noteworthy development was a strong upsurge of confidence in science and research. In April, 73% of survey respondents "completely" or "rather" trusted science and research. In the previous three years this value had oscillated around 50%.[57] This rise of confidence in science corresponds to the prominent role that experts, particularly virologists and epidemiologists, played in public. In late February, NDR public radio began an almost daily 30- to 40-minute podcast with Berlin coronavirus expert, Christian Drosten. It soon became the most widely downloaded podcast in Germany.[58] In this podcast, Drosten communicated the latest scientific insights and provided his opinions on questions debated in public. Soon after the Drosten podcast was launched, MDR public radio began a similar podcast with University of Halle epidemiologist and virologist, Alexander Kekulé. It became the second most popular podcast in Germany.[59] These two and a number of other experts were also frequently invited to talk shows and cited in the news media.

The overall wide acceptance of government measures does not imply a lack of public debate. Due to Germany's federal structure, the responsibility for most anti-pandemic measures lies with the states. The Federal Government took the lead in suggesting measures and initiating legislation for economic relief packages. However, it had to moderate agreements between the federal level and the states in terms of anti-epidemic interventions. Different heads of states positioned themselves with slightly different nuances regarding the scope of restrictions and the speed of reopening. The epidemic policy-making process had many "veto points",[60] providing openings for virologists, economists and other scientists to weigh in with position papers and opinions from their respective disciplinary perspectives. Mainstream opinions differed on the detailed configurations and the timing of the measures. However, they largely converged on the risk of COVID-19 to public health and the need for anti-pandemic measures to control its spread.

This consensus was challenged by a vocal minority. This dissenting camp was composed of a hodgepodge of groups, ranging from libertarians, vaccine sceptics, members of the alternative medicine and esoteric scene, adherents of various conspiracy narratives to hard-core right-wing

---

56 In May, 62% of AfD supporters demanded further relaxations of social distancing measures, but 38% rather wanted to maintain existing restrictions. www.infratest-dimap.de/umfragen-analysen/bundesweit/ard-deutschlandtrend/2020/mai/, accessed July 24, 2020.

57 www.wissenschaft-im-dialog.de/fileadmin/user_upload/Projekte/Wissenschaftsbarometer/Dokumente_20/2020_WiD-Wissenschaftsbarometer_Corona_Spezial_Ergebnispraesentation.pdf, accessed July 24, 2020.

58 https://meedia.de/2020/03/26/ueber-15-mio-abrufe-der-gewaltige-erfolg-des-coronavirus-update-mit-professor-christian-drosten/, accessed July 10, 2020.

59 www.mdr.de/nachrichten/ratgeber/gesundheit/neuer-podcast-corona-verstehen-kekule-100.html, accessed July 10, 2020.

60 Ellen M. Immergut, "Institutions, Veto Points, and Policy Results: A Comparative Analysis of Health Care," *Journal of Public Policy* 10, no. 4 (1990): 391–416.

extremists. According to German security organs, the latter have gained increasing influence over the camp.[61] Dissenters have often used the absence of a high number of deaths and an overstretched healthcare system in Germany to cast doubts on the threat posed by COVID-19 and thereby to question the rationale for the government's anti-epidemic policies. The political, media and scientific elite in Germany have remained relatively united in rejecting such claims as unscientific and extremist. A retired physician and a virologist professor emeritus, who have argued that the threat of the virus has been overblown, have been largely shunned by the mainstream media.[62] The only serving university professor who openly joined the opposition camp—an economist—has been publicly denounced and ostracised by his peers.[63]

"Anti-corona" protests took place in various German cities since late March. In August, two rallies in Berlin drew between 30,000 and 40,000 participants each.[64] In mid-May, 16% of the population approved of these protests, while 81% disapproved. By August, these patterns of public opinion had remained largely stable,[65] although the protests received substantial media attention. The demonstrations are disapproved of by large majorities of supporters of all political parties, except those of the far-right AfD. 61% of AfD supporters approved them in May.[66] However, a sizable minority of the party's voter base does not approve of the protests and supports strict anti-pandemic measures.[67] The AfD's signalling on the issue has therefore remained lukewarm.[68] Attempts at organising a so-called "Resistance 2020" party appear to have collapsed.[69] Hence, although the members of the "corona-opposition" are united in their disapproval of the mainstream consensus and the government's anti-pandemic measures, they do not yet seem to share a common ideology or organisation.[70] Nonetheless, the issue links right-wing extremists with other fringe groups, which could open pathways for a broader anti-establishment coalition. So far, however, the extent of political polarisation over the pandemic in Germany has remained limited.

Conclusion

Germany emerged from the first wave of the pandemic in comparatively good shape. Although decision makers were—similar to most Western European countries—initially caught off-guard, the Merkel government quickly turned around and provided decisive crisis management. The country was able to

---

61   www.spiegel.de/politik/deutschland/verfassungsschutz-stellt-starke-rechtsextremistische-komponente-fest-a-e5700a4f-b600-4e21-8f37-9dcb78cac3e9, accessed September 8, 2020.

62   www.zdf.de/nachrichten/panorama/coronavirus-bhakdi-wodarg-check-100.html, accessed July 10, 2020.

63   www.tagesspiegel.de/politik/der-fall-des-stefan-homburg-ein-wirtschaftsprofessor-als-raunender-corona-kritiker/25866032.html, accessed July 10, 2020.

64   www.tagesspiegel.de/berlin/polizei-korrigiert-zahlen-nach-oben-auf-der-ersten-corona-demo-in-berlin-waren-doch-30-000-menschen/26136252.html, accessed September 10, 2020.; www.spiegel.de/politik/deutschland/zehntausende-menschen-bei-kundgebung-an-siegessaeule-a-4238778c-9e90-4914-8680-2084c6773a4d, accessed September 10, 2020.

65   www.spiegel.de/politik/deutschland/demos-gegen-corona-politik-grosse-mehrheit-der-deutschen-hat-kein-verstaendnis-a-2e920864-7f07-420f-b46c-6dbf55c05aac, accessed Septmber 10, 2020.

66   www.zdf.de/nachrichten/politik/politbarometer-coronavirus-grenzoeffnung-eu-100.html?slide=1589461853968, accessed September 10, 2020.

67   See footnote 57.

68   www.tagesschau.de/inland/afd-corona-demonstrationen-101.html, accessed September 7, 2020.

69   www.spiegel.de/politik/deutschland/corona-protestbewegung-widerstand-2020-eine-moechtegern-partei-zerlegt-sich-selbst-a-dd92766e-275c-4086-9323-ca072ec53203, accessed Septmber 7, 2020.

70   www.zdf.de/nachrichten/politik/coronavirus-demos-protest-100.html, accessed Septmber 10, 2020.

draw on its scientific infrastructure to enable widespread testing early on and effectively communicate knowledge to the public. Moreover, Germany came into the crisis with a strong fiscal position and was, therefore, able to enact large economic support packages. Nonetheless, luck may have played a significant role as well. The first local cluster was detected due to a test conducted in China. Had Germany experienced local hotspots with longer covert transmission similar to Italy, Spain or France, the public health crisis could easily have become much more critical.

To an extent, Germany became a victim of its relative success in the containment of the virus. The absence of an acute public health crisis played into the hands of actors pushing conspiracy narratives that cast doubt on COVID-19's threat to public health. However, such voices remained marginal and did not find an effective political broker. The political, scientific and media elites were relatively united in their assessment of the threat and the necessity for counter-measures. Even the right-wing populist AfD supported dissenting views only reluctantly. Hence, the country has, so far, largely avoided intense political polarisation over the pandemic.

As of late August, the spread of the virus appears to be relatively under control and its immediate economic fall-out has been cushioned by government support packages. Nevertheless, local outbreaks and gradually rising infection numbers across the board over the summer clearly suggest that the epidemic is far from over. Recurring "anti-corona" protests since March, as well as clashes between frustrated youngsters and the police,[71] signal that latent popular discontent is present. It remains to be seen whether Germany's relative stability will hold when COVID-19's economic damage begins to be felt more broadly and the country possibly experiences a second surge of infections over the winter months.

---

71 www.zeit.de/gesellschaft/zeitgeschehen/2020-06/krawalle-stuttgart-ausschreitungen-pluenderungen-polizei-randale-innenstadt, accessed July 24, 2020.

GERMANY

H. Christoph Steinhardt

16.01–29.10 Total 242,381 cases / 9,298 deaths

01

Key events and public health policies

16.01 Christian Drosten and his team at Charité Hospital Berlin, developed and publicized the first diagnostic test for the novel coronavirus on January 16, 2020,[1] and distributed the test protocol to a large network of government and private labs in Germany.[2]

22.01 On 22 January, Health Minister, Jens Spahn, declared that the virus posed "a very minor" risk to public health in Germany, that there was "no reason for alarm"[3] and that the country was "well prepared" for COVID-19.[4] The director of the Robert-Koch Institut (RKI), Lothar Wieler, declared that the RKI did not expect that the virus "will not spread very widely." Virologist and epidemiologist, Alexander Kekulé, challenged this assessment.[5]

28.01 Minister of Health Jens Spahn declared Germany "well prepared" for Covid-19.[6]

The first confirmed cases of infection at car component manufacturer Webasto near Munich qas detected. The index case was a Chinese employee who came in from Shanghai. The virus spread to 13 others, but the outbreak was contained. The cases were extensively studied by scholars.[7]

30.01 A tourist returning from Austrian Tyrol was tested positive.

02

Key events and public health policies

02.02 100 German returnees from Wuhan were tested positive and isolated.

23.02 Virologist Drosten stated that a pandemic is now unavoidable and will affect Germany.[8]

Mid to late February
Carnival parties, mostly in western and southern Germany, are being celebrated.

25.02 First infections diagnosed among participants of a carnival party (15.01) of around 300 participants in Heinsberg county, Western Germany. All participants were asked to quarantine themselves. Heinsberg turned into Germany's first Covid-19 hotspot.[9]

Virologist Alexander Kekule criticized the Federal Government for

** where shown, the number in brackets is the accumulated number of confirmed cases and death cases respectively.

1 www.charite.de/en/service/press_reports/artikel/detail/researchers_develop_first_diagnostic_test_for_novel_coronavirus_in_china/

2 www.bbc.com/news/health-52234061

3 https://rp-online.de/panorama/ausland/bundesregierung-coronavirus-nur-geringes-gesundheitsrisiko-in-deutschland_aid-48488333, accessed September 10, 2020.

4 www.welt.de/regionales/bayern/article205400853/Spahn-nach-Coronavirus-Fall-in-Bayern-Sind-gut-vorbereitet.html, accessed September 10, 2020.

5 www.merkur.de/welt/corona-rki-robert-koch-institut-hopkins-zahlen-infektionen-statistik-kritik-wieler-deutschland-zr-13602916.html.

6 www.welt.de/regionales/bayern/article205400853/Spahn-nach-Coronavirus-Fall-in-Bayern-Sind-gut-vorbereitet.html

7 See, e.g. Camilla Rothe et al., "Transmission of 2019-NCoV Infection from an Asymptomatic Contact in Germany," *New England Journal of Medicine* 382, no. 10 (March 5, 2020): 970–71, https://doi.org/10.1056/NEJMc2001468; Roman Wölfel et al., "Virological Assessment of Hospitalized Patients with COVID-2019," *Nature*, April 1, 2020, 1–10, https://doi.org/10.1038/s41586-020-2196-x.

8 www.zdf.de/nachrichten/panorama/italien-coronavirus-pandemie-gefahr-100.html

9 www1.wdr.de/nachrichten/rheinland/corona-virus-zusammenfassung-donnerstag-100.html

misjudging the risk of the virus, not adopting sufficient measures.[10]

26.02 Health Minister Spahn declared that Germany was at the beginning of an epidemic.[11]

A growing number of infections were detected among business travellers and tourists, mostly those returning from Italy, Austria and Switzerland.

NDR public radio began a podcast with coronavirus expert Christian Drosten. It became the most widely downloaded podcast in Germany.[12]

27.02 Ministries of Health and Interior Affairs formed a crisis group.[13]

Travelers from Covid-19 hotspot countries had to fill in registration forms upon arrival. A travel ban similar to measures adopted elsewhere was explicitly rejected.[14]

Germany temporarily stopped intake of refugees from UN resettlement program and for humanitarian reasons. Asylum seeking remained principally possible.[15]

The RKI called on people with symptoms to stay home.[16]

03

Key events and public health policies

Early March A growing number of infections could not be traced back to travel history. Community transmissions were established in multiple locations.

02.03 The RKI increased its risk assessment for Germany from low to medium.

04.03 In reaction to shortages in the health care system, the federal government began to procure Personal Protective Equipment (PPE) for medical personnel.[17]

PPE exports were temporally banned (leading to tensions with neighbouring countries).[18] The ban was later suspended.

08.03 Health minister Spahn recommended cancelling events above 1000 participants.[19]

09.03 The first two Covid-19 deaths occurred in North-Rhine Westphalia.[20]

12.03 Chancellor Merkel recommended everyone to stay home, reduce social contacts, wherever possible, and to cancel all unnecessary events.[21]

12.03 Halle in Easter Germany became the first city to close all schools and kindergartens.[22]

13–18.03 Federal states closed schools, kindergartens and universities.[23]

Socio-Economic Policy Packages

14.03 Parliament passed law to expand short-time work.[24]

10 www.welt.de/vermischtes/article206114643/Jens-Spahn-unterschaetzt-das-Coronavirus-glaubt-ein-Virologe.html

11 www.welt.de/vermischtes/article206136215/Coronavirus-Spahn-sieht-Deutschland-am-Beginn-einer-Epidemie.html

12 https://meedia.de/2020/03/26/ueber-15-mio-abrufe-der-gewaltige-erfolg-des-coronavirus-update-mit-professor-christian-drosten/

13 www.spiegel.de/politik/deutschland/coronavirus-in-deutschland-bundesregierung-fuehrt-registrierung-von-reisenden-aus-betroffenen-laendern-ein-a-d718ed8d-6d3c-4acd-9cf7-98fdba4bce68

14 www.spiegel.de/politik/deutschland/coronavirus-in-deutschland-bundesregierung-fuehrt-registrierung-von-reisenden-aus-betroffenen-laendern-ein-a-d718ed8d-6d3c-4acd-9cf7-98fdba4bce68< www.tagesschau.de/ausland/eu-coronavirus-101.html

15 www.tagesschau.de/inland/fluechtlinge-2185.html

16 www.derwesten.de/panorama/vermischtes/coronavirus-covid-19-symptome-desinfektion-news-zahlen-tote-id228522951.html

17 www.deutsche-apotheker-zeitung.de/news/artikel/2020/03/04/medizinische-schutzausruestung-wird-jetzt-zentral-beschafft

18 http://web.archive.org/web/20200316000031/www.bafa.de/DE/Aussenwirtschaft/Ausfuhrkontrolle/Coronavirus_Schutzausruestung/coronavirus_schutzausruestung_node.html

19 www.n-tv.de/panorama/Spahn-Alle-Grossveranstaltungen-absagen-article21627196.html

20 www.dw.com/de/erste-corona-todesf%C3%A4lle-in-deutschland/a-52597027

21 www.wa.de/deutschland-welt/coronavirus-sars-cov-2-corona-epidemie-suedkorea-dramatisch-merkel-aeussert-sich-zr-13560844.html; www.bundeskanzlerin.de/bkin-de/aktuelles/pressekonferenz-von-bundeskanzlerin-merkel-ministerpraesident-soeder-und-dem-ersten-buergermeister-tschentscher-1730300

22 www.mz-web.de/halle-saale/wegen-corona-halle-schliesst-als-erste-deutsche-grossstadt-alle-schulen-und-kitas-36404152

23 www.spiegel.de/panorama/coronavirus-wo-schulen-und-kitas-geschlossen-werden-a-30dc65e6-b6bc-4787-9113-f8a4945005bb

24 www.buzer.de/s1.htm?g=Gesetz+zur+befristeten+krisenbedingten+Verbesserung+der+Regelungen+f%C3%BCr+das+Kurzarbeitergeld&f=1

Key events and public health policies

16.03 Germany closed the border to most neighbouring countries.[25]

Bavaria declared the state of emergency.[26]

MDR public radio started a coronavirus podcast with epidemiologist and virologist Alexander Kekulé.[27] It became the second most popular podcast in Germany.

17.03 The Ministry of Foreign Affairs declared a worldwide travel warning.[28]

The RKI raised its risk assessment to "high".

Bavaria ordered 400 civil servants to support local health departments.[29]

Psychotherapists were allowed to treat patients via video.[30]

Socio-Economic Policy Packages

19.03 The federal government announced 40 billion EUR rescue package for self-employed and small businesses.[31]

Key events and public health policies

20.03 The federal government ordered large quantities of additional ventilators from German producers.[32]

Hesse health minister called for students and retired doctors to volunteer in hospitals.[33]

22.03 An internal federal government document, which estimated over 1 million deaths if no anti-epidemic measures are taken, was leaked to the public.[34]

The federal government and states agreed on nationwide social distancing measures. These included:

- A recommendation to reduce close social contacts as much as possible
- To entering the public space only alone of with members of one's household
- To keep a minimum distance of 1.5 m to people outside of one's household
- Going to work, exercise or walks outside remained permitted
- Public gatherings were banned
- Restaurants were closed except for take-away
- Hygiene measures in all work places
- Etc.

- Mandatory mask wearing was not included.[35]

Some federal states mandated stricter stay at home orders.

Socio-Economic Policy Packages

23.03 Federal government announced crises relief package of 122.5 billion EUR, including: [36]

- 50 billion EUR for small companies and self-employed, including direct subsidies[37]
- Further expansion of short-time work programme[38]
- Support measures for hospitals and clinics
- 55 billion for anti-pandemic measures
- 3.5 billion for PPE procurement and vaccine research
- Support for families with children

25 www.tagesschau.de/inland/corona-grenzschliessung-deutschland-101.html

26 www.merkur.de/bayern/coronavirus-soeder-bayern-katastrophenfall-tote-massnahmen-schliessung-geschaefte-news-sars-cov-2-zr-13599530.html

27 www.mdr.de/nachrichten/ratgeber/gesundheit/neuer-podcast-corona-verstehen-kekule-100.html

28 www.spiegel.de/panorama/gesellschaft/coronavirus-bundesregierung-spricht-weltweite-reisewarnung-aus-a-9209a1d9-ec60-4619-84e1-c25318d676a5

29 www.frankenpost.de/region/bayern/Coronavirus-400-Beamte-in-Gesundheitsbehoerden-abgeordnet;art2832,7180770

30 www.bptk.de/begrenzung-von-videobehandlungen-aufgehoben/

31 www.spiegel.de/wirtschaft/soziales/corona-krise-bundesregierung-will-40-milliarden-euro-fuer-kleinstunternehmen-bereitstellen-a-ca1f6b3f-8156-4258-a31b-ff335095c9f2

32 www.faz.net/aktuell/wirtschaft/coronavirus-hersteller-von-beatmungsgeraeten-arbeiten-am-anschlag-16688797.html

33 www.faz.net/aktuell/rhein-main/hessen-medizinstudenten-sollen-in-krankenhaeusern-aushelfen-16688501.html

34 https://fragdenstaat.de/dokumente/4123-wie-wir-covid-19-unter-kontrolle-bekommen/

35 www.bundesregierung.de/breg-de/themen/coronavirus/besprechung-der-bundeskanzlerin-mit-den-regierungschefinnen-und-regierungschefs-der-laender-1733248

36 www.bundesfinanzministerium.de/Content/DE/Standardartikel/Themen/Schlaglichter/Corona-Schutzschild/2020-03-13-Milliarden-Schutzschild-fuer-Deutschland.html

37 www.bundesregierung.de/breg-de/themen/coronavirus/soforthilfen-beschlossen-1733604

38 www.bundesregierung.de/breg-de/themen/coronavirus/kurzarbeitergeld-1729626

The federal government introduced an addition economic stabilization package of 600 billion EUR in credit and guarantees for larger companies.[39]

Parliament cleared a temporary raise of the debt ceiling by 100 billion EUR for 2020.[40]

Key events and public health policies

26.03 The RKI raised its risk assessment to "very high"

The president of German association of medical doctors called for universal surgical or DIY face mask wearing — contradicting the RKI's position, which then recommended masks only for the sick and medical personnel.[41]

31.03 All incoming travel from Iran was banned.[42]

04

Socio-Economic Policy Packages

06.04 The Ministry of Finance announced new fast-track credit program for small and medium enterprises.[43]

Key events and public health policies

09.04 Virologist Hendrik Streek released intermediary results from a community study in Covid-19 hotspot Heinsberg; reports that 15% of the population have developed anti-bodies.

The press conference announcement caused a stir and fuelled the debate over "re-opening".[44]

The RKI announced the beginning of a representative, nationwide immunity study. First results were expected in June.[45]

Socio-Economic Policy Packages

09.04 EU finance ministers agree on a first 500 billion EUR rescue package.[46]

Ministry of Commerce expert panel projected the economy to shrink by 4.2% in 2020.[47]

Key events and public health policies

10.04 All incoming travellers were required to go in 14 days quarantine.[48]

15.04 The federal government and the states agreed on a gradual loosening of social distancing measures.[49]

- Distancing and stay at home orders extended to 03.05
- Gradual reopening of schools from 04.05
- Large events banned until 31.08

- Shops up to 800 m2 sales area, and all book shops, bike shops, and care sellers were allowed to reopen from 20.04.

Some states announced additional loosening measures or restrictions.

The federal government "strongly" recommended mask wearing in public transport and in shops. In the following days, most federal states issued mandatory mask rules.[50]

19.04 The German Academy of Sciences, Leopoldina released a report with policy recommendations on how to manage the Covid-19 crisis.[51]

30.04 Chancellor Merkel and state prime ministers agreed on a further loosening of anti-pandemic measures during a telephone conference.[52]

39 www.bundesregierung.de/breg-de/themen/coronavirus/wirtschaftsstabilisierung-1733458

40 www.faz.net/aktuell/wirtschaft/wegen-des-coronavirus-die-schuldenbremse-faellt-16688082.html

41 www.faz.net/aktuell/rhein-main/hessen-medizinstudenten-sollen-in-krankenhaeusern-aushelfen-16688501.html

42 www.bundesgesundheitsministerium.de/fileadmin/Dateien/3_Downloads/C/Coronavirus/Anordnung_BMG_31._Maerz_2020.pdf

43 www.bundesfinanzministerium.de/Content/DE/Pressemitteilungen/Finanzpolitik/2020/04/2020-04-06-gemeinsame-pm-bmf-bmwi-kfw.html

44 www.rundschau-online.de/region/corona-pressekonferenz-mit-laschet--der-lockdown-hat-auch-viele-schaeden-verursacht--36439428

45 www.rki.de/DE/Content/Service/Presse/Pressemitteilungen/2020/05_2020.html

46 www.bundesfinanzministerium.de/Content/DE/Video/2020/2020-04-09-eurogruppe-pk-april/2020-04-09-eurogruppe-pk-april.html

47 www.bmwi.de/Redaktion/DE/Pressemitteilungen/2020/20200408-altmaier-rechnen-mit-deutlichen-einschnitten-in-wirtschaftsentwicklung-gemeinschaftsdiagnose-stellt-fruehjahrsgutachten-vor.html

48 www.tagesschau.de/inland/corona-reisende-quarantaene-101.html

49 www.spiegel.de/politik/deutschland/corona-krise-bund-und-laender-einigen-sich-auf-erste-schritte-aus-dem-lockdown-a-42d774df-b457-4cf4-9b2e-6d3baf164c20

50 www.mdr.de/brisant/maskenpflicht-bayern-sachsen-100.html

51 www.leopoldina.org/uploads/tx_leopublication/2020_04_13_Coronavirus-Pandemie-Die_Krise_nachhaltig_%C3%BCberwinden_final.pdf

52 www.bundesregierung.de/resource/blob/975226/1749804/353e4b4c77a4d9a724347ccb688d3558/2020-04-30-beschluss-bund-laender-data.pdf?download=1

05

Key events and public health policies

06.05 Chancellor Merkel and state prime ministers agreed on further loosening of anti-pandemic measures during a telephone conference.

The agreement also included an "emergency break" of 50 new infections per 100,000 individuals at the city/county level, in seven days above which renewed local anti-epidemic measures become necessary.[53]

06

Key events and public health policies

03.06 Parliament passed another record-breaking economic growth programme (Konjunkturprogramm) of EUR 130 billion, aimed at strengthening economic demand, supporting local government investments as well as investments in strategic areas of modernisation (environmental sustainability, digitalisation, pandemic protection, education and research).[54]

05.06 EU interior minister agreed to reopen border within the Schengen area until the end of June.[55]

The federal government announced the cancellation of travel warnings for all EU members plus the UK, Switzerland, Liechtenstein, Norway and Iceland from June 15.[56]

Since 15 June, the government designated high-risk areas. Incoming travellers from these regions are subject to quarantine rules.

16.06 The federal government released a Corona warning app and appeals to the public to install it on their smart phones. Its use is voluntary.[57]

21.06 Hundreds of frustrated youngsters and the police clashed in Stuttgart.[58]

07

Key events and public health policies

01.07 Germany opened its borders for the first 11 non-EU countries.[59]

24.07 Federal and state health ministers agreed to offer free Sars-Cov-2 tests to returning travellers from abroad.[60]

08

Key events and public health policies

01.08 30,000 protested against the government's anti-pandemic policies in Berlin.[61]

12.08 The RKI released a new national Sars-Cov-2 testing strategy, offering public-insurance paid tests for those with any respiratory, COVID-19 typical symptoms; those with contact to a confirmed COVID-19 case; patients and staff in hospitals and other care institutions; individuals in shared facilities (schools, asylum seekers centres, prisons etc.); parts or the complete population in the case of severe local outbreaks; incoming travellers from risk regions (mandatory) and non-risk region (voluntary).[62]

27.08 Chancellor Merkel and state prime ministers agreed on further measures including a common minimum penalty of EUR 50 for violations of mask mandates (Saxony-Anhalt opted out); a continuation of a testing requirement for incoming travellers from risk regions.[63]

Socio-Economic Policy Packages

27.08 Chancellor Merkel and state prime ministers agreed on another 500 million EUR for digital school teaching and additional days of childcare sick leave for parents.[64]

Key events and public health policies

29.08 38,000 protested against the government's anti-pandemic policies

53 www.tagesschau.de/inland/lockerungen-bund-laender-101.html

54 www.bundesfinanzministerium.de/Content/DE/Standardartikel/Themen/Schlaglichter/Konjunkturpaket/2020-06-03-eckpunktepapier.pdf?__blob=publicationFile.

55 www.nzz.ch/international/reisefreiheit-zurueck-in-europa-ld.1560082

56 www.tagesschau.de/inland/kabinett-reisewarnung-aufhebung-101.html

57 www.bundesregierung.de/breg-de/themen/corona-warn-app

58 www.zeit.de/gesellschaft/zeitgeschehen/2020-06/krawalle-stuttgart-ausschreitungen-pluenderungen-polizei-randale-innenstadt

59 www.tagesschau.de/inland/einreise-deutschland-kabinett-101.html

60 www.gmkonline.de/documents/final_gmk-beschluss-nach-tsk-2407_reinschrift_1595838561.pdf

61 www.tagesspiegel.de/berlin/polizei-korrigiert-zahlen-nach-oben-auf-der-ersten-corona-demo-in-berlin-waren-doch-30-000-menschen/26136252.html.

62 www.rki.de/DE/Content/Service/Presse/Pressemitteilungen/2020/08_2020.html

63 www.bundesregierung.de/resource/blob/975232/1780568/2f9c77a8e8a549bcac8123fbeff4ee27/2020-08-27-beschluss-mpk-data.pdf?download=1

64 www.bundesregierung.de/resource/blob/975232/1780568/2f9c77a8e8a549bcac8123fbeff4ee27/2020-08-27-beschluss-mpk-data.pdf?download=1

in Berlin. Clashes erupted after the police cancelled the demonstration permit due to violations of hygiene requirements.[65] A few hundred hardcore protesters attempted to storm the parliament.[66]

09

Key events and public health policies

29.09 Chancellor Merkel and state prime ministers agreed that due to the epidemic development no further opening measures are possible. Additional measures in hotspot regions (50 new infections per 100,000 individuals at the city/county level per seven days) shall be further taken more decisively.[67]

10

Key events and public health policies

07.10 The Chancellor's Chief of Staff and his state counterparts agreed that more attention must be paid to hotspot regions. The federal and state governments will provide support to safeguard contact tracing in hotspots. The state will require domestic travellers from hotspots to provide a negative Sars-Cov-2 test in order to be allowed to stay in overnight accommodations. Several state governments protocol additional opinions.[68]

14.10 Chancellor Merkel and state prime ministers agreed to further expand and tighten the "hotspot strategy". At a seven-day rate of 35 new infections per 100,000 individuals at the city/county level additional restrictions are recommended. At a seven-day rate 50 new infections per 100,000 individuals at the city/county level a list of measures become mandatory. If the rate of infections further increase after 10 days, additional contact restrictions are mandated.[69]

15.10 The National Academy of Sciences, Leopoldina issued a statement recommending stricter contact restrictions, warning of an "escalating" growth of infections and an imminent loss of control over the epidemic. The Academy further publishes a list of recommendations for fall and winter.[70]

16.10 The head of the domestic intelligence service (Bundesamt für Verfassungsschutz) and his two deputies were tested positive for SARS-CoV-2.[71]

21.10 Minister of Health Jens Spahn was tested positive for SARS-CoV-2.[72]

27.10 The presidents of the six largest German research institutions the German Research Foundation Association, the Fraunhofer Association, the Helmholtz Association, the Leibnitz Association, The Max Planck Association and the National Academy of Sciences, Leopoldina released a position paper entitled "Coronavirus pandemic: the situation is serious." It recommended a decisive, timely reduction of social contacts to 1/4 and a sustainable continuation of hygiene measures afterwards in order to prevent the epidemic from getting out of control.[73]

28.10 Chancellor Merkel and state prime ministers agreed to mandate another nationwide package of social distancing measures to break the accelerating rate of COVID-19 infections and prevent an overwhelm of the health care system. They begin from 2 November, will be evaluated two weeks later and are set to expire at the end of the month.[74] The package included:

- A mandate to enter the public space with at most one other household and groups of at most 10 people

---

65 www.spiegel.de/politik/deutschland/zehntausende-menschen-bei-kundgebung-an-siegessaeule-a-4238778c-9e90-4914-8680-2084c6773a4d

66 www.rnd.de/politik/sorgen-wurden-wahr-corona-demo-mit-sturm-auf-den-reichstag-QF6VWMMHHJA7ZPXRNG4KORCKWA.html

67 www.bundeskanzlerin.de/bkin-de/suche/videoschaltkonferenz-der-bundeskanzlerin-mit-den-regierungschefinnen-und-regierungschefs-der-laender-am-29-september-2020-1792240

68 www.bundeskanzlerin.de/bkin-de/aktuelles/telefonschaltkonferenz-des-chefs-des-bundeskanzleramts-mit-den-chefinnen-und-chefs-der-staats-und-senatskanzleien-der-laender-am-7-oktober-2020-1796770

69 www.bundesregierung.de/resource/blob/997532/1798920/9448da53f1fa442c24c37abc8b0b2048/2020-10-14-beschluss-mpk-data.pdf?download=1

70 www.leopoldina.org/presse-1/nachrichten/leopoldina-fordert-konsequenteres-handeln/

71 www.tagesspiegel.de/politik/corona-trifft-den-nachrichtendienst-gesamte-leitung-des-bundesamtes-fuer-verfassungsschutz-infiziert/26281806.html

72 www.tagesschau.de/inland/coronavirus-spahn-107.html

73 www.helmholtz.de/fileadmin/user_upload/01_forschung/03_Gesundheit/2020_Gemeinsame_Erklaerung_zur_Coronavirus-Pandemie.pdf

74 www.bundesregierung.de/resource/blob/997532/1805024/5353edede6c0125ebe5b5166504dfd79/2020-10-28-mpk-beschluss-corona-data.pdf?download=1

- A recommendation to reduce close social contacts to an absolute minimum, to refrain from private travel, and ban of hotel accommodation for private travel
- A closure of recreational institutions and events including theatres, cinemas, exhibitions, brothels and prostitution, amateur sports, swimming pools, fitness centres, restaurants, night clubs, etc.
- A closure of businesses that require close physical contact such as tattoo shops, beauty salons and massage salons
- Exempted are retail and whole sale business, industry, craft trade, hairdressers, and medically required physical treatments
- Schools and Kindergartens stay open

Socio-Economic Policy Packages

28.10 The federal government released another 10 billion EUR in emergency aid to businesses, associations and self-employed individuals affected by the renewed temporary closures.

The aid covers 75% of the revenue during the same time last year for businesses of up to 50 employees, as well as to be determined amounts for larger businesses.[75]

Key events and public health policies

29.10 The National Association of Statutory Health Insurance Physicians ("Kassenärztliche Bundesvereinigung") together with leading virologists Hendrik Streeck and Jonas Schmidt-Chanasit released a position paper. It argues against a renewed suppression of infections through mandatory social distancing, highlighting the negative side effects of such measures. The authors argue for a principle of recommendations instead of mandates, a more systematic and organized protection of risk groups, a focus of contact tracing on super spreading events, health care workers and risk groups, and a nationally unified "signal light" system to communicate the regional epidemic risk to the population.[76]

---

75 www.bundesregierung.de/resource/blob/997532/1805024/5353edede6c0125ebe5b5166504dfd79/2020-10-28-mpk-beschluss-corona-data.pdf?download=1

76 www.kbv.de/media/sp/2020-10-29_KBV-Positionspapier_COVID-19.pdf

COVID-19 in Hong Kong:
Pulling Together amidst Divisions[1]

Linda Chelan Li[2], assisted by Cleo Wong, Jeffrey Chung and Xin Yan

Against the backdrop of unprecedented political polarization since June 2019, the city's response to the COVID-19 pandemic tells the depth of social resilience and the strength of its institutions. Bottom-up initiatives of individuals and groups — including many small-medium-sized companies — made up the bulk of interconnected networks of community responses from social distancing to local production of face masks, and contributed to significant policy lobbies.

Up till 5 September 2020, cumulative confirmed COVID-19 cases in Hong Kong have reached 4,858, with deaths of 94 and total recoveries of 4,492. (See Figures 5.1 and 5.2) It took 80 days since 23 January to reach 1,000 cases in Hong Kong and 101 days to double, while only 18 days were taken to double again reaching 4,000 cases in total. As of August 2020, Hong Kong's economy has contracted 9% over a year earlier, and the seasonally adjusted unemployment rate in July has reached 6.1%.

Figure 5.1 Daily confirmed cases, deaths and recoveries from 23 January 2020 to 5 September 2020[3]

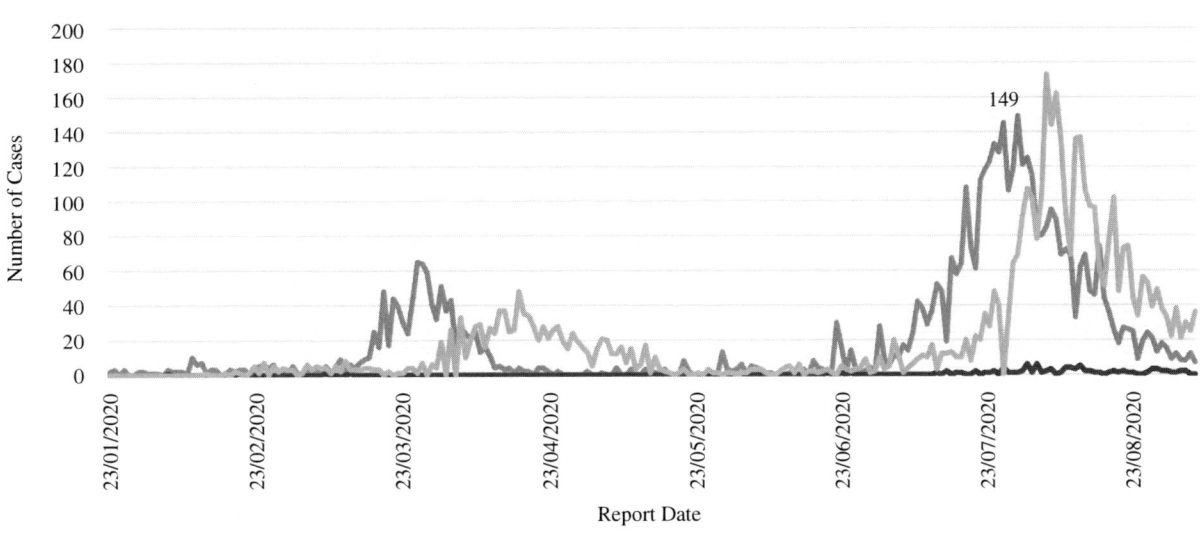

1 An early version of this Hong Kong account appears as CSHK Working Paper No.4 released in May 2020

2 Linda Chelan Li is professor of political science at Department of Public Policy, and director of Research Centre for Sustainable Hong Kong (CSHK), City University of Hong Kong; contact email: salcli@cityu.edu.hk.

3 The data is drawn from Hong Kong Center for Health Protection and database of WorldoMeters, at www.worldometers.info/coronavirus/country/china-hong-kong-sar/

Figure 5.2 Cumulative cases from 23 January to 5 September 2020

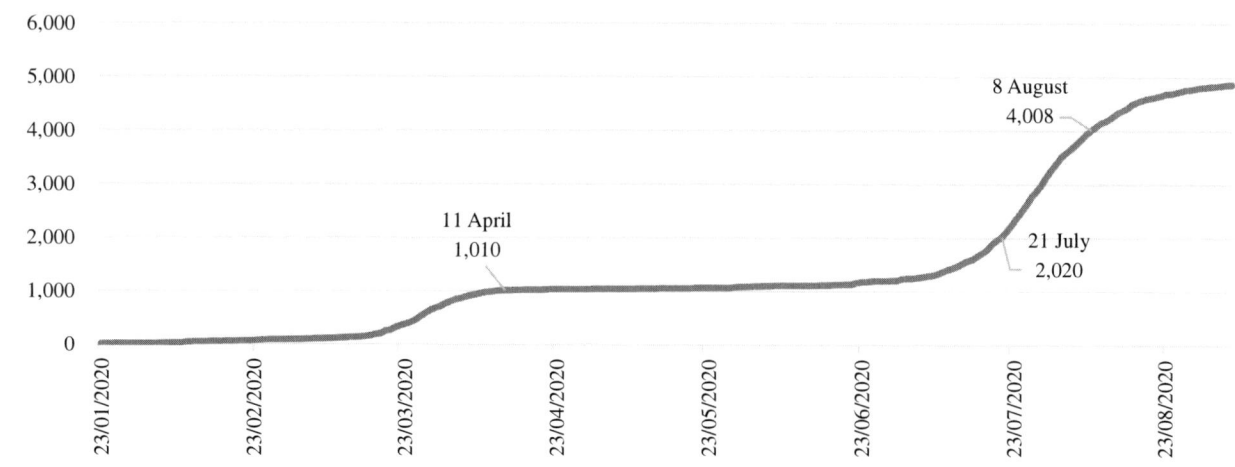

Source: HK Centre for Health Protection

A Society-Driven Response

Hong Kong's strategies on COVID-19 have appeared in international media and scientific reports.[4] The city has contained the community spread of the virus relatively successfully despite its proximity with Mainland China and function as a regional and international transport hub. Hong Kong has also not had the blanket "lock down" of social activities as in other parts of China, or parts of Europe and many other regions. Instead a selective approach targeting premises of higher risks was adopted. Notwithstanding the recent heightening of social and political tensions in the city, the Hong Kong SAR Government has displayed a high degree of caution in mandating instructions to the market, reflecting the deep-seated influence of the free market ethos on the city governance.

A conspicuous feature of Hong Kong's response to the pandemic is the almost universal voluntary use of surgical face masks from the early days. Surveys by a group of epidemiologists in University of Hong Kong found that masks were worn regularly by 74.5% as early as 20-23 January, ahead of the commencement of lockdown of Wuhan on 23 January. The coverage rose to 97.5% and 98.8% by 11-14 February and 10-13 March respectively. Also, many of the surveyed had voluntarily avoided crowded places to reduce risks of infection.[5] Another study by Hong Kong Polytechnic University found 95% of people wore face masks in public areas between February and April 2020, while one-eighth of them appeared not wearing the masks properly.[6] Unlike in some cities, e.g. Singapore, where people are fined

---

4   A few examples are: The Guardian, Test and trace: lessons from Hong Kong on avoiding a coronavirus lockdown, 17 April 2020 (www.theguardian.com/world/2020/apr/17/test-trace-lessons-hong-kong-avoiding-coronavirus-lockdown); Bloomberg, Hong Kong Shutdown a Lesson to the World in Halting Virus, 16 March 2020 (www.bloomberg.com/news/articles/2020-03-16/hong-kong-shutdown-is-a-lesson-to-the-world-in-halting-the-virus); *Nature*, Whose coronavirus strategy worked best? Scientists hunt most effective policies, 27 April 2020 (www.nature.com/articles/d41586-020-01248-1); Cowling, Benjamin J., et al (2020), Impact assessment of non-pharmaceutical interventions against coronavirus disease 2019 and influenza in Hong Kong: an observational study, *The Lancet*, Vol. 5 (May 2020), e279-e288. (www.thelancet.com/journals/lanpub/article/PIIS2468-2667(20)30090-6/fulltext).

5   Cowling, Ali and Ng et al., "Impact assessment of non-pharmaceutical interventions against coronavirus disease 2019 and influenza in Hong Kong: an observational study", *Lancet*, vol. 5 (2020), pp. e279-e288.

6   The Hong Kong Polytechnic University Press Release, (28 April 2020), "PolyU Study Shows One in Eight Not Wearing Face Masks Properly • Almost 80% of People Reusing Them • Experts Urge Users to Wear Face Masks Correctly and Formulate Guidelines on Reuse to Minimise Contagion Risks," https://www.polyu.edu.hk/media/media-releases/2020/0428_polyu-study-shows-one-in-eight-not-wearing-face-masks-properly-almost-80-of-people/

for noncompliance of mandatory orders, wearing face masks has acquired a status of social convention in Hong Kong, making legislation almost redundant. Government eventually legislated in mid-July 2020, during the third wave of outbreak, to make the wearing of masks mandatory, initially in public transport only and later in all public open-air places (See Government Measures).

Since January 2020, securing sufficient supply of surgical masks to meet the demand for everyone has preoccupied discussion in society. Leading local medical experts have supported the use of surgical masks to reduce infection as early as the first week of the outbreak.[7] The Hong Kong Legislative Council raised the issue with the Secretary for Food and Health of the HKSAR Government as early as 8 January.[8] Senior government officials, from bureau ministers to the Chief Executive, were grilled daily over their effectiveness in ensuring an adequate supply of face masks at the government press briefing sessions. Government leaders briefly attempted to discourage the use of face masks by the general public by downplaying their utility in protection, in order to conserve the supplies to medical staff, but their appeal failed to win public support.[9] Since surgical masks are part of the personal protective equipment recommended for medical staffs in taking care infectious disease patients, the reasoning of the popular wisdom is that they must be useful in offering protection in public places. A preferred strategy, from this perspective, should be to secure as much supply of these essential protective items as possible, and then determine priority in allocation, rather than uphold a conflicting message of useful for medics but not useful for the general public.

In view of the continuing shortage, citizens developed multiple means from bottom up to secure supply of face masks. First, on an individual level, personal networks of families and friends residing overseas were mobilized to buy and mail back to Hong Kong the face masks in small parcels. This strategy worked briefly in February, but global supply soon tightened up. Then many organizations, from medium-to-small sized companies to NGOs, leveraged on their overseas connections from own branches to clients to purchase in bulk for their staffs and business contacts. Some even sent their overseas staff to oversee the overseas production lines to ensure the product quality and timely delivery.[10] Free masks were distributed to vulnerable groups (e.g. elderlies, homeless, residents in care homes) through NGOs and community organizations. To secure local supply, some enterprises set up, from scratch, face mask production lines in Hong Kong. Others dwelt into the option of reusable masks in collaboration with local universities and research institutions.

New public policies have emerged out of strong demands from society. A controversial strike in early February 2020 by 5,100 staff in public hospitals, about 8% of total Hospital Authority (HA) workforce, in part led to government actions to reduce border traffic from February, which proved critical in containing imported infection (see Government Measures). The calls within the community to develop local production of face masks and other personal protection equipment led to the government's decision in late February to roll out funding support for 20 local production lines to manufacture face masks for local use. A total $44.5 million of public funds were approved as of 24 April.[11]

---

7   For one example, "Government not to drop appeal over anti-facemask law" (25 January 2020), RTHK, https://news.rthk.hk/rthk/en/component/k2/1504818-20200125.htm; RTHK (Chinese only): https://news.rthk.hk/rthk/ch/component/k2/1504801-20200125.htm

8   "「政情網上行」戴口罩的學問" (8 January 2020), Now, https://news.now.com/home/local/player?newsId=375966

9   Chung, Kimmy (4 February 2020), "Coronavirus: Carrie Lam orders Hong Kong officials not to wear masks to save stocks for medical workers," *South China Morning Post*, www.scmp.com/news/hong-kong/health-environment/article/3048883/coronavirus-carrie-lam-warns-hong-kong-officials

10 See Facebook posts by Thailand Immigration Services Limited, www.facebook.com/ThaiImmigrationLtd/?epa=SEARCH_BOX

11 HKSARG press release (28 February 2020), "Mask production plan to launch," www.news.gov.hk/eng/2020/02/20200228/20200228_160013_539.html; www.hkpc.org/en/our-services/additive-manufacturing/latest-information/hkpc-mask-production-support

Two Waves of Imported Outbreaks

The first two cases in Hong Kong were recorded on 23 January 2020, with both having a travel history to/from Wuhan, the initial epicentre of the outbreak. After a dozen other imported cases from Mainland, local cases first emerged in early February. Transmission channels at the time were mainly religious[12] and family gatherings[13]. Until 17 March, daily new cases had mostly remained at a single digit level. Then cases doubled during the week of 22 March. There were a few local transmission clusters, for example in popular nightlife district Lan Kwai Fong,[14] and fitness clubs.[15] On 27 March, daily new cases reached a new high of 65, with mostly imported cases from students returning home from Europe and North America where the virus was spreading.

This second wave turned out to be, somewhat unexpectedly, more severe than the first wave outbreak from Mainland. During the first wave, from 23 Jan to 16 March, Hong Kong registered a total of 158 confirmed cases, an average of 2.93 cases per day. From 17 March to 29 April, there were a total of 880 cases, an average of 20.47 cases per day (Figure 5.3). If we cut the "tail" of the second wave from 12 April, when the daily new cases dropped to a consistent single digit, the daily average for the main part of the second wave of outbreak from 17 March to 11 April was 32.4 cases. This is 11 times of the first wave average. The death toll had been stable and at a low level. After a fourth death registered on 13 March, there were no further fatalities until late June, suggesting the relative success of treatment of the patients during the first and second wave (See The "cocktail" approach to treatment and scientific advice). The "tail" of the second wave lasted for about a month from April to end of June.

Figure 5.3 Cumulative confirmed cases in 2 waves

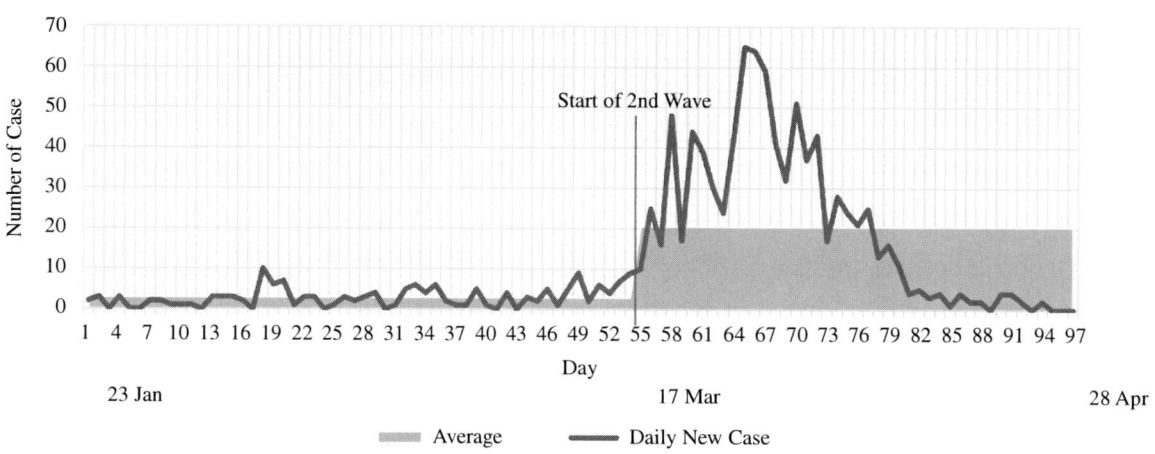

Source: Graph constructed with data from HK Centre for Health Protection

12 Lum, Alvin (11 March 2020), "Coronavirus: Hong Kong Buddhist temple linked to COVID-19 cluster 'sincerely sorry'". *South China Morning Post*, www.scmp.com/news/hong-kong/health-environment/article/3074640/coronavirus-hong-kong-buddhist-temple-linked

13 Rahhal, Natalie (10 February 2020), "Nine members of a Hong Kong family contracted coronavirus after a hotpot meal together as officials warn against 'gatherings' and utensil sharing," *Daily Mail*, www.dailymail.co.uk/health/article-7988815/Nine-family-members-shared-hotpot-meal-Hong-Kong-contract-coronavirus.html

14 Low, Zoe, and Tsang, Denise (20 March 2020), "Hong Kong nightlife hub of Lan Kwai Fong hit by coronavirus scare as business plunges, but owners say area is taking unfair blame". *South China Morning Post*, www.scmp.com/news/hong-kong/hong-kong-economy/article/3076202/hong-kong-nightlife-hub-lan-kwai-fong-hit

15 Cheung, Lilian, and Tsang, Denise (19 March 2020), "Coronavirus: Hong Kong fitness chain Pure Group to close all venues for cleaning after two cases linked to gyms". www.scmp.com/news/hong-kong/health-environment/article/3075899/coronavirus-hong-kong-fitness-chain-pure-group

The Third Wave

The third wave from early July reports a steep slope of soaring cases, the most serious of the three outbreaks since January. Figure 5.4 shows the two peaks of the second and third waves. Compared to the second wave, the third wave sees a sharper and longer spike of cases. In comparison, the initial, first wave of outbreak during January and February appears like a "ripple". The peak of the second wave lasted for 26 days (17 March to 11 April), with daily confirmed cases peaking at 65 cases on 27 March, whilst the third wave has lasted for 61 days since 7 July up to 5 September, with daily confirmed cases peaking at 149 cases on 30 July. There was a consecutive 12 days (19 July to 2 August) with over 100 daily new cases, of which over 90% were locally transmitted cases. A total of 3,528 cases were added to the total toll up to 5 September. On 18 July, the number of cumulative confirmed cases of COVID-19 (at 1,778) surpassed the 1,755 record of SARS in 2003. As of 5 September, the total cumulative cases reached 4,858, against 1,283 at the end of the tail of second wave on 6 July. More elderlies were infected due to the breakout clusters in care homes. The number of deaths soared from 7 at the beginning of third wave to 94 by 5 September, with the latest death rate approaching 2% (1.93%), significantly up from 0.55% at the end of second wave.

Figure 5.5 shows the preponderance of local cases in the third wave, unlike the previous two waves which are dominated by imported cases. The ratio of locally transmitted cases jumps from 0% to 64.3% during the first week of July. It then rises to over 90% during the 6 weeks between 7 July to 17 August, and fluctuates between 58.3% and 100% after 17 August. Considerable evidence points to loopholes in the infection control measures causing the community outbreak: categories of people e.g. air crews and sailors who stop by Hong Kong on transit but are exempted from infection control measures. In a study, Professor Malik Peiris from University of Hong Kong found at least four sources of virus, and that only one type of virus that was imported had caused large scale infection in the third wave.[16] 34 members of sea or air crew were tested positive during the initial days of the third wave, before the government moved to tighten up quarantine and testing requirements for this group on 26 July.[17] During the third wave, elderly homes, dormitories for foreign domestic helpers, and workplace for port workers are amongst the hardest hit sectors.

The daily new cases returned to double digit level from 3 August and kept an overall downward trend. On 24 August, the daily confirmed number fell to under 10 for the first time since third wave outbreak and stabilized thereafter, marking the beginning of the third wave tail.

16 University of Hong Kong press release (30 July 2020), "病毒學權威裴偉士：第三波疫情病毒基因幾乎完全相同", https://fightCOVID19.hku.hk/zh/病毒學權威裴偉士：第三波疫情病毒基因幾乎完全/ Another HKU research team (Professor Yuen KY et al) arrived at similar conclusions in an epidemiological study that point towards an imported origin of the third wave outbreak. See https://hk.appledaily.com/local/20200809/ZOYCQUCVGGAAC26E7WKBCON2NE/.

17 Ting, Victor and Cheung, Elizabeth (21 July 2020), "Hong Kong third wave: how did city's scariest surge in COVID-19 cases start, and what did authorities miss?", *South China Morning Post*, www.scmp.com/news/hong-kong/health-environment/article/3093978/hong-kong-third-wave-how-did-citys-scariest-surge

Figure 5.4 The Second and Third Waves of COVID-19, as of 5 September

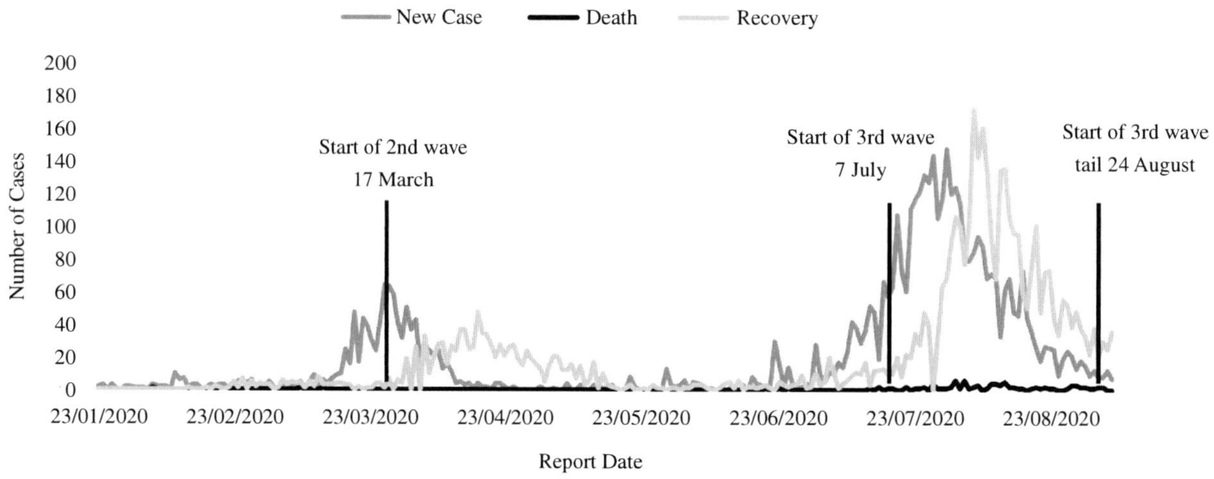

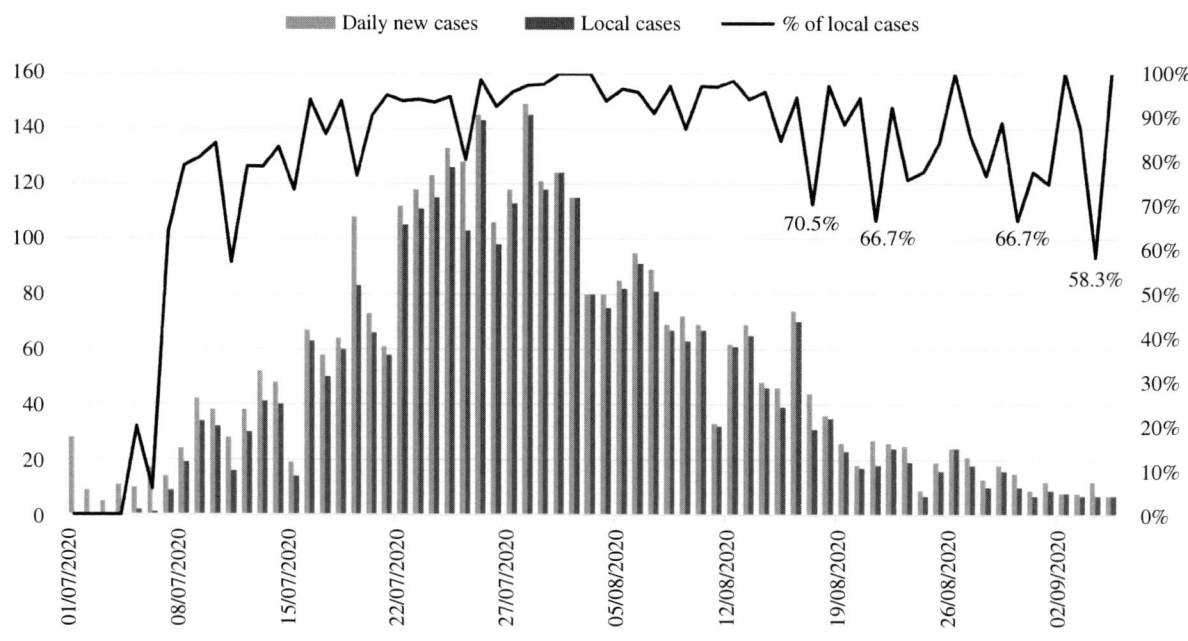

Source: Constructed from data from HK Centre for Health Protection

Figure 5.5 Percentage of local cases in the Third Wave, as of 5 September

Source: Constructed from data from HK Centre for Health Protection

Also on 24 August, Hong Kong registered the first case evidence worldwide that COVID-19 will likely continue to circulate in human population. A 33-year-old man in Hong Kong who recently travelled back from Spain was confirmed to be infected again, four and a half months after he first caught the disease.[18] The patient did not show symptoms but tested a high level of inflammation. Viral genome tests by University of Hong Kong show substantial differences between the first and second

---

18   Siu, Phila, Choy, Gigi, Cheng, Lilian and Chan, Ho-him (24 August 2020), "World's first coronavirus reinfection case confirmed in University of Hong Kong study," *South China Morning Post*, www.scmp.com/news/hong-kong/health-environment/article/3098551/hong-kongs-third-wave-losingmomentum-city

episodes of infections. This finding suggests that any natural immunity acquired in infections is short lasting and that future vaccination programs will need to include people recovered from previous infections.[19] The existence of different strains of SARs-CoV-2 across countries increases the risks of large-scale reinfection once the global transportation resumes normal operation.

The "Cocktail" Approach to Treatment and Scientific Advice

A number of medical scientists have played a conspicuous role in advising the government and the public on anti-infection matters. A 4-member medical expert team was appointed as government advisers early during the development of the epidemic, which included Professors Keiji Fukuda, Yuen KY and Gabriel Leung of University of Hong Kong, and Hui Shu-cheung of the Chinese University of Hong Kong. Their advice is instrumental to the government decisions to tighten up border controls with Mainland China in the last week of January and early February.[20] Yuen and Leung are also active in COVID-19 research and have held multiple media briefings to timely disseminate their scientific findings to the general public. In addition, Dr Ho Pak-leung of University of Hong Kong has been proactive in providing behavioural advice to citizens from the early stage of the pandemic, including on the correct way of washing hands and other detailed guidance on personal and household hygiene. For months he held daily media briefings to update the public on various aspects of concern, a practice which he halted in late August amidst controversies around the new government program of community testing.[21] Ho was also vocal in advocating an early closure of border with Mainland China to better contain the infections during the first wave outbreak.

The success of the local medical treatment approach adds to public confidence in the medical science sector in Hong Kong. Early diagnosis and quarantine (in isolation wards), as well as early medication, are critical to the remarkably low death rate.[22] The objective has been to hospitalize all patients tested positive, and to release them after patients successively have two negative tests and display no symptom. The patients are assessed by an expert panel. Compound treatment consisting of protease inhibitor, interferon, and Ribavirin are prescribed to most patients to suppress the virus at an early stage. For patients with milder symptoms, they might be treated by only the protease inhibitor, with or without the supportive measures. The effectiveness of the three-in-one cocktail approach has been proved clinically and scientifically.[23] The latest treatment encouraged in Hong Kong is transfusion of the blood plasma of recovered COVID-19 patients, which scientists have found to contain antibodies

19   University of Hong Kong, "HKU documents the world's first case of COVID-19 reinfection," 25 August, 2020, https://fightCOVID19.hku.hk/hku-documented-the-worlds-first-case-of-COVID-19-reinfection/

20   "Debate heats up over calls to shut border crossings" (26 January 2020), *RTHK*, https://news.rthk.hk/rthk/en/component/k2/1504967-20200126.htm; HKSARG press release (28 January 2020), "行政長官抗疫記者會開場發言（只有中文），" www.info.gov.hk/gia/general/202001/28/P2020012800741.htm

21   "COVID-19: Expert who criticised Hong Kong's mass testing project quits radio show about pandemic", 28 August, 2020, *HK Free Press*, https://hongkongfp.com/2020/08/28/COVID-19-expert-who-criticised-hong-kongs-mass-testing-project-quits-radio-show-about-pandemic/

22   See "「和你抗疫」港用雞尾酒療法助患者更快康復出院 藥劑師：或因症狀輕微時已用藥有關" (24 March 2020), *Apple Daily*, https://hk.appledaily.com/lifestyle/20200324/HOMR222HE24XNVO3LTQDA6LQZ4/.

23   Cheung, Elizabeth (9 May 2020), "Coronavirus: Hong Kong researchers find three-drug combination suppresses virus nearly twice as fast as drug held up as major hope against pandemic," *South China Morning Post*, www.scmp.com/news/hong-kong/health-environment/article/3083612/coronavirus-hong-kong-researchers-find-three-drug. For full report of the study published in *Lancet*, led by Professor KY Yuen, see www.thelancet.com/journals/lancet/article/PIIS0140-6736(20)31042-4/fulltext.

that can kill 99% of the virus in patients still fighting the disease.[24] More recovered patients are being appealed to come forward to donate blood plasma to help those still in sick.[25]

University of Hong Kong researchers have been working on vaccine research since January 2020, through modifying a nasal spray influenza vaccine which the team previously invented with part of the surface antigen of the novel coronavirus. Permission to perform clinical testing from national authorities was secured in early September, with human clinical testing set to start in November 2020. Further testing and production of the vaccine would be conducted in collaboration with Xiamen University and Beijing Wantai Biological Pharmacy.[26]

Government Measures

Public Health and Prevention

On 31 December 2019, Hong Kong health authorities received information about a viral pneumonia outbreak in Wuhan with unknown sources. The government immediately issued warnings to public hospitals and enhanced border screening, taking the lessons of SARS and bird flu outbreaks in previous years.[27]

On 8 January, Hong Kong's Centre for Health Protection (CHP) added "Severe respiratory disease associated with a novel infectious agent" to their list of notifiable diseases to expand their authority on quarantine. Hospital visitors were required to wear face masks. Screening was tightened at airports and train stations with connections to Wuhan. On the same day when the first two "highly suspected cases" emerged, on 23 January 2020, the Government designated Lady MacLehose Holiday Village in Sai Kung as a quarantine centre. Major events to celebrate the Lunar New Year, which started on 25 January, were cancelled.

On 25 January, the Hong Kong government declared the viral outbreak an "emergency", the highest warning tier. Public hospitals ceased visit arrangements. Popular theme-parks which normally attract large crowds, including Hong Kong Disneyland Resort, Ocean Park Hong Kong, and Madame Tussauds Hong Kong, were closed from 26 January.

Since early to mid-January, there was strong urge from society to "close the border" with the mainland immediately in order to better contain the risk. After 8 new confirmed cases with a previous travel history to the mainland on the day of 28 January, Chief Executive of Hong Kong Carrie Lam announced on the same day the suspension of the high-speed rail service between Hong Kong and

---

24 University of Hong Kong, "Plasma can kill 99 per cent of virus, HKU teams says", May 9, 2020, https://fightCOVID19. hku.hk/plasma-can-kill-99-per-cent-of-virus-hku-teams-says/

25 Siu, Phila (15 May 2020), "Coronavirus: call for Hong Kong COVID-19 survivors to donate plasma, which tests show kills infection," *South China Morning Post*, www.scmp.com/news/hong-kong/health-environment/article/3084440/ coronavirus-call-hong-kong-COVID-19-survivors

26 University of Hong Kong press release (9 September 2020), "HKU State Key Laboratory for Emerging Infectious Diseases co-developed COVID-19 vaccine candidate approved for clinical trial in humans", www.hku.hk/press/news_ detail_21583.html

27 Zuo, Mandy, Cheng Lilian, Yan Alice and Yau Cannix (31 December 2019), "Hong Kong takes emergency measures as mystery 'pneumonia' infects dozens in China's Wuhan city," *South China Morning Post*. www.scmp.com/news/china/ politics/article/3044050/mystery-illness-hits-chinas-wuhan-city-nearly-30-hospitalised

mainland China starting from 30 January.[28] New visas to individual mainland tourists and all cross-border ferry services were also suspended. Civil servants started to work from home, while classes in schools and universities went online. Museums and public amenities such as swimming pools and beaches were closed.

In February, public services were reduced as many civil servants continued to work from home. On 3 February, thousands of Hong Kong public hospital workers started a 4-day strike to demand that the government step up its measures and "close the border" with mainland China completely to fend off the coronavirus.[29] On 8 February, as the strike subsided and the first case of local transmission was confirmed, all border crossings with Mainland China were closed, except for the Hong Kong-Zhuhai-Macau Bridge, Shenzhen Bay Port and the international airport. All travellers from mainland China entering Hong Kong, including local residents, were required to go into quarantine for 14 days. A newly completed public housing estate with 4,800 flats, Chun Yeung Estate in Fo Tan area of Shatin, was announced to become Hong Kong's fifth quarantine site, as the existing facilities were near full capacity. Hong Kong Arts Festival 2020 due to take place in 8-17 February was cancelled.[30] Due to the reduction in air travel demand, Cathay Pacific slashed 30% of its global flights. Hospital Authority (HA) announced personal protective equipment (PPE) in its reserves could last only a month. Anticipating unstable supply of PPE, non-essential services would be shut down or reduced.[31] The Chief Executive (CE) announced a HK$30 billion relief package on 20 February. Over half of it would finance one-off cash injections to retailers, food and drink service providers, transport companies, students, the arts and culture sector, guest houses and travel agents. The rest would go to HA to cushion its budget to fight the virus.

On 24 February, due to the escalation of the outbreak in Korea, a Red Outbound Travel Alert to Korea was issued, the first travel alert issued since the COVID-19 outbreak in Hong Kong. Starting from 1 March the entry of non-HK citizens from Korea would be banned and returning HK citizens from Korea would need to have mandatory quarantine for 14 days. On 28 February, similar border restrictions were applied to arrivals from Iran and the regions of Emilia-Romagna, Lombardy and Veneto in northern Italy. The CE announced herself, her cabinet and other top officials were donating one month's salary to support the city's battle with the deadly coronavirus.[32]

On 10 March, the CE announced a tightening of border restrictions: anyone (regardless of citizenship) arriving from Italy, parts of France, Germany, Japan and Spain would be placed on a

28 Cheung, Tony, Lum, Alvin, Cheung, Elizabeth and Sum, Lok-kei (28 January 2020), "China coronavirus: Hong Kong scrambles to roll out containment plan stopping short of total closure, with cuts on cross-border travel and reduced transport services with mainland", *South China Morning Post*, www.scmp.com/news/hong-kong/health-environment/article/3047907/china-coronavirus-hong-kong-government-deny-entry

29 Lau, Chris (3 February 2020), "Hong Kong hospital strike kicks off as top doctor backs mainland China border closure calls amid coronavirus fears," *South China Morning Post*, www.scmp.com/news/hong-kong/politics/article/3048705/hong-kong-hospital-strike-kicks-top-doctor-backs-mainland

30 Chik, Holly and Kwong, Kevin (10 February 2020), "Coronavirus: entire Hong Kong Arts Festival cancelled over outbreak; arts fans say it's disappointing but understandable", *South China Morning Post*, www.scmp.com/lifestyle/arts-culture/article/3049799/coronavirus-entire-hong-kong-arts-festival-cancelled-over

31 Mok, Danny and Low, Zoe (8 February 2020), "Coronavirus: Hong Kong government scrambles to buy more masks after revealing it only has 12 million left". *South China Morning Post*, www.scmp.com/news/hong-kong/health-environment/article/3049631/hong-kong-government-goes-global-search-face

32 Cheung, Lilian (28 February 2020), "Coronavirus: Carrie Lam, cabinet, other top Hong Kong officials to donate one month's pay to charity amid city's battle with epidemic". *South China Morning Post*, www.scmp.com/news/hong-kong/politics/article/3052944/coronavirus-carrie-lam-top-hong-kong-ministers-donate-one

mandatory quarantine in government facilities for 14 days starting 14 March.[33] On 15 March, a red travel alert was issued to Ireland, the U.K., and the U.S. Anyone arriving from the 3 countries should undergo a mandatory home quarantine period for 2 weeks.

On 17 March, the government issued red travel alert to all countries and regions, except mainland China, Taiwan and Macao. All arrivals from 19 March would undergo 2-week home quarantine, except from those coming from Macao and Taiwan. The DSE examination scheduled for late March would be deferred until the end of April. Civil servants would resume work from home after a brief spell of normality. On 23 March, the border control was further tightened: all non-Hong Kong citizens arriving by flights would be denied entry for 2 weeks starting 25 March. All air transfer services would cease. At the same time, pockets of local outbreaks in pubs led the Government to contemplate a shut down of the city's 8,600 restaurants, bars and clubs which with liquor licences to enforce better social distancing measures. Due to strong opposition from industry, this plan was dropped and new measures to limit the size of social gatherings to 4 or below were executed instead. Public entertainment venues including games centres, party rooms, cinemas, and bathhouses, fitness centres, places of amusement — such as skating rings and bowling alleys — were closed. Restaurants must enact social distancing measures: could fill up to 50 per cent capacity, and each table of customers is separated by at least 1.5 metres.

The Department of Health also stepped up health quarantine and COVID-19 testing arrangements for all inbound travellers. Testing was initially applied to a sample of incoming travellers. Starting from 29 March, all returning citizens were required to be tested, either at home or centrally upon arrival at the Temporary Specimen Collection Centre at AsiaWorld-Expo next to the airport, and from April 8, only centrally. On 22 April, the Hospital Authority began rapid tests which could produce results in one to two hours.

Cases started to dwindle from mid-April. The Government confirmed that Hong Kong (DSE) Examination would be held on 24 April as scheduled.

As the situation stabilized, social distancing measures were gradually relaxed. Civil servants stopped working from home from 4 May, and public services and amenities resumed normal hours on a phased schedule. Restaurants could entertain up to 8 guests in a table from 8 May and discussions started on relaxing the social distancing measures and streamlining the cross-border quarantine arrangements.[34]

During the "tail" of the second wave, the government adjusted the public health policies according to the latest situation, described as a strategy of "Suppress and Lift". In May, the government announced a series of measures to allow an increase in human flow between Hong Kong and China Mainland for specified needs. On 21 May onwards, personnel of enterprises relating to logistics, port or shipping business with an operating base in the Mainland may apply for exemption from compulsory quarantine. A mechanism for directors of listed companies or listing applicants to apply for exemption was introduced. Social distancing measures were relaxed. The size of group gathering in

---

33 Cheung, Lilian, Lum, Alvin and Siu, Phila (10 March 2020), "Hong Kong to quarantine arrivals from Italy and parts of France, Germany, Japan, Spain as world braces for coronavirus spread and city cases hit 120", *South China Morning Post*, www.scmp.com/news/hong-kong/politics/article/3074380/coronavirus-hong-kong-planning-extend-travel-restrictions

34 For example, Ting, Victor and Guo, Rui (26 May 2020), "Coronavirus: China's 'Sars hero' Zhong Nanshan urges Hong Kong to relax border controls with mainland and Macau', *South China Morning Post*, www.scmp.com/news/hong-kong/health-environment/article/3086021/coronavirus-chinas-sars-hero-zhong-nanshan-urges

public places was extended to eight people from 4 June. Bathhouses, party rooms, clubs or night clubs and karaoke establishments could resume normal operation from 29 May. Cross-boundary students resumed classes from 15 June.

The process was quickly reversed as third wave struck, however. On 9 July, the limit of gathering for party rooms, karaoke and fitness centres was reduced from 16 to eight. On July 13, The Hospital Authority announced that due to the larger number of new patients, patients tested positive might need to wait for a few days at home before admission to a hospital. Group gathering was tightened drastically from 50 to four people, then further down to 2 on 29 July. Secretary for Education Kevin Yeung announced to allow all schools and kindergartens to advance the beginning of summer holiday to 13 July. Wearing masks on public transport became mandatory from midnight of 15 July, which was extended to all indoor public places on 22 July and to all outdoor public places from 29 July. Meanwhile, catering business could only provide take-away service from 6 p.m. to 4:59 a.m. of subsequent day. Also, from 15 July, all leisure and cultural facilities were closed until further notice.

From 15 to 20 July, free COVID-19 testing were expanded for high-risk groups: communities with links to recently confirmed cases, staffs of catering business, frontline property workers, etc.

As the daily new cases spiked over 100 in late July, the government once banned all dine-in services. The ban immediately sparked a public outcry as many labourers doing outdoor work could not find a place to have lunch. In less than 24 hours since the ban took effect the government announced that the ban would be retracted the next day. The Chief Executive and a few medical experts advocating the ban apologized in order to allay the public anger at the poorly conceived ban.[35]

As the daily confirmed cases continued to surge, the Chief Executive appealed for public support, in particular to follow strictly the social distancing measures and stay at home as far as possible. At this point, the limited testing capacity in the public health sector and its slow development since January increasingly came under public scrutiny. Medical experts from Hong Kong reiterated their earlier calls to speed up testing.[36] Figure 5.6 shows the number of tests in Hong Kong per month increased gradually from a low base of under 10,000 in January to exceed 100,000 in June (109,388). Just under 300,000 tests were conducted in July during the third wave outbreak, close to triple the June total. Due to the limited testing capacity, the testing targeted eight high-risk groups: taxi and public light bus drivers, catering premises with seating area, frontline property management workers, residents in Tsz Wan Shan (an area with a number of clusters), staffs in wet markets, residents in other communities with local cases, pregnant women, and foreign domestic helpers in boarding facilities. On 30 July, Prof Zhong Nanshan, an influential medical expert in mainland China, urged Hong Kong to conduct universal coronavirus testing and have more exchange of experience with respiratory experts in the mainland.[37]

---

35 Cheng, Lilian (30 July 2020). "Hong Kong third wave: officials scrap coronavirus-related ban on eating in restaurants after just 24 hours," *South China Morning Post*, www.scmp.com/news/hong-kong/health-environment/article/3095283/hong-kong-third-wave-government-changes-mind

36 "袁國勇商台訪問足本重溫：全民檢測是好政策，但採樣方法一定要正確", University of Hong Kong, August 17, 2020, https://fightCOVID19.hku.hk/zh/袁國勇商台訪問足本重溫：全民檢測是好政策，但/

37 Lo, Kinling (30 July 2020), "Hong Kong needs citywide coronavirus testing, China's 'SARS hero' Zhong Nanshan says", *South China Morning Post*, www.scmp.com/news/china/society/article/3095277/hong-kong-needs-citywide-COVID-19-testing-chinas-sars-hero-zhong

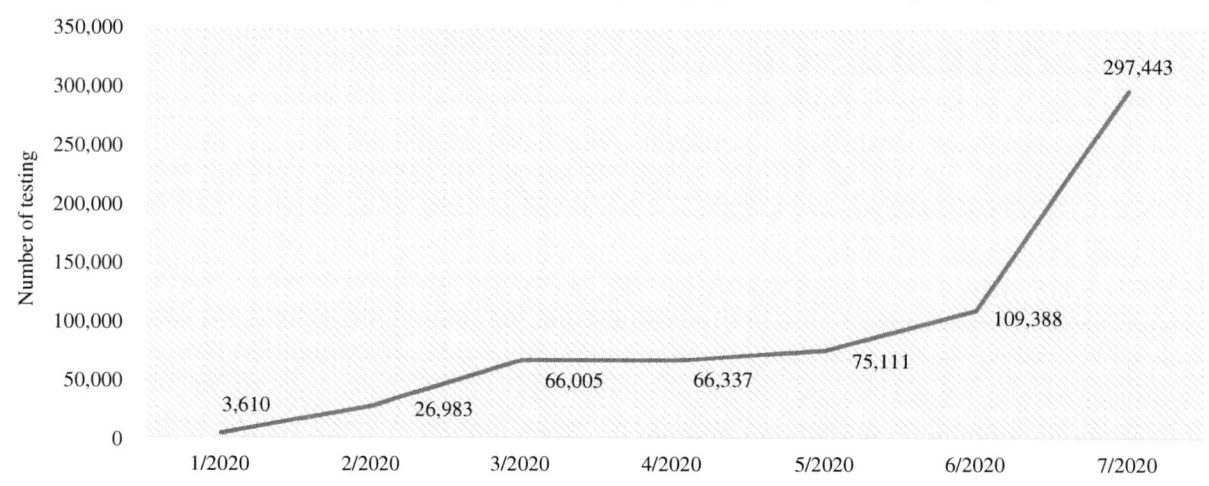

Figure 5.6 Coronavirus testing in Hong Kong by month (January – July 2020)

Source: Department of Health and Hospital Authority

On 30 July, the Hospital Authority announced a plan to convert the Asia World-Expo facility to a COVID-19 community treatment facility with 500 beds, and a new quarantine facility in Lei Yue Mun with 350 beds would soon be ready for use. The next day, the government announced in the daily COVID-19 briefing that a seven-member nucleic acid test support team was arriving the same day from mainland to help raise the city's virus testing capacity. Another 60-member team would arrive soon to set up more temporary treatment facilities, or "cabin hospitals" for Hong Kong. The sudden announcement, and short notice — the team were arriving in hours after the official announcement — immediately caused concerns in society. Questions were raised on the scope of the work, qualifications of the personnel, possible gaps in accountability and so on. A Department of Public Health spokesman on COVID-19 admitted she only learned of the decision through the news.[38]

On 5 August, four days after the mainland support team arrived, the government sketched its plan on large-scale testing. A temporary laboratory would be set up at Sun Yat Sen Memorial Park in the western district of Hong Kong Island, and 2,000 beds were to be set up at Asia World-Expo centre. The government would directly procure the testing services from three mainland-related providers with the Anti-Epidemic Fund, namely Sunrise Diagnostic Centre established by BGI, China Inspection Company's subsidiary China Dragon Inspection and Certification (Hong Kong), and Prenetics. Work started immediately, and over 90,000 tests for high-risk groups were completed by 4 August. In view of the mounting concerns over privacy and accountability, the Chief Executive stressed that any collection of personal data would be strictly for the execution of the testing and must meet the requirements under the Personal Data (Privacy) Ordinance. All mainland health workers participating in the program would also have to meet the relevant local registration or exemption requirements.

On 7 August, the government announced further details of the universal testing program: the test would be voluntary and provided to residents free of charge. It was also considered that any community movement restrictions would not be practically feasible and thus lockdown measures were ruled out.

---

38   Cheung, Elizabeth, Zhuang, Pinghui, Cheng, Lilian and Chan, Ho-him (1 August 2020), "Hong Kong third wave: free COVID-19 tests for residents as mainland Chinese clinical teams head to city", *South China Morning Post*, www.scmp. com/news/hong-kong/health-environment/article/3095646/hong-kong-third-wave-mainland-clinical-teams; "張竹君：看 新聞才得知中央派員來港展開實驗室工作" (1 August 2020), 881903, www.881903.com/news/local/2350125/張竹君看新 聞才得知中央派員來港展開實驗室工作

The test has aroused mixed response from society. Whilst the enhancement of testing capacity was welcome, the lack of prior consultation and transparency over execution arrangements continued to draw criticisms.[39] There were concerns, for example, over the ways of taking samples for testing,[40] and the background of the outsourced laboratories.[41] In response, the Government announced 5 principles: (1) start testing as soon as possible, (2) observe social distancing rules, (3) make the pick-up and return of specimen bottle as convenient as possible, (4) separating the collection and distribution points to enhance safety, and (5) protect personal data.

On 13 August, the government emphasized, yet again, that the Universal Community Testing Programme had the sole objective of conducting tests on COVID-19, and that all the specimen collected would not leave Hong Kong and would be destroyed after testing. Responding to various circulating rumours, it was stressed that the collected specimens would only be identified by a serial number.

The test program continued to draw controversies, however, including association to the proliferation of "false positive cases" in tests done by one of the contracted laboratories in Sweden.[42] Another worry among Hong Kong people was about privacy in the proposed "Health Code" programme. Alfred Sit, Secretary for Innovation and Technology, explained that the Health Code would not track citizens' locations or limit access to public places.[43]

The Universal Community Testing Programme was scheduled, initially, to run for seven days from 1 September, allowing for extension to up to fourteen days, in 141 specimen collection centres set up across 18 districts. As of 30 August, 420,000 people have registered to take part. A day later, Hospital Authority expressed its support to the Programme. Interest and participation grew gradually, reaching 1,058,000 as of 5 September (Table 5.1), but fell short of the original target to cover several millions as suggested by the medical sector. The testing capacity was also improving daily, with three batches of Mainland nucleic acid test support teams involving 420 members joining the work. Attributing to issues of logistics and coordination, just about half of the collected specimens as of 5 September were tested, while the pace picked up subsequently in the following days. The testing identified only a handful of positive cases, 16 as of 8 September, largely falling short of the expected range of 1500 asymptomatic patients.[44] On 9 September, the government announced to extend the programme for three days to September 14.[45]

---

39 Cheng, Lilian and Cheung, Gary (8 August 2020), "Hong Kong third wave: why mainland China's help in fighting COVID-19 has sparked anxiety rather than appreciation," *South China Morning Post*, www.scmp.com/news/hong-kong/health-environment/article/3096562/hong-kong-third-wave-why-mainland-chinas-help

40 University of Hong Kong press release (10 August 2020), "HKU expert stresses the importance of taking coronavirus samples correctly," https://fightCOVID19.hku.hk/hku-expert-stresses-the-importance-of-taking-coronavirus-samples-correctly/

41 Siu, Jasmin and Cheung, Gary (17 August 2020), "Coronavirus third wave: US biotech firm accuses Chinese laboratory helping to test Hongkongers of infringing on patent," *South China Morning Post*, August 17, 2020, www.scmp.com/news/hong-kong/health-environment/article/3097681/coronavirus-third-wave-us-biotech-firm-accuses

42 "「華大基因」核酸檢測套裝有問題 致瑞典出現3,700個「假陽性」個案," (26 August 2020), *Apple Daily*, https://hk.appledaily.com/international/20200826/5OTSBPMAOBA7NPRGAZ3S7PZI2E/

43 "薛永恒聲稱「冇諗過」用健康碼追蹤市民 民協：名為檢測 實為監控," (24 August 2020), https://hk.appledaily.com/local/20200824/UDP5YN7YPVFD3HQYRSZMKFTVMI/

44 "普檢找出16名確診者　林鄭月娥稱比例很低", (8 September 2020) *RTHK*, https://news.rthk.hk/rthk/ch/component/k2/1548421-20200908.htm

45 HKSARG press release (9 September 2020), "Universal Community Testing Programme extended for three days to September 14", www.info.gov.hk/gia/general/202009/09/P2020090900639.htm?fontSize=1

Table 5.1 A snapshot of universal community testing (1 Sept to 9 Sept 2020)

Date	Total registration number	Testing capacity (Total persons received)	Testing capacity (Total specimens tested)
1 Sept.	674,000	126,000	—
2 Sept.	798,000	278,000	49,000
3 Sept.	884,000	470,000	138,100
4 Sept.	953,000	656,000	284,800
5 Sept.	1,058,000	847,000	439,000
…	…	…	…
9 Sept.	1,273,000	1,423,000	1,268,000

Source: Press Releases of Hong Kong Government

Further relaxation of social distancing measures continued into September, with dine-in service hours extended and more exercise premises re-opened. Face-to-face classes in schools were resumed gradually, starting from 23 September.

Economic Support to the Needy

As the economy sees a downturn, unemployment reached 6.2% in June. Two rounds of Anti-Epidemic Fund involving 30 billion HKD and 137.5 billion HKD are approved by the Legislative Council on 21 February and 18 April. In addition, a 120 billion relief package is included in the 2020-21 Budget, announced on 26 February. As of 5 August, reliefs for 24 sectors in the first round and 42 sectors in the second round have been rolled out. Table 5.2 shows the amount of funding in the three rounds. The largest scheme focusing on saving employment are divided into eight parts, in which the top three are: "Employment Support Scheme" (ESS) (81,151.3 million HKD), "Job Creation" (6,000 million HKD) and "Distance Business Programme" (1500 million HKD). A total of 1.87 million employees have received subsidies of 43.2 billion HKD under the ESS as of 11 August.

To help small and medium sized enterprises (SMEs), the Hong Kong Monetary Authority in April 2020 instructed 162 banks in Hong Kong to grant unprecedented six-month loan repayment holiday and released one trillion HKD lending support.[46] During this period, companies need to pay the interest but not the principal of their loans. On 2 September, the maximum duration for principal moratorium was extended for 6 more months, from October 2020 to April 2021. Firms with annual turnover of less than HKD800 million and without serious overdue loans will qualify for the scheme. Of the 130,000 firms that qualify, about 15,000 have applied since May.[47]

---

46 Yiu, Enoch (17 April 2020), "Hong Kong orders banks to grant unprecedented six-month loan repayment holiday to help small businesses survive slump," *South China Morning Post*, www.scmp.com/business/banking-finance/article/3080467/hong-kong-orders-banks-grant-unprecedented-six-month-loan.

47 Yiu Enoch (3 September 2020), "Banks told to extend SMEs' loan break", *South China Morning Post*, www.scmp.com/business/banking-finance/article/3099927/hong-kong-extends-payment-holidays-until-april-2021-give.

On 18 August, the Chief Executive announced a new round of Anti-Epidemic Fund to target the hardest-hit industries including hospitality, catering, tourism and personal services. A support fund was set up to provide up to HKD 300,000 to each business to support development of IT and other business solutions to fit the needs for social distancing. Within government, 3,000 time-limit jobs were open for application between late August and early September. These are amongst the total of 30,000 time-limit jobs to be created in the public and private sectors in the coming two years to relieve the crucial unemployment situation under the 'Job retention, job creation and job advancement' fund.

On 23 August, the government first introduced a penalty clause in the coming second tranche of ESS. The disbursed wage subsidies, up to HKD 9,000 per employee, will be clawed back in full or part if staffs are laid off.

On 15 September, the government announced the third round of Anti-epidemic Fund, with a new assistance package totalling HKD 24 billion. The reduced scale of support, relative to the first 2 rounds, led to complaints from industries including the catering,[48] tourism,[49] performing arts,[50] and vulnerable groups such as the unemployed.[51] Financial Secretary pleaded for prudence, stressing an expanding deficit (to over $300 billion), and decline in fiscal reserves to $800 billion (on par of fiscal reserve in 2003 when SARS hit Hong Kong).[52]

Conclusion

The COVID-19 pandemic is posing new questions to the old art of governing worldwide. Not only are governments under the most severe stress test of decades, with the quality of their policy response placed under critical scrutiny, but many accustomed behaviours and taken-for-granted beliefs are challenged. How different societies manage effective communications and decision-making in the uncertainties of a pandemic carries high stakes. The burden often falls unevenly, moreover. The elderly, the sick, the minorities and those with less means are often the hardest hit in many societies. Given the severe shocks the city had recently suffered during the protracted protests in 2019, when public trust in government dived, it is amazing how Hong Kong has managed to pull itself together. But it has. Facing a dire threat to public and individual health, bottom-up self-help initiatives sprung up. Medical scientists applied their efforts not only in laboratories but also in press rooms and in the local community, playing both a role of researcher as well as communicator and educator. The vibrant social media sped up the flow of information. Where and when government measures converged with the emergent social consensus,

48 "中小企食店聯盟指第三輪防疫抗疫基金未能補漏拾遺" (17 September 2020), *RTHK*, https://news.rthk.hk/rthk/ch/component/k2/1550146-20200917.htm

49 "抗疫基金｜旅遊業界調查指逾500旅行社擬結業　斥內地拒港健康碼" (22 September 2020), *HK01*, www.hk01.com/%E7%A4%BE%E6%9C%83%E6%96%B0%E8%81%9E/526836/%E6%8A%97%E7%96%AB%E5%9F%BA%E9%87%91-%E6%97%85%E9%81%8A%E6%A5%AD%E7%95%8C%E8%AA%BF%E6%9F%A5%E6%8C%87%E9%80%BE500%E6%97%85%E8%A1%8C%E7%A4%BE%E6%93%AC%E7%B5%90%E6%A5%AD-%E6%96%A5%E5%85%A7%E5%9C%B0%E6%8B%92%E6%B8%AF%E5%81%A5%E5%BA%B7%E7%A2%BC

50 "出席活動及演藝製作界記者會　回應抗疫基金　馬逢國多次哽咽一度落淚" (22 September 2020), *Standnews*, www.thestandnews.com/culture/%E5%87%BA%E5%B8%AD%E6%A5%AD%E7%95%8C%E5%9B%9E%E6%87%89%E6%8A%97%E7%96%AB%E5%9F%BA%E9%87%91%E8%A8%98%E8%80%85%E6%9C%83-%E9%A6%AC%E9%80%A2%E5%9C%8B%E5%A4%9A%E6%AC%A1%E5%93%BD%E5%92%BD%E4%B8%80%E5%BA%A6%E8%90%BD%E6%B7%9A/

51 "胡志偉及鄭泳舜俱指第三輪基金對失業及基層支援不足" (17 September 2020), *RTHK*, https://news.rthk.hk/rthk/ch/component/k2/1550078-20200917.htm

52 Paul Chan (20 September 2020), Financial Secretary of HKSARG Blog, "Progress ahead steadily", 20 September 2020, www.fso.gov.hk/eng/blog/blog20200920.htm

they thrived. The importance of forging a robust private-public partnership for a successful response to COVID-19, and by extension for the effective governance of the city, cannot be over-emphasised in the political context of Hong Kong of 2020, and beyond.

Table 5.2 The Anti-Epidemic Fund by Hong Kong Government

	Major Measures	Funding (million HKD)	SUB-TOTAL (Billion HKD)	%
First Round	1. Enhancing anti-epidemic capability	10,190*	30	15.7
	2. Providing reliefs to enterprises and individuals	16,900*		
Second Round	1. Job retention, job creation, job advancement	87,800**	137.5	71.8
	2. Provision of one-off relief for specific sectors	21,044**		
	3. Easing the cash flow and burden of businesses and individuals	800**		
	4. Other measures, such as "implementation of a six-month unemployment support scheme under the CSSA framework", "loan guarantee commitment under the Special 100% Guarantee Product" and "one-off interest-free deferral of loan repayment for schools and Students"	17,000		
Third Round	1. Enhancing anti-epidemic capability	13,000	24***	12.5
	2. Providing relief to sectors and individuals directly affected by Government's anti-epidemic measures	4,500		
	3. Rental concessions, waivers of fees and charges and enhanced rates concession	5,000		
	Total		191.5	100

* *10% contingency was added to these figures in the calculation of their resulting rounded-off sub-total (see page 8 of LegCo "Item for Finance Committee" on 21 February 2020[53])*

** *10% contingency was added to these figures in the calculation of their resulting rounded-off sub-total (see page 16 of LegCo "Item for Finance Committee" on 17 April 2020[54])*

*** *To implement the whole set of measures, the government claimed it amounts to $24 billion (see slide 14 of "Powerpoint presentation at press conference" on 15 September 2020[55])*

53 HKSARG (21 February 2020), "Item for Finance Committee," www.legco.gov.hk/yr19-20/english/fc/fc/papers/f19-46e.pdf

54 HKSARG (7 April 2020), "Item for Finance Committee," www.coronavirus.gov.hk/pdf/fund/FCR(2020-21)2e.pdf

55 HKSARG (15 September 2020), "Fight the Virus Together with Confidence," www.coronavirus.gov.hk/pdf/fund/20200915-pressreleaseppt_en.pdf

Fighting COVID-19 in Hong Kong:
The Effects of Community and Social mobilization[1]

Kin-Man Wan, Lawrence Ka-ki Ho, Natalie W. M. Wong and Andy Chiu

The globalized world economy has been affected by the COVID-19 pandemic since early February 2020. In the midst of this global public health crisis, a prompt review of the counterinsurgencies that have occurred in different jurisdictions is helpful. This article examines the experience of Hong Kong (HKSAR), which successfully limited its number of confirmed cases to approximately 1100 until mid-June 2020. Considering the limited actions that the government has taken against the pandemic, we emphasize the prominent role of Hong Kong's civil society through highlighting the strong and spontaneous mobilization of its local communities originating from their experiences during the SARS outbreak in 2003 and the social unrest in 2019, as well as their doubts regarding the pandemic assessments and recommendations of the HKSAR and WHO authorities. This article suggests that the influence of civil society should not be overlooked in the context of pandemic management.

Introduction

Conventional wisdom acknowledges the crucial role of the state in sustaining health services and reducing the risk of epidemics (Dionne, 2011; Lieberman, 2007; Bollyky et al., 2019; Wigley and Akkoyunlu-Wigley, 2011). Most governments view regional lockdowns, social distancing and massive screening as rational responses to the COVID-19 pandemic, and some state-centric approaches provide a model for the rest of the world (Wang, Ng, and Brook 2000). However, it is worth studying the roles of public personnel in the COVID-19 situation and the ways in which society responds to this pandemic. In this article, we examine the experience of the Hong Kong Special Administrative Region (HKSAR) to explain the importance of civil society and social mobilization as decisive elements of the fight against the pandemic.

In the time between the outbreak of COVID-19 in mainland China during the month of January to mid-June, there have been approximately 1100 confirmed cases of the virus in Hong Kong, which is densely populated with over 8 million people (Fig. 5.7). In addition to the government's efforts to limit the spread of the virus,[2] the role of civil society is prominent to combat the surge of infection. Paradoxically, the strong and spontaneous mobilization observed in Hong Kong was a consequence of the population's devastating memories of the SARS outbreak in 2003 and the social unrest in 2019, as well as of their skepticism of the pandemic figures, assessments and recommendations given by the authorities of HKSAR, mainland China, and the World Health Organization (WHO). The lesson that can be learned from Hong Kong is that of an alternative approach to ensuring the effectiveness of pandemic management.

---

1   This chapter is originally published in Wan, Kin-Man, Lawrence Ka-ki Ho, Natalie W. M Wong, and Andy Chiu, 2020, Fighting COVID-19 in Hong Kong: The Effects of Community and Social Mobilization. *World Development, 134*: 105055, https://www.sciencedirect.com/science/article/abs/pii/S0305750X20301819, with minor adaptations for this volume.

2   For details regarding the measures taken by the HKSAR government, please refer to Appendix A.

Figure 5.7 Confirmed cases of COVID-19 in Hong Kong (as of June 15, 2020)

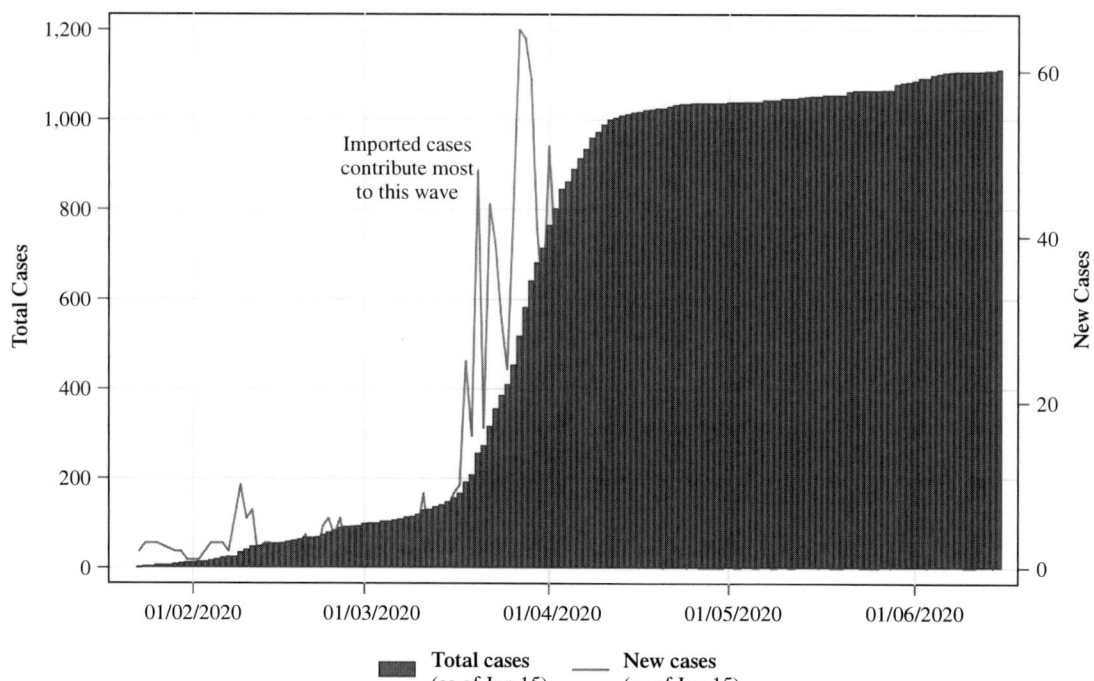

Community Response: Anxiety, Distrust and Social Mobilization

Anxiety: Lesson from SARS 2003

The advent of COVID-19 (also known as SARS2 by HKU and the public) reminded the public of their experience during the SARS outbreak in 2003, which led to 1,755 cases and 299 deaths as well as economic depression in Hong Kong. As a result of this experience, the public learned the importance of social distancing, personal hygiene, and the use of surgical masks in the context of SARS-like pandemics (Lau et al., 2010). Among their Asian neighbors, Hong Kong citizens were the first to react to the pandemic. Using Apple mobility trend data, Fig. 5.8 shows that Hong Kong citizens rapidly reduced their frequency of walking out of their homes by over 40% (from 100 to approximately 50) after the first reported case in Hong Kong on Jan 23.[3] This trend continued even during the Lunar New Year public holiday occurring days after.[4]

---

3 A survey also found that approximately 61.3% respondents avoiding going to crowded places (Cowling et at. 2020), which is highly consistent with the Apple mobility trend data.

4 Driving data from Apple also exhibits a similar trend as does the walking data. For these similar results using data drawn from the Google community mobility report, please see Appendix B.

Figure 5.8 Mobility trends during the COVID-19 period. Source: Apple, 2020

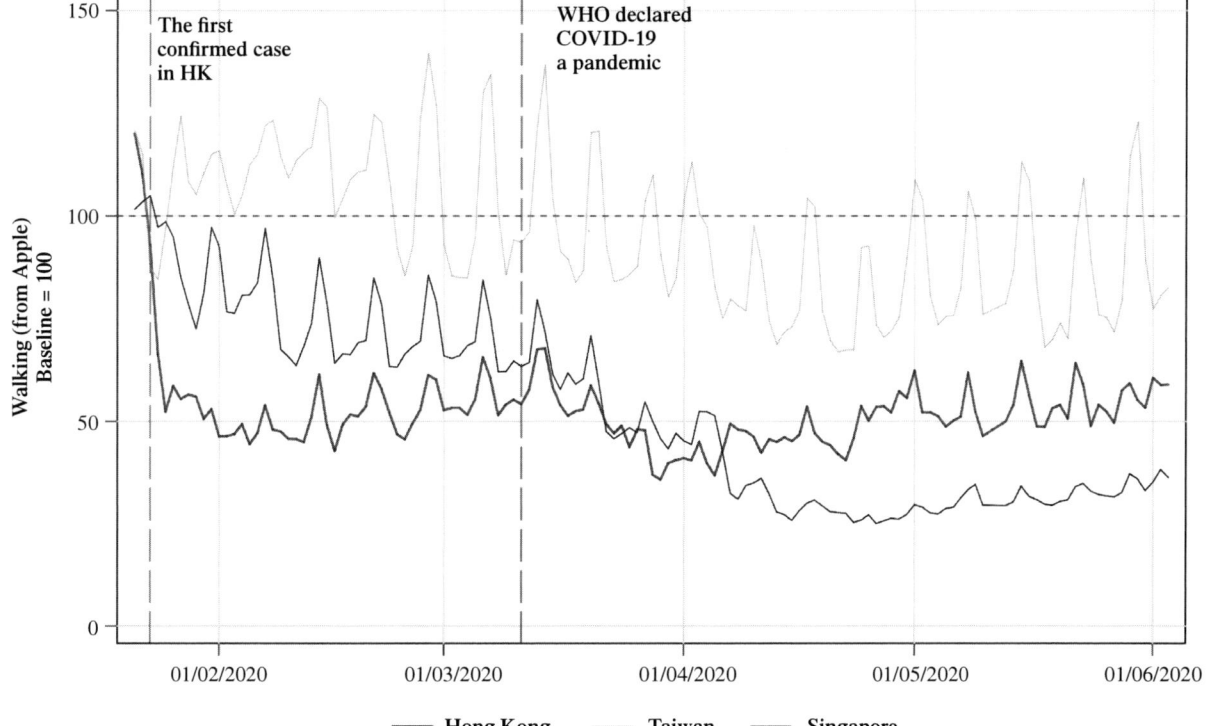

In addition to social distancing, Hong Kong citizens began using surgical masks at the beginning of the pandemic, even when it was not recommended by the WHO officers. Approximately 74.5% of the adults in Hong Kong used surgical masks in public areas in late January, and 95% of the people used surgical masks in February and March (Cowling et at. 2020); this proved to be an effective in limiting the spread of COVID-19 (Cheng et al., 2020; Chan et al., 2020). The experience of devastation of the SARS outbreak in 2003 led to Hong Kong society being self-disciplined and experienced in its fight against COVID-19, which prevented a large-scale community outbreak during the early stages of this pandemic.

Distrust: Legacies of the Anti-Extradition Bill movement

Extant works have suggested the crucial role of the state in the context of a pandemic; however, its effectiveness is dependent on the public's perception of the legitimacy of the government (Wallner, 2008; Gibson, Caldeira and Spence, 2005). Initially, the public demand for preventive measures from the government was high, and these measures included a full closure of the border between Hong Kong and Mainland China and a sustainable supply of surgical masks. However, the HKSAR government was reluctant to act proactively and thus exacerbated the tension and distrust that had already been deeply established during the Anti-Extradition Bill movement of 2019.

Figure 5.9 Attitudes regarding the HKSAR government's performance in addressing coronavirus disease

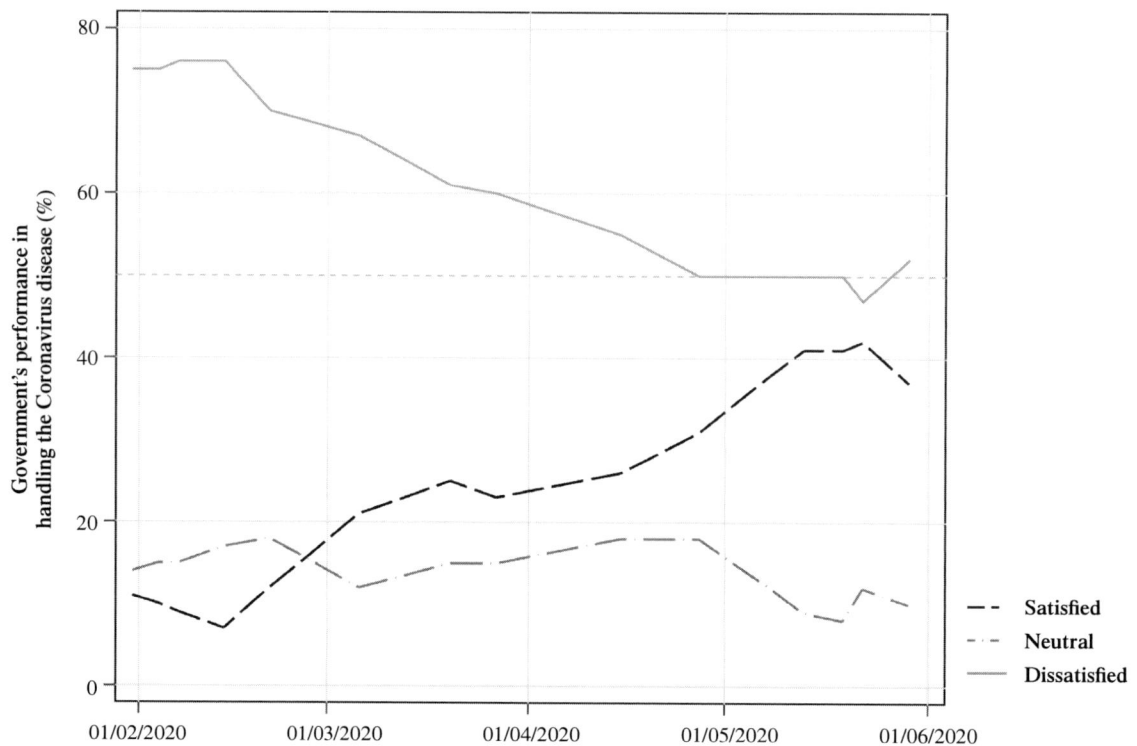

Source: Hong Kong Public Opinion Research Institute, 2020a.

Fig. 5.9 shows that over 70% of the public was dissatisfied with the government's performance in addressing the COVID-19 pandemic before March, which was a crucial period for the containment of the pandemic. Simultaneously, a media-conducted survey suggested that most respondents believed that Hong Kong citizens should be credited for the success achieved regarding the containment of the pandemic instead of the government (Cheung and Wong, 2020).

Indeed, the prominent dissatisfaction of Hong Kong citizens is accompanied by declining trust towards the government. In Fig. 5.10, we can observe a dramatic decline in the government trust from June 2019, when the Anti-extradition Bill movement began. In the early stages of the pandemic (January to March), the rate of support for the Chief Executive was also recorded below 20 over 100, and less than 30% of the population trusted the government and were satisfied with the police force (Hong Kong Public Opinion Research Institute, 2020d; Ho, 2020). It was argued that this attitude towards the police force has become a major divide between the citizens of Hong Kong and the HKSAR government (Chau and Wan, 2020). These attitudes have led to considerable public doubts about the measures that the government has taken and the policies that it has implemented in response to COVID-19. For instance, the Prevention and Control of Disease Ordinance, which prohibits all public gatherings of more than eight people, is perceived as a double standard, as police officers cited the ordinance for crowd control purposes in March[5] but the government permitted the reopening of amusement parks and the Hong Kong Book Fair 2020 in June.

---

5   This gathering is a monthly event held to commemorate the protesters and commuters who were injured in a confrontation with riot police at a metro station. Over half (55%) of the people of Hong Kong believe that the social distancing rule is a means for political suppression rather than for fighting against the pandemic (Hong Kong Public Opinion Research Institute, 2020a).

**Figure 5.10 Attitudes towards and trust of the HKSAR government,
the Chief executive, and the police force**

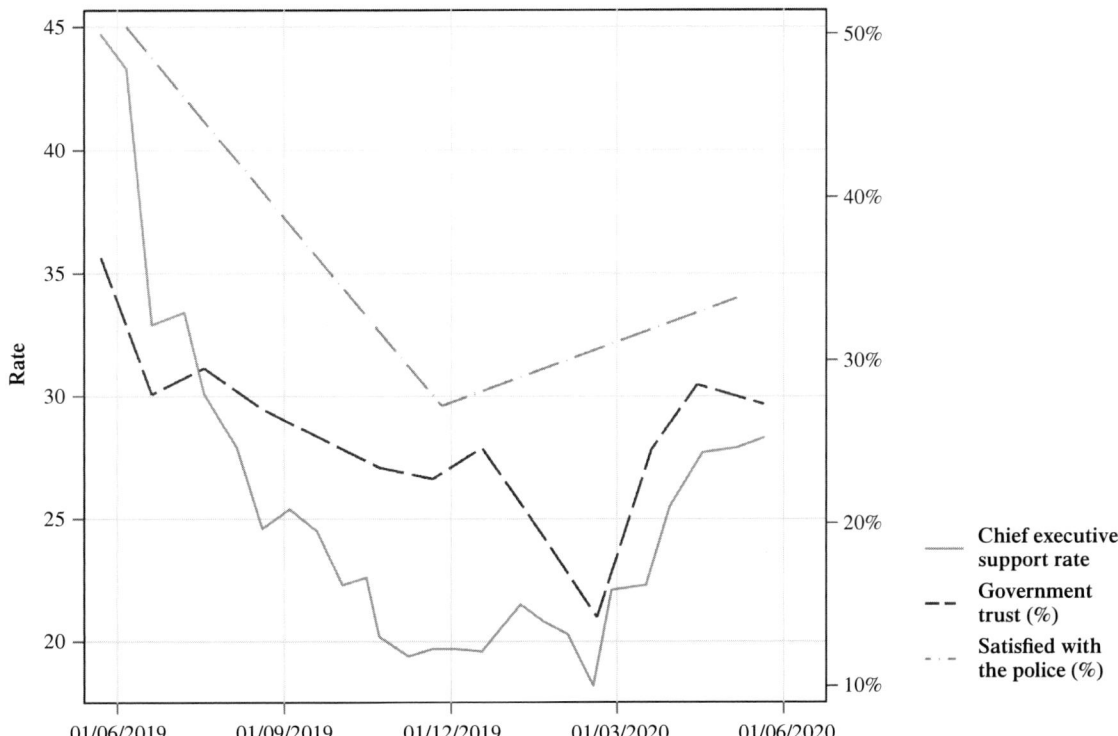

Source: Hong Kong Public Opinion Research Institute, 2020b; 2020c; 2020d.

Social Mobilization: Community Network and Self-help Model

The HKSAR government's reluctance to fully shut down its border and the deeply rooted distrust between society and the government have raised questions regarding the rationale and priorities behind the government's policy-making process. Some believe that the government has placed national interest and pride over public safety and local interest, which resulted in the following actions and responses from society. A community-based mobilization of mutual assistance was implemented instead of full reliance on governmental actions.

The most salient case is the sharing and distribution of community-based personal protective equipment (PPE), particularly surgical masks and hand sanitizers.

The supply of surgical masks was limited due to the export bans implemented by other countries and the public's considerable demand as influenced by their experience during the SARS outbreak. While the WHO officers insisted that it was not recommended for healthy individuals to use surgical masks, the Chief Executive refused to respond to the public demand for surgical masks and mandated that government officials and civil servants take off their surgical masks at work. The supply of surgical masks (both purchased and donated) in Hong Kong was sustained by the efforts of the District Councilors, local organizations and shop owners through mask sharing events. Figs. 5.11 and 5.12 show the mask distribution densities of 432 district councilors from January to early February.[6] Over 40% of the District Councilors held at least one sharing activity in January, and this number increased to 65% and 82% in early and late February, respectively. These mask distributions were prioritized to serve the disadvantaged and groups with a high level of exposure risk[7], as these groups are the most vulnerable to COVID-19 (Jordan, Adab, and Cheng 2020).

Figure 5.11 Mask sharing in Hong Kong (January)

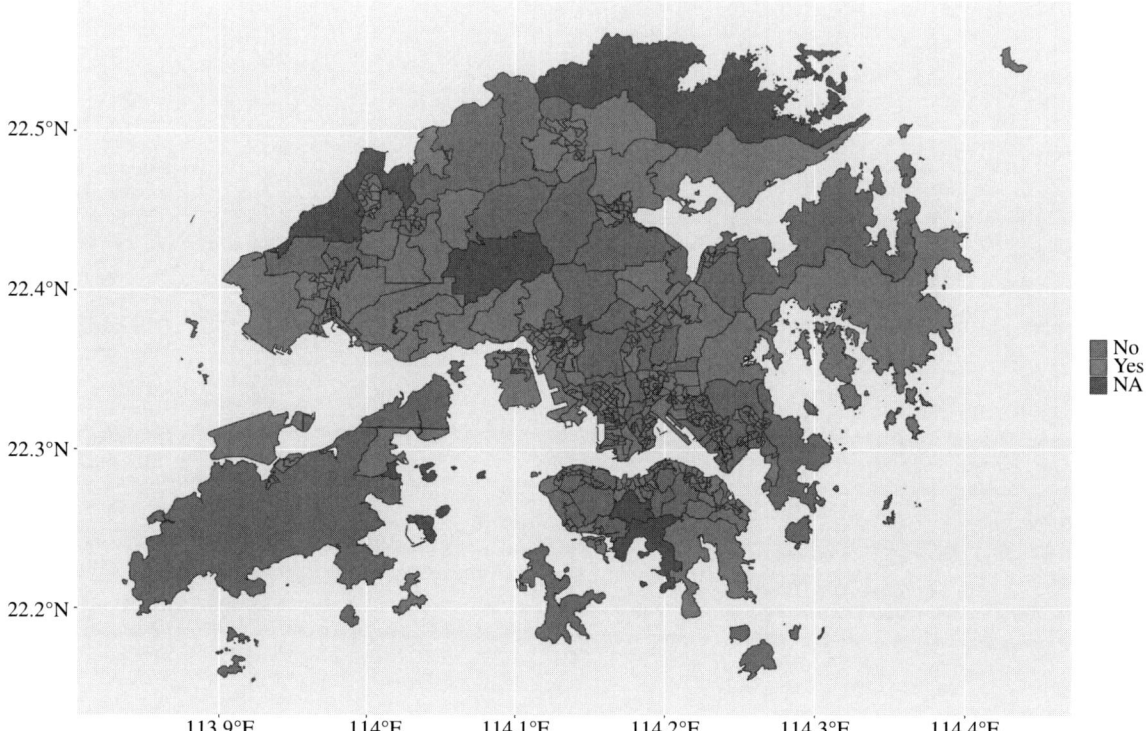

---

6   The graph shows each reported event's frequency. We developed a novel dataset by collecting data from each district councilors' Facebook fan page or personal public account. We excluded all institutional-supported resources and events. For the coding rules and data details, please see Appendix C. We only consider the density of mask sharing rather than including all PPE sharing, because the demand for masks was contradictory to the government's advice; thus, this factor can better to show the how distrust determines people's behavior, and thus reduces transmission.

7   For instance, lower socioeconomic status groups, elderly people, patients with chronic illnesses, medical workers, building security guards, and cleaning workers.

Figure 5.12 Mask sharing in Hong Kong (February: first half)

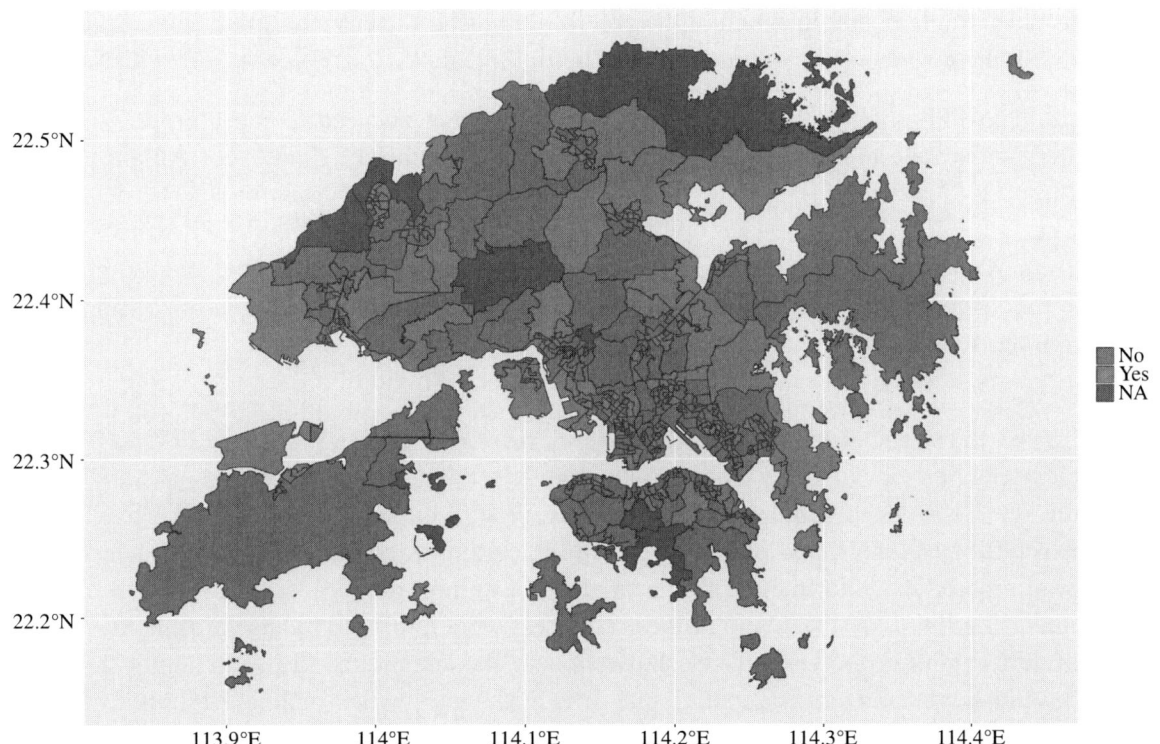

Figure 5.13 The density of mask sharing frequency of the pro-democratic and pro-Beijing districts

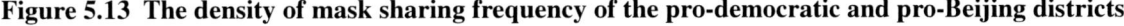

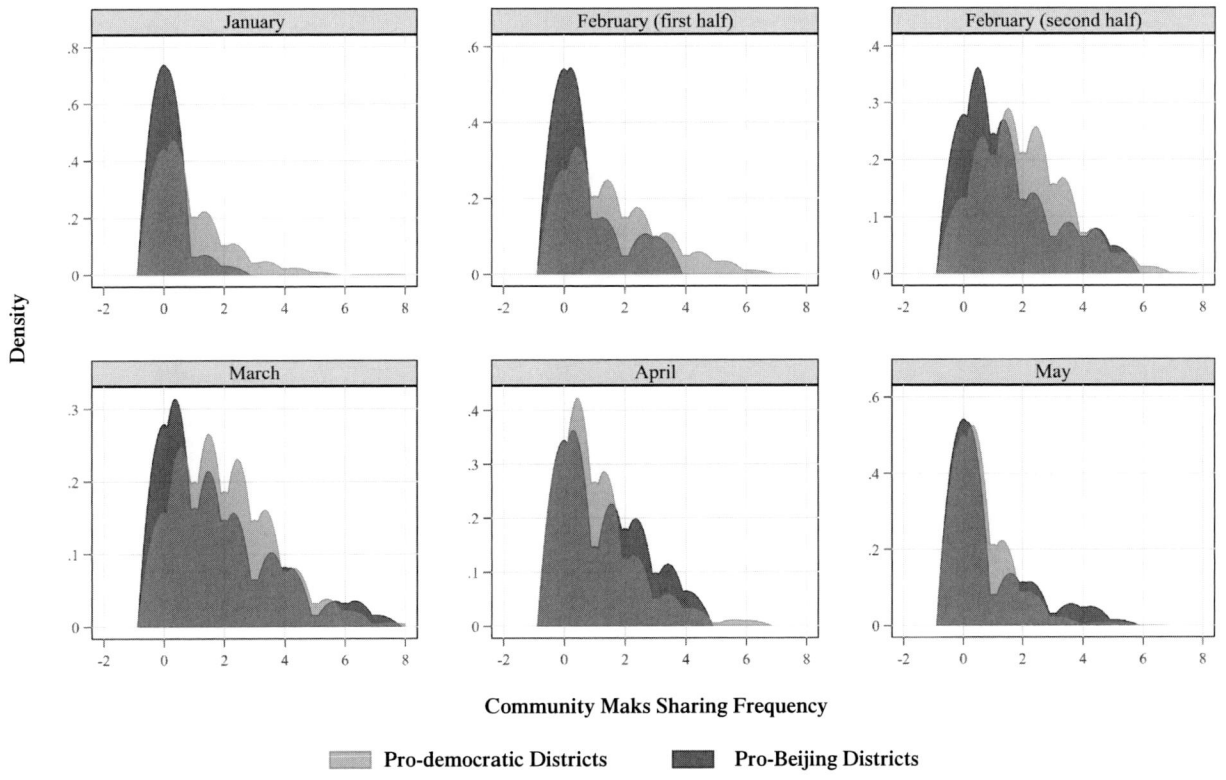

It is argued that the pro-democratic councilors, as a proxy representing a higher level of government distrust, were the first to act. Fig. 5.13 shows that the density of mask sharing in these pro-democratic districts is considerably higher than that of the pro-Beijing districts before March.[8] This implies that the higher the distrust towards the government is in a district, the faster the response of this district was.

In addition to PPE sharing, this distrust of the government also led to more progressive actions against government measures. In late January, the Hospital Authority Employees Alliance (HKEA), a union formed by medical professionals, organized a strike to demand a complete border shutdown after the Chief Executive refused to shut down the high-speed railway to China and restricted incoming travelers from Wubei. Over 60% of the public consistently supported this strike, and the government eventually announced that it would be partially shutting down the high-speed railway to China in early February (Hong Kong Public Opinion Research Institute, 2020a). Thus, the strike of HKEA prevented a potential large-scale outbreak caused by travelers from infected regions.

Furthermore, the public distrust and social unrest occurring since the summer of 2019 have reshaped the public communications in Hong Kong. As the public remained doubtful of the official figures and advice from the HKSAR government, China and the WHO,[9] citizens accessed social media such as Facebook, YouTube channels, and public or private Telegram groups to exchange the latest COVID-related news, reports and information; this was also a common practice during the Anti-Extradition Bill movement (Lee et al., 2019). Users of these channels were reminded to check residential pipes and drainage systems, prompted to verify facts, shown how to test unqualified PPE, and taught how to make cloth masks and hand sanitizers at home. A real-time dashboard, which included details regarding the cases, high-risk areas, questionable pharmacies, etc.[10], was established far before the government official dashboard was established. These platforms provided public-friendly access to COVID-19-related information; this was essential in the fight against COVID-19, since unequal access to information due to differences in socioeconomic status would impede the effectiveness of the society's response to this public health crisis (Lin et al., 2014).

A social and community-based network formed by these self-help models has promoted the protection of the public, especially that of disadvantaged groups and high-risk workers. The fast and transparent circulation of information has enabled citizens to overcome the collective challenges that have faced them (Putman 1993).

Conclusion

An important discussion regarding successful pandemic management centers on governance capacity, including information transparency and timely responses to potential threats. Taiwan and Hong Kong are identified as outstanding cases regarding the containment of the deadly COVID-19 virus due to the low number of confirmed cases and deaths in these places. While Taiwan's success was identified as a model of high governance capacity, this article presented Hong Kong's success as a case supported by civic society and social mobilization.

---

8   The pro-Beijing councilors are much more resourceful than the pro-democratic (Wong 2015). We also provide more supportive evidence and placebo test in appendix, please refer to Tables A2 to A5, and Fig. A8.

9   Over 55% respondents dissatisfied with WHO works on the COVID-19 (Hong Kong Public Opinion Research Institute, 2020a).

10   Please visit COVID-19 in HK https://wars.vote4.hk/en.

Existing studies have suggested that trust between society and the government is crucial in responding to epidemics (Blair et al., 2017), and it is possible that the public gained a higher approval of leadership and a higher sense of national unity during this crisis, as the "rally-round the flag" concept suggested (Mueller 1970; Baum 2002). In this article, we demonstrated that public distrust of the government may not necessarily lead to a failure of pandemic control. In contrast, skepticism of ineffective policies and the presence of a strong civic society driven by state society tensions may contribute positively to pandemic management. The case of Hong Kong exhibits a sharp deviation from the mainstream discourse that places a dual emphasis on capacity and accountability in effective crisis management.

However, it should be made clear that our findings should not be interpreted to undermine the important role of the state in pandemic management. We are rather suggesting that the influence of civil society should be taken into serious consideration in the context of public health crisis-related studies (Eimer and Lutz, 2010).

References

Apple. (2000). Apple Mobility Trends Reports. www.apple.com/covid19/mobility.

Baum, M. A. (2002). The constituent foundations of the rally-round-the-flag phenomenon. *International Studies Quarterly*, 46(2), 263–298.

Blair, R. A., Morse, B. S., & Tsai, L. L. (2017). Public health and public trust: Survey evidence from the Ebola Virus Disease epidemic in Liberia. *Social Science & Medicine*, 172, 89–97.

Bollyky, T. J., Templin, T., Cohen, M., Schoder, D., Dieleman, J. L., & Wigley, S. (2019). The relationships between democratic experience, adult health, and cause-specific mortality in 170 countries between 1980 and 2016: an observational analysis. *The Lancet*, 393(10181), 1628–1640.

Chan, J. F. W., Yuan, S., Zhang, A. J., Poon, V. K. M., Chan, C. C. S., Lee, A. C. Y., ... & Tang, K. (2020). Surgical mask partition reduces the risk of non-contact transmission in a golden Syrian hamster model for Coronavirus Disease 2019 (COVID-19). *Clinical Infectious Diseases.*

Chau, T. H., & Wan, K. M. (2020). Pour (Tear) Gas on Fire? Violent Confrontations and Anti-Government Backlash in Hong Kong. Available at SSRN: https://ssrn.com/abstract=3557130.

Cheng, V. C., Wong, S. C., Chuang, V. W., So, S. Y., Chen, J. H., Sridhar, S., ... & Yuen, K. Y. (2020). The role of community-wide wearing of face mask for control of coronavirus disease 2019 (COVID-19) epidemic due to SARS-CoV-2. *Journal of Infection.*

Cheung, T., & Wong, N. (2020, April 01). Most Hongkongers unhappy with official Covid-19 response, Post poll shows. Retrieved June 09, 2020, from www.scmp.com/news/hong-kong/politics/article/3077761/coronavirus-post-poll-shows-hong-kong-residents-unhappy

Cowling, B. J., Ali, S. T., Ng, T. W., Tsang, T. K., Li, J. C., Fong, M. W., ... & Wu, J. T. (2020). Impact assessment of non-pharmaceutical interventions against coronavirus disease 2019 and influenza in Hong Kong: An observational study. *The Lancet Public Health*, 5, e297–288.

Dionne, K. Y. (2011). The role of executive time horizons in state response to AIDS in Africa. *Comparative Political Studies*, 44(1), 55–77.

Eimer, T., & Lütz, S. (2010). Developmental states, civil society, and public health: Patent regulation for HIV/AIDS pharmaceuticals in India and Brazil. *Regulation & Governance*, 4(2), 135–153.

Gibson, J. L., Caldeira, G. A., & Spence, L. K. (2005). Why do people accept public policies they oppose? Testing legitimacy theory with a survey-based experiment. *Political Research Quarterly*, 58(2), 187–201.

Ho, L. K. K. (2020). Legitimization & De-legitimization of Police: In British Colonial & Chinese SAR Hong Kong. *Journal of Inter-Regional Studies: Regional and Global Perspectives*, 3, 2–13.

Hong Kong Public Opinion Research Institute. (2020a) "Community health module" research report (Chinese only). www.pori.hk/research-reports.

Hong Kong Public Opinion Research Institute. (2020b) Popularity of Chief Executive. www.pori.hk/pop-poll/chief-executive/a003/rating.

Hong Kong Public Opinion Research Institute. (2020c) People's trust in the HKSAR government. www.pori.hk/pop-poll/hksarg/k001.

Hong Kong Public Opinion Research Institute. (2020d) People's satisfaction with the disciplinary force- Hong Kong Police Force. www.pori.hk/pop-poll/disciplinary-force/x001/satisfaction.

Jordan, R. E., Adab, P., & Cheng, K. K. (2020). Covid-19: risk factors for severe disease and death. *BMJ*.

Lau, J. T., Griffiths, S., Choi, K. C., & Tsui, H. Y. (2010). Avoidance behaviors and negative psychological responses in the general population in the initial stage of the H1N1 pandemic in Hong Kong. *BMC Infectious Diseases*, 10(1), 139.

Lee, F. L., Yuen, S., Tang, G., & Cheng, E. W. (2019). Hong Kong's Summer of Uprising. *China Review*, 19(4), 1–32.

Lieberman, E. S. (2007). Ethnic politics, risk, and policy-making: A cross-national statistical analysis of government responses to HIV/AIDS. *Comparative Political Studies*, 40(12), 1407–1432.

Lin, L., Jung, M., McCloud, R. F., & Viswanath, K. (2014). Media use and communication inequalities in a public health emergency: A case study of 2009–2010 pandemic influenza A virus subtype H1N1. *Public Health Reports*, 129(6_suppl4), 49–60.

Mueller, J. E. (1970). Presidential Popularity from Truman to Johnson. *American Political Science Review*, 64(1), 18–34.

Putnam, R.D. (1993). M*aking democracy work: Civic traditions in modern Italy*. Princeton: Princeton University Press.

Wallner, J. (2008). Legitimacy and public policy: Seeing beyond effectiveness, efficiency, and performance. *Policy Studies Journal*, 36(3), 421–443.

Wang, C. J., Ng, C. Y., & Brook, R. H. (2020). Response to COVID-19 in Taiwan: big data analytics, new technology, and proactive testing. *JAMA*, 323(14), 1341–1342.

Wigley, S., & Akkoyunlu-Wigley, A. (2011). The impact of regime type on health: Does redistribution explain everything? *World Politics*, 63(4), 647–677.

Wong, S. H. W. (2015). *Electoral politics in post-1997 Hong Kong*. Singapore: Springer.

Appendix

A   Anti-Pandemic Measures Taken by the HKSAR Government

B   COVID-19 Community Mobility Tracking

C   Community Mask Sharing Behavior

    C1. Constructing the mask-sharing frequencies

    C2. Coding rules

    C3. The rationale behind dividing February into two halves

    C4. Empirical evidence of the effects of pro-democratic districts on mask sharing

    C5. The addition of control variables

    C6. Estimation by matching

    C7. Placebo test

A. Anti-Pandemic Measures Taken by the HKSAR Government

Table A1 Chronology of the Anti-Pandemic Measures taken by the HKSAR Government

Dates	Anti-epidemic Measures
30 Jan	1. Activated emergency response level 2. Suspended cross boundary intercity railways, immigration clearance services, cross-boundary private cars, and cross-boundary ferry services
4-5 Feb	1. Closed four boundary control points 2. Suspended cross-border passenger railway and checkpoints 3. Imposed a 14-day mandatory quarantine on all inbound passengers from Mainland China
19 Mar	1. Implemented a compulsory quarantine requirement for individuals arriving in Hong Kong from foreign places
25 Mar	1. Further limited social contacts and gatherings 2. Closed the border to all incoming nonresidents arriving from overseas 3. Banned transit through Hong Kong 4. Imposed a 14-day compulsory quarantine order on all returning residents
11 Apr	1. Expanded the health tests required of arrivals. Asymptomatic inbound travelers arriving on flights from the US and other areas in Europe required to proceed to the Temporary Specimen Collection Centre for deep-throat saliva sample collection and to wait for their COVID-19 test results.
28 Apr	1. Extended the compulsory quarantine to include travelers from Mainland China, Macao and Taiwan until 7 June
5 May	1. Extended the requirement regarding social-distancing measures until 21 May 2. Increased the number of individuals allowed to attend group gatherings from four to eight 3. Allowed amusement game centers, fitness centers, cinemas, and beauty parlors to reopen. Bars and pubs could resume operations subject to compliance with additional stringent requirements 4. Announced the distribution of reusable masks (CuMask) to every Hong Kong citizen; ten disposable masks were distributed to each household
12 May	1. Conducted viral testing of samples collected from asymptomatic patients in care homes and nursing homes as well as patients admitted to psychiatric wards
19 May	1. Extended the requirement regarding social-distancing measures to 4 June (religious gatherings exempted) 2. Adjusted anti-epidemic requirements for gyms and places of public entertainment 3. Increased the viral testing capacity to 7000 tests per day

Sources: Government Information Services, Government of Hong Kong SAR, 2020

B. COVID-19 Community Mobility Tracking

The Apple Mobility Trend data used the mobility count at 13 Jan 2020 as its baseline and setting this baseline to 100.

Google Community Mobility Reports show movement trends by region across different types of places. Collection of the Google data collection began later than that of the Apple data. The baseline day was set to on February 6, and it is the median value of the 5-week period spanning from January 3 to February 6, 2020. Thus, we can see that the declining margin of Hong Kong citizens in the Google data is slightly lower than it is in the Apple data because the population of Hong Kong started to walk out of their homes less frequently in late January.

Figure A1 Mobility trends derived from Apple and Google from January to June of 2019

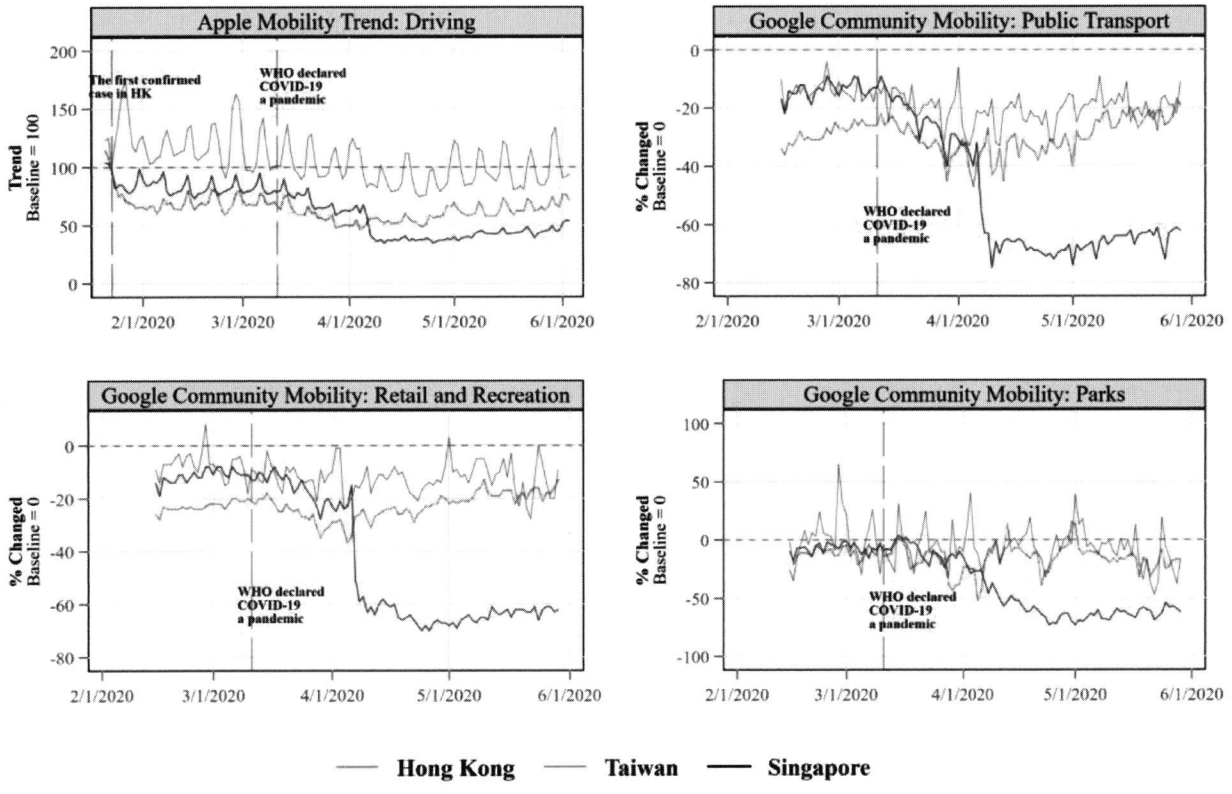

C. Community Mask-Sharing Behavior

C1. Constructing the mask-sharing frequencies

We collect mask-sharing activities directly from each councilor's Facebook fan page or personal public account. There are 452 constituencies within 18 districts in the 2019 Hong Kong District Council, and 20 constituency councils (~5%) do not have a public Facebook page or an account. As a result, our dataset covers 432 (95.5%) of the constituencies in Hong Kong.

Once we have a list of the district councilors and have searched their Facebook fan pages or public accounts, we search for the specific word "mask" (口罩) and then search for the phrase "epidemic prevention" (防疫) as a supplement. After searching for the word "mask", we read every post in the search results.

C2. Coding rules

The aim of this analysis is to use this dataset to show how the community self-help model works. We encountered a problem in that some may argue that the District Council is part of a formal institution, and thus may use institutionally supported or sponsored materials and resources to deliver PPE or masks to the public.

To address this issue, we exclude all institutionally sponsored mask-sharing activities, as some districts approved the use of institutional funding to purchase masks for the public; those materials typically arrived in HK after mid-March. Thus, we only include masks that are delivered or sold from the following sources:

1. Voluntary donations;

2. Private purchases of councilors;

3. Private purchases of political parties;

4. Platforms enabling constituencies to collectively purchase masks from overseas or local companies.

Overcalculation represents the most challenging difficulty that we encountered during the process of data construction. To address this issue, we employ an activity-day as the unit examined. First, if the councilor uses a pack of masks and then delivers or sells it to place A, place B, place C, and place D within a day, we see this as 1 event and record it as such, although it seems to be composed of 4 activities. This rule prevents the overcalculation of doorstep deliveries.

Second, to prevent another type of repeated calculation regarding mask sharing or selling, we also record 1 event if a constituent received or picked up a mask that had been registered on the buying platform earlier.

C3. The rationale behind dividing February into two halves

We divide February into two different periods because the WHO officials and Chief Executive, the government, and even the government advisory expert panelists suggested that the public use of masks was not recommended in January and early February, which contradicted the understanding and demands of the public. Later, an advisory expert panelist issued a public apology for his recommendation against using masks. Thus, we attempt to see if any variation exists between the first and second halves of February.

Figure A2 Mask sharing frequency (January)

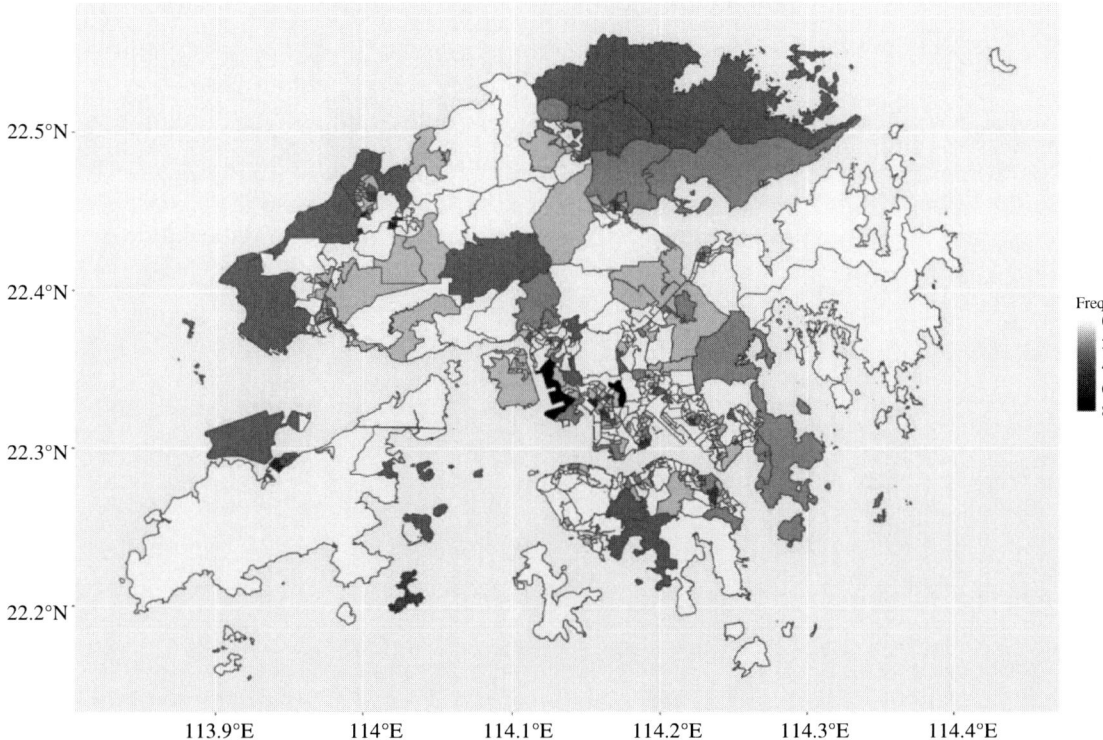

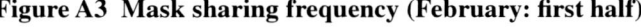

Figure A3 Mask sharing frequency (February: first half)

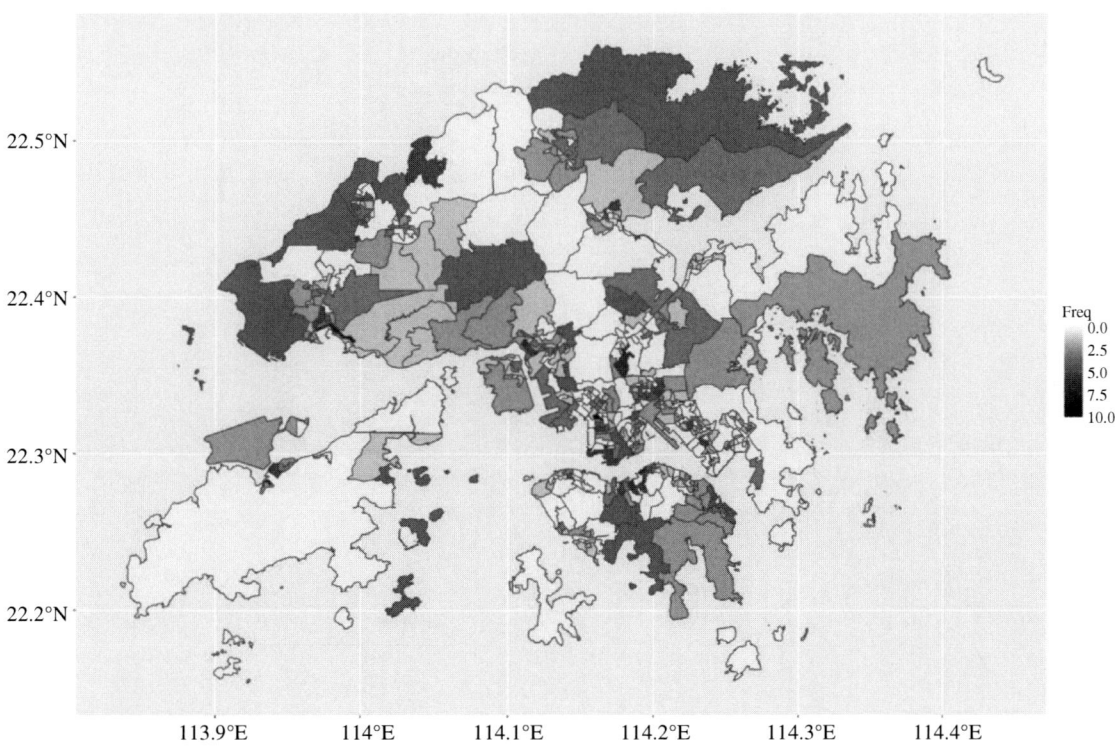

Figure A4 Mask sharing frequency (February: second half)

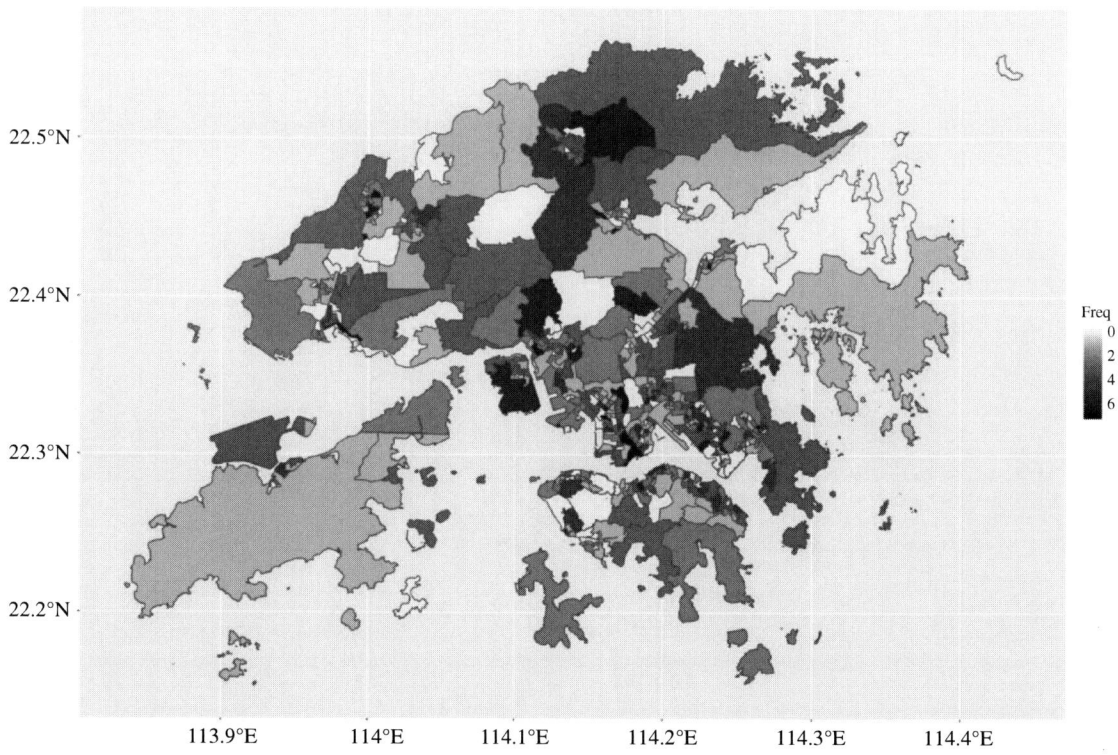

Figure A5 Mask sharing frequency (March)

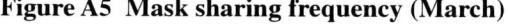

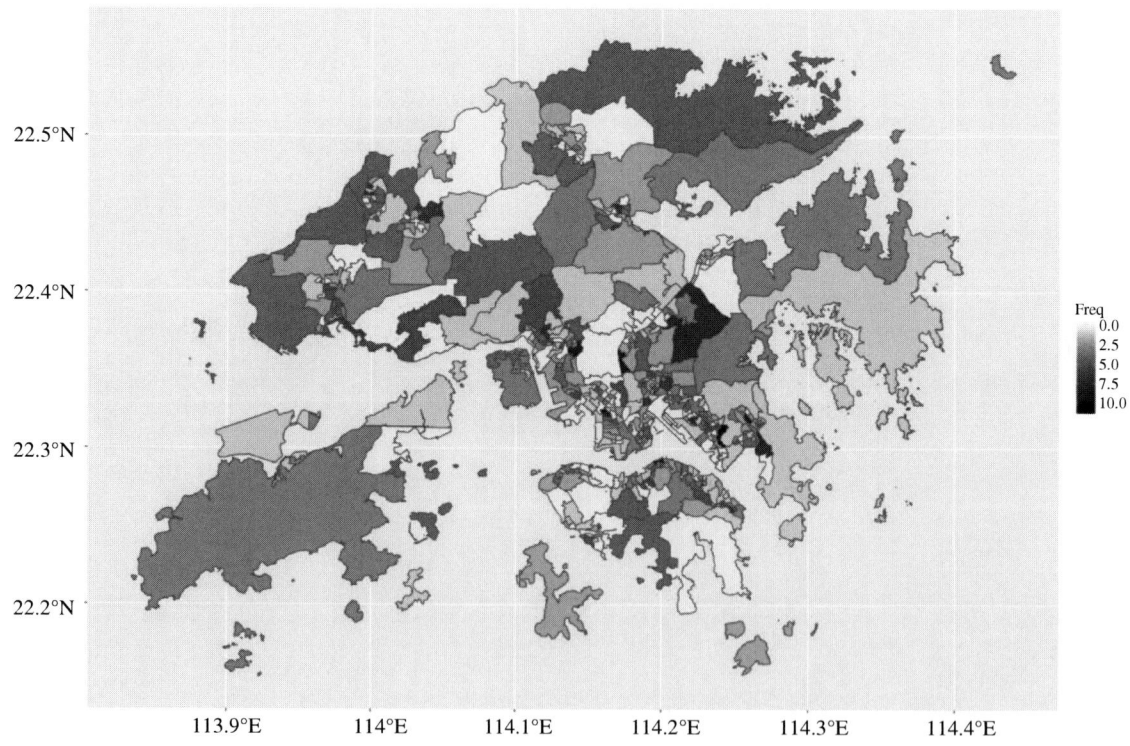

Figure A6 Mask sharing frequency (April)

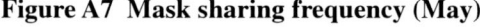

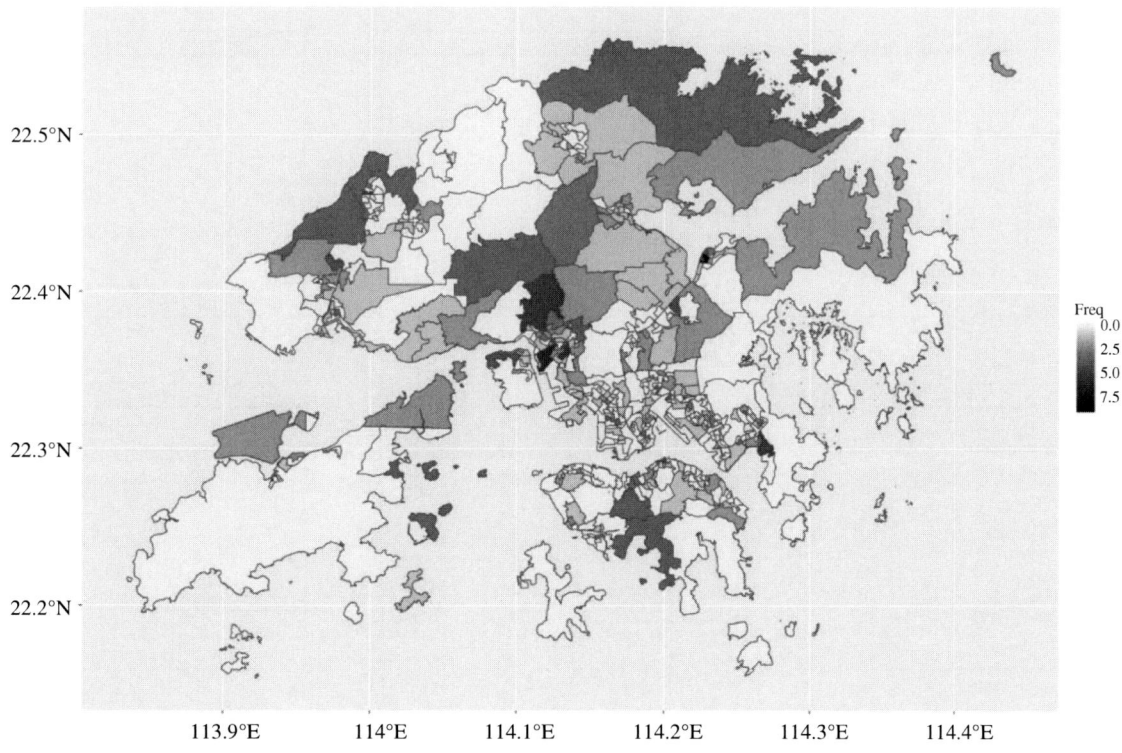

Figure A7 Mask sharing frequency (May)

C4. Empirical evidence of the effects of pro-democratic district on mask sharing

We provide more supportive evidence that the pro-democratic districts (representing a proxy for the level of distrust towards the government) acted faster than did the pro-Beijing camp districts that followed the advice of the government. We use the mask-sharing frequency and construct a binary variable (a mask-sharing frequency > 0 is coded as 1), which is used as the outcome variable in Table A2 and Table A3.

Then, we code the pro-democratic seats as 1 using the following rules: If, in the 2019 District Council Election, a councilor included "Five demands, not one less" in his or her platform, which represents the consensus of the 2019 protest, or if he or she was endorsed by the "Democratic Coalition for the DC Election" (民主派區選聯盟), he or she is determined to be pro-democratic. The other councilors who support the government are coded as 0. Thus, we observe that our sample contains 388 pro-democratic districts and 62 pro-Beijing districts. We include the Legislative Council (LegCo: 5) fixed effects and the District Council (District: 18) fixed effects in the models to account for the unobserved factors. Additionally, we use the District Council fixed effects to fix the neighboring effects within the 18 districts. For instance, a councilor may use a neighboring district as a reference point. This councilor may be more motivated to share masks if his or her neighboring councilor continues to deliver masks to his or her constituents.

The empirical findings shown in Tables A2 and A3 show that the pro-democratic districts exhibit a significantly higher frequency of mask sharing than do the pro-Beijing districts during the months of January and February. However, there were no significant differences between these groups during March and April. The pro-Beijing camp seems to exhibit a higher frequency of mask sharing in May once the pandemic was relatively under control in Hong Kong.

Figure A8 Marginal effects of the pro-democratic districts on mask sharing with 95% CI

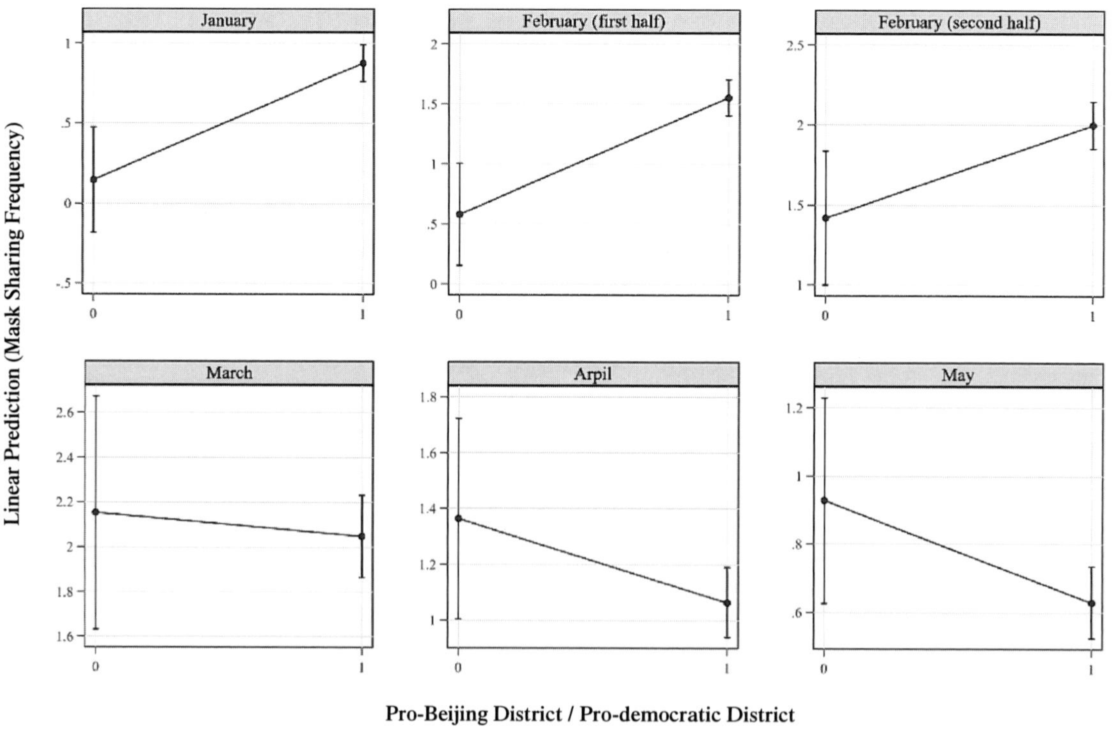

Pro-Beijing District / Pro-democratic District

162

Table A2 Baseline model of the effects of the pro-democratic districts on mask sharing (Frequency)

| | Mask Sharing (Frequency) | | | | | | | | | | | |
| | Jan | | Feb (first half) | | Feb (second half) | | Mar | | Apr | | May | |
	(1)	(2)	(3)	(4)	(5)	(6)	(7)	(8)	(9)	(10)	(11)	(12)
Pro-democratic	0.724***	0.732***	0.970***	0.976***	0.583**	0.581*	0.034	-0.105	-0.262	-0.300	-0.282#	-0.299#
	(0.176)	(0.180)	(0.229)	(0.233)	(0.222)	(0.229)	(0.274)	(0.284)	(0.190)	(0.196)	(0.160)	(0.165)
LegCo FE	✓		✓		✓		✓		✓		✓	
District FE		✓		✓		✓		✓		✓		✓
R2	0.066	0.133	0.075	0.145	0.020	0.067	0.007	0.045	0.040	0.082	0.053	0.102
Observations	432	432	432	432	432	432	432	432	432	432	432	432

Note: Standard errors are reported in parentheses.
 # $p < 0.1$, * $p < 0.05$, ** $p < 0.01$, *** $p < 0.001$ (two-tailed test).

Table A3 Baseline model of the effects of the pro-democratic districts on mask sharing (Binary, Yes=1)

| | Mask Sharing (Binary: Yes = 1) | | | | | | | | | | | |
| | Jan | | Feb (first half) | | Feb (second half) | | Mar | | Apr | | May | |
	(1)	(2)	(3)	(4)	(5)	(6)	(7)	(8)	(9)	(10)	(11)	(12)
Pro-democratic	0.354***	0.340***	0.343***	0.354***	0.178**	0.173**	0.152*	0.128*	-0.026	-0.038	0.007	0.005
	(0.072)	(0.075)	(0.070)	(0.073)	(0.058)	(0.060)	(0.061)	(0.062)	(0.074)	(0.077)	(0.073)	(0.074)
LegCo FE	✓		✓		✓		✓		✓		✓	
District FE		✓		✓		✓		✓		✓		✓
R2	0.078	0.124	0.081	0.126	0.026	0.048	0.022	0.089	0.031	0.048	0.044	0.114
Observations	432	432	432	432	432	432	432	432	432	432	432	432

Note: Standard errors are reported in parentheses.
 # $p < 0.1$, * $p < 0.05$, ** $p < 0.01$, *** $p < 0.001$ (two-tailed test).

C5. The addition of control variables

It is possible that the frequency of mask sharing depends on a district's demographics. For instance, districts with a high number of elderly people or a high number of people with a lower socioeconomic status may experience a higher demand for mask sharing than do other districts; similarly, districts with high average income levels may experience a lower demand for mask sharing. To address this issue, we added the median age, median income, and the percentage of degree holders of each district as control variables in Table A4. These data are collected from the 2016 Population By-census of Hong Kong. Reassuringly, the results of this analysis are highly consistent with those of the baseline model shown in Tables A2 and A3.

Table A4 Adding demographic control variables

	Jan	Feb 1st	Feb 2nd	Mar	Apr	May
Pro-Democratic	0.658**	0.974***	0.499#	-0.377	-0.165	-0.326#
	(0.209)	(0.270)	(0.260)	(0.329)	(0.227)	(0.191)
Degree holders	0.911	1.588	2.776#	4.374*	-0.138	-0.276
	(1.246)	(1.612)	(1.552)	(1.965)	(1.354)	(1.139)
Median age	0.012	0.012	-0.010	0.056#	-0.007	-0.010
	(0.020)	(0.026)	(0.025)	(0.032)	(0.022)	(0.019)
Median income	-0.000	-0.000#	-0.000#	-0.000*	-0.000	-0.000
	(0.000)	(0.000)	(0.000)	(0.000)	(0.000)	(0.000)
District FE	✔	✔	✔	✔	✔	✔
R2	0.119	0.146	0.074	0.065	0.094	0.114
Obversions	400	400	400	400	400	400

Note: Standard errors are reported in parentheses.
*# $p < 0.1$, * $p < 0.05$, ** $p < 0.01$, *** $p < 0.001$ (two-tailed test).*

C6. Estimation by matching

Various district demographic covariates can influence electoral results (we use the difference of pro-Beijing vs. pro-democratic as a proxy for the level of trust of the government). We match treated districts that have pro-democratic councilors with controlled districts based on a set of observed covariates: (1) median income level; (2) median age; and (3) percentage of degree holders. Observations that lack matches are discarded, and the remaining matched cases share very similar characteristics.

We apply a coarsened exact matching procedure (cem in STATA) to select treatment and control observations that are exactly matched based on the coarsened values of the matching variables (Iacus, King, and Porro, 2012). There are 432 original observations. There are 45 controlled districts and 216 treated districts (total: 261). Table A5 presents the average treatment effects (ATE) estimated by this matching process.

**Table A5 Effect of the pro-democratic districts on mask sharing
and the average treatment effects using CEM**

	ATE	ATE
January	0.652**	0.731**
February (first half)	0.996***	1.227***
February (second half)	0.545*	0.583*
March	-0.181	-0.162
April	-0.231	-0.245
May	-0.192	-0.285
District FE		✔
Observations	261	261

*Note: * p < 0.05, ** p < 0.01, *** p < 0.001 (two-tailed test).*

C7. Placebo test

We also conducted a placebo test to determine whether our findings were valid. We use pro-democratic t-1 (based on the camps of district councilors during the year 2015) as the independent variable to be regressed on the mask sharing frequency. These results completely different from our main findings.

Table A6 Placebo test: Using pro-democratic districts in 2015

	Jan	Feb 1st	Feb 2nd	Mar	Apr	May
Pro-democratic t-1	-0.442***	-0.317#	-0.556***	-0.583**	-0.302*	-0.197#
	(0.126)	(0.172)	(0.162)	(0.204)	(0.140)	(0.116)
District FE	✔	✔	✔	✔	✔	✔
R2	0.139	0.117	0.081	0.063	0.099	0.124
Observations	390	390	390	390	390	390

Note: Standard errors are reported in parentheses.
*# p < 0.1, * p < 0.05, ** p < 0.01, *** p < 0.001 (two-tailed test).*

References

Apple. Apple Mobility Trends Reports. www.apple.com/covid19/mobility Accessed: <8 June, 2002>.

Google LLC. Google COVID-19 Community Mobility Reports. www.google.com/covid19/mobility/ Accessed: <8 June, 2020>.

Iacus, S. M., King, G., & Porro, G. (2012). Causal inference without balance checking: Coarsened exact matching. *Political Analysis*, 20(1), 1–24.

HONG KONG

Linda Chelan Li, Cleo Wong, Xin Yan and Jeffrey Chung
19.01–14.11 Total 5,445 cases / 108 deaths

19.01 – 25.01 (5; all imported)**

Public Health Policies

19.01 Restricted visiting arrangements imposed in all public hospitals.

23.01 Lady MacLehose Holiday Village was converted as quarantine centre and close contacts would be transferred to the village for quarantine.

Health declaration form system was extended to Hong Kong West Kowloon Station starting from January 24.

25.01 Hospital Authority (HA) announced the activation of Emergency Response Level in public hospitals to tie in with the Government raising the response level from 'Serious' to 'Emergency'.

Education Bureau (EDB) announced that all schools (including kindergartens, primary schools, secondary schools and special schools) would extend their Chinese New Year holidays to February 16.

26.01 – 01.02 (14; 13 were imported or close contacts of the infected, 1 might be local case)**

Public Health Policies

26.01 The response level under the Preparedness and Response Plan would be raised to Emergency level and CE would chair a Steering Committee cum Command Centre with a view to formulating relevant strategies and measures.

Indefinitely suspended flight and high-speed train services to and from Wuhan of the Hubei Province.

Expanded the arrangements of health declaration by in-coming travellers from the Mainland as soon as possible to all boundary control points, and gradually piloted the use of e-health declaration system.

Speeded up the procurement process for protective gears as far as possible to ensure adequate supply for government departments.

28.01 Starting from 9am 29 Jan, all inbound traveller by air from the Mainland were required to complete and submit a health declaration form.

Major cross-border arrangements:

1. The services of Hong Kong section of the Guangzhou-Shenzhen-Hong Kong Express Rail Link and the Intercity Through Train would be suspended from January 30.

2. Immigration clearance service for passengers and cross boundary coaches, private cars and hired cars at Sha Tau Kok and Man Kam To Control Points were suspended.

3. From January 30, four local airlines would gradually reduce their scheduled passenger flights between Hong Kong and 24 Mainland destinations by half until further notice.

4. From January 30, the cross-boundary ferry services of China Ferry Terminal at Tsim Sha Tsui and Tuen Mun Ferry Terminal of the Marine Department would be suspended until further notice.

Special work arrangement (work from home) for government departments (except emergency services and essential public services) would be implemented after the Lunar New Year holidays starting from January 29.

29.01 The Government contacted more than 140 suppliers from over 10 countries to procure surgical masks to cope with the epidemic.

30.01 Correctional Services Department would try to extend production to 24 hours, increasing the production from 1.1 million to 1.8 million per month.

02.02 – 08.02 (26)**

Public Health Policies

03.02 Control point services at four control points - Lo Wu, Lok Ma Chau Spur Line, Lok Ma Chau and Macau Ferry Terminal - would be suspended with effect from February 4 until further notice.

People who have been to the Hubei Province in the past 14 days and do not have symptoms would

---

*   Source: HKSARG Press Release: www.info.gov.hk/gia/general/

\#   Source: News.gov.hk: www.news.gov.hk/eng/categories/covid19, unless otherwise specified

*"   where shown, the number in brackets is the accumulated number of confirmed cases and death cases respectively. And in following brackets, the number for the recovered or discharged is also displayed.

be put under mandatory home quarantine. The existing quarantine centres would also reserve units for those in need of home quarantine but not suitable to stay at home.

The Government would increase quarantine facilities as soon as possible and was looking for existing sites suitable for quarantine purposes.

Any person concerned who leave home without permission may commit a criminal offence, and would be subject to a maximum penalty of $5,000 and imprisonment of six months on conviction. The Government would use electronic wristbands to monitor the location of those people under quarantine.

For civil servants who were utilizing government issued surgical masks:

Heads of departments should ensure that those masks are only provided to staff members for use if (i) he/she would have frequent contact with members of the public as part of his/her duties (e.g. counter staff) or work in crowded places; or (ii) it is for meeting essential operational needs; or (iii) it is for meeting special needs

of the staff members concerned (e.g. medical conditions).

04.02 As a large number of staff members were absent from duty, emergency services in public hospitals have been affected to a certain extent.

05.02 The Government imposed a 14-day mandatory quarantine on all the people entering Hong Kong from the Mainland, including Hong Kong residents, Mainland residents as well as other visitors.

06.02 The Government Logistics Department (GLD) claimed that it had been exercising maximum flexibility to procure directly from suppliers through different channels and means in order to secure the supply of masks and other protective items promptly to meet the urgent needs of government departments.

EDB announced that all schools would resume class no earlier than 2 March.

All DSE examinations taking place before 27 March would be postponed.

07.02 Starting from February 8, the Department of Health (DH) would

issue quarantine orders to all people entering Hong Kong from the Mainland, including Hong Kong residents, Mainland residents and visitors from other places.

The following categories of persons were exempted from the compulsory quarantine requirement with effect from the commencement of the Regulation:

1. cross-boundary goods vehicle drivers and necessary accompanying personnel;

2. cross-boundary coach and shuttle drivers and necessary crew members;

3. air crew disembarking from planes at Hong Kong International Airport and entering Hong Kong;

4. crew members of aircrafts of air freight operators who need to commute to and from the Mainland for performance of necessary duties related to freight forwarding;

5. government officials carrying out governmental duties;

6. government agents and contractors supporting the operation of cross-boundary functions;

7. crew members of goods vessels; and

8. crew members of fishing vessels and fish collectors (including mainland fishermen deckhands).

Major Development

03.02 More than 2,400 Hong Kong public hospital workers staged a strike on Monday morning as a top microbiologist agreed with their central demand that the government close the border with mainland China to fend off the deadly coronavirus.[1]

04.02 Thousands of medical workers in Hong Kong joined a second day of strikes on Tuesday to put pressure on the government to impose a full shutdown of the Chinese border to curb the coronavirus outbreak.[2]

05.02 A union for public hospital workers on Wednesday rejected the Hong Kong leader's plan to implement mandatory quarantine measures on travellers arriving from mainland China rather than a full closure of the border to combat the new coronavirus, vowing to take its strike into the fourth day.

The HAEmployees Alliance said 7,000 took part

1   *SCMP*: www.scmp.com/news/hong-kong/politics/article/3048705/hong-kong-hospital-strike-kicks-top-doctor-backs-mainland

2   *HKFP*: https://hongkongfp.com/2020/02/04/coronavirus-hong-kong-medics-escalate-strike-demand-full-shutdown-chinese-border/

in the third day of the strike – about the same as on Tuesday.[3]

07.02 Hong Kong's striking hospital workers have voted down a plan to extend their industrial action but insisted they would continue to fight for better protection against the deadly new coronavirus and the full closure of the city's border with mainland China.

The HA Employees Alliance on Friday announced it would vote to decide whether to press ahead with the work boycott until next Wednesday. It garnered only 3,000 votes, short of the 6,000 vote – 30 per cent of its total membership – the union called for, while 4,000 voted against a further strike.[4]

09.02 – 15.02 (56/1; 1 discharged)**

Public Health Policies

12.02 Apart from those being transferred to the Tso Kung Tam Outdoor Recreation Centre, if the persons under compulsory quarantine failed to share their real-time locations with their mobile phones at the boundary control points, the government would immediately request

them to wear electronic wristbands with a view to monitoring whether they were staying at the dwelling places.

13.02 EDB decided that schools would not resume classes before March 16.

In view of the latest situation, the special work arrangement for government departments would be extended until February 23.

14.02 An additional allocation of $4.7 billion would be mobilized to support HA in implementing various measures to enhance public hospitals' capability to respond to the new coronavirus epidemic.

Land sports facilities, aquatic and cultural facilities would be temporarily closed.

The Legislative Council (LegCo) Secretariat announced special arrangements for meetings of LegCo and its Committees.

15.02 Government was arranging chartered flight to take the Hong Kong residents under quarantine on board the Diamond Princess cruise ship back to Hong Kong free of charge soonest possible after they are permitted to disembark and land.

Socio-Economic Policy Packages

11.02 Hong Kong Monetary Authority (HKMA) convened a special teleconference of the Banking Sector SME Lending Coordination Mechanism on February 11 to discuss ways for the industry to extend greater support to their small and medium-sized enterprise (SME) customers in light of the latest developments.

14.02 The Government would set up a $25 billion fund to help local residents and businesses tide over the coronavirus situation.

16.02 – 22.02 (68/2; 10 recoveries)**

Public Health Policies

18.02 The HA said it would enhance surveillance of patients at general out-patient clinics and accident and emergency departments from February 19 to boost the early detection of novel coronavirus infections.

20.02 The special work arrangement for government departments would be extended until March 1.

21.02 The Global Logistics Department (GLD) closed the open tender and indicated that a

total of three offers were received for procuring 57 million masks.

The Centre for Health Protection (CHP) would like Police to activate its Major Incident Investigation & Disaster Support System to assist them with contact tracing and identifying clusters.

Socio-Economic Policy Packages

20.02 The Secretary for Home Affairs, Mr Lau Kong-wah, met the representatives from the property management ("PM"), cleansing and security sector to introduce relevant details of the "Property Management Sector Support Scheme" under the Anti-epidemic Fund. The total funding required would be about $1 billion. Upon the approval of the Finance Committee of the Legislative Council, the scheme should be open for application in March 2020.

EDB announced the provision of additional subsidies to kindergartens (KGs), primary and secondary schools and their students to alleviate the burden of schools and parents in defraying extra expenses during the fight against the epidemic and class suspension.

---

3   *SCMP*: www.scmp.com/news/hong-kong/health-environment/article/3049166/hospital-workers-strike-organisers-threaten

4   *SCMP*: www.scmp.com/news/hong-kong/health-environment/article/3049512/hong-kong-medical-workers-strike-goes-level

21.02 The funding application for the Anti-epidemic Fund by the LegCo Finance Committee was passed.

22.02 The Secretary for Innovation and Technology, Mr. Nicholas Yang indicated under the anti-epidemic fund, the government would provide 6-month rent free period for the 1,800 tenants at Cyberport and Science Park

23.02 – 29.02 (94/2; 30 recoveries)**
Public Health Policies

24.02 The government issued a red travel warning (Red Outbound Travel Alert) in regard to visit to Korea.

To address the concern that the prescription medications taken by the Hong Kong residents who are currently located in Guangdong and Fujian Provinces may soon be running out, the HKSAR Government introduced the special scheme to deliver prescription medications to them.

The Government would arrange for chartered flights to bring back Hong Kong people stranded in Hubei Province in batches.

25.02 EDB decided that classes of all schools would continue to be suspended until end of the schools' Easter holidays.

The Territory-wide System

Assessment (TSA) (including all oral and written assessments) would be suspended for the current school year.

26.02 To facilitate epidemic prevention work, the Government has stepped up access control at Chung Ying Street located in Sha Tau Kok FCA.

27.02 Targeted measures would be implemented to reduce social contact and infection control measures and gradually resume more public services from March 2 in an orderly manner.

28.02 Red Outbound Travel Alert is issued on Emilia-Romagna, Lombardy and Veneto regions in Italy which cover Bologna, Milan, Venice and Verona.

Socio-Economic Policy Packages

23.02 In response to media enquiries regarding details of the Local Mask Production Subsidy Scheme under the Anti-epidemic Fund, a spokesman for the Commerce and Economic Development Bureau said:

1. To be eligible for a subsidy from the Government, a production line must satisfy a number of stringent conditions.
2. A subsidy of up to $3 million may be given to each production line and up to $2 million to each additional produc-

tion line in the same factory.

24.02 The Government established the Travel Agents Subsidy Scheme under the Anti-epidemic Fund. Each eligible travel agent might receive a one-off subsidy of $80,000.

The Government has established the Licensed Guesthouses Subsidy Scheme under the Anti-epidemic Fund. Each eligible guesthouse might receive a one-off subsidy of either $50,000 or $80,000.

HA Board approved a special allowance for staff working in high-risk COVID-19 areas during the special emergency response period.

26.02 The Budget Speech by the Financial Secretary announced numerous relief measures for enterprises, employees, the underpriviledged, the general public (e.g. the cash payout) and the HA.

01.03 – 07.03 (105/2; 58 recoveries)**
Public Health Policies

05.03 4 government-chartered flights brought back a total of 469 Hong Kong residents stranded in Hubei Province.

06.03 Queen Mary Hospital, Princess Margaret Hospital and Prince of Wales Hospital would start clinical trials of an

antiviral drug (which was still an investigational drug)

Socio-Economic Policy Packages

02.03 Housing Authority would extend 50% rent concession for its retail and factory tenants for six months from April 1 to September 30.

04.03 Food Licence Holders Subsidy Scheme: (i) A one-off subsidy of $200,000 for holders of general restaurants, marine restaurants and factory canteens; (ii) A subsidy of $80,000 for holder of light refreshment restaurants, fresh provision shops, food factories, bakeries and siu mei and lo mei shops.

Licensed Hawkers Subsidy Scheme: A $5,000 subsidy to each eligible licensee of a hawker license.

06.03 Carrie Lam and 43 officials donated $10,805,250 (a month's salary) to Community Chest of Hong Kong

08.03 – 14.03 (142/4; 84 recoveries)**
Public Health Policies

08.03 The HA announced that one more GOPC would be covered by the Enhanced Laboratory Surveillance Programme from March 9, making for a total of 64 GOPCs and 17 A&E Departments.

The Innovation & Technology Commission

launched a special call under the Public Sector Trial Scheme for projects to support product development and application of technologies for the prevention and control of COVID-19. The target funding recipients were local R&D centres, universities and other designated public research institutes, as well as all technology companies conducting R&D activities in Hong Kong.

10.03 Red Outbound Travel Alert was issued on the whole of Italy, France (Bourgogne-Franche-Comte and Grand Est), Germany (North Rhine-Westphalia), Japan (Hokkaido) and Spain (La Rioja, Madrid and Pais Vasco) in response to the latest situations of COVID-19. The DH also strengthened health quarantine arrangements on inbound travellers arriving from these countries/regions.

12.03 With the approach of the Ching Ming Festival (April 4), Government appealed to members of the public to stagger grave-sweeping activities over a wider period before and after the Ching Ming Festival to prevent the spread of COVID-19.

13.03 Red Outbound Travel Alert was issued on certain European countries (Schengen Area), including Austria, Belgium, Czech Republic, Denmark, Estonia, Finland, France, Germany, Greece, Hungary, Iceland, Italy, Latvia, Principality of Liechtenstein, Lithuania, Luxembourg, Malta, the Netherlands, Norway, Poland, Portugal, Slovak Republic, Republic of Slovenia, Spain, Sweden, and Switzerland. The DH strengthened health quarantine measures on people arriving from these countries and demand them to undergo compulsory home quarantine.

HA said they were trying to purchase any PPE items from across the world - to try to buy directly without tendering, and claimed they tried their best to make sure the logistics and supply chain were effective in delivering PPE to Hong Kong.

14.03 Office of the Government Chief Information Officer (OGCIO) was in contact with different developers to source other technology solutions that can complement the current monitoring system and enhance the effectiveness of monitoring. The OGCIO was in collaboration with Compathnion Technology Limited which is a local startup in the Science Park. Developed by the startup and a local university, the mobile app paired with the electronic wristbands can help analyse the change in communication signals with artificial intelligence and big data to ascertain people under quarantine are staying at their dwelling places.

15.03 – 21.03 (274/4; 103 recoveries)**

Public Health Policies

15.03 Red Outbound Travel Alert (OTA) issued on the Ireland, the United Kingdom and the United States.

16.03 Persons staying in temporary accommodation provided by the Government would be charged a daily fee of $200 for accommodation and meal arrangements from March 17 in order to combat abuse of the facilities and reserve places for people with genuine need.

The Government announced that it would arrange the second batch of chartered flights to take Hong Kong residents currently stranded in Xiaogan, Xianning, Huangshi and Wuhan in Hubei Province back to Hong Kong.

17.03 Red Outbound Travel Alert (OTA) has been issued on all overseas countries/territories based on public health considerations, the DH would extend health quarantine arrangements on inbound travellers arriving from all countries/territories accordingly and demand them to undergo compulsory quarantine.

Government arranged 67,000 surgical masks to be distributed by Cathay Pacific by proxy to passengers boarding at UK and USA, in regard to the difficulty in purchasing surgical masks in these countries.

18.03 Compulsory Quarantine of Persons Arriving at Hong Kong from Foreign Places Regulation would commence at 0.00am on March 19.

Chief Secretary for Administration exempted the following categories of persons from the quarantine requirement with effect from the commencement of the Regulation:

1. crew members of aircrafts who need to commute to and from foreign places for performance of necessary duties;

2. crew members of goods vessels;

3. government officials carrying out governmental duties;

4. Public officers at or above the level of Executive Directors (or equivalent) in the Hong Kong Monetary Authority, the Securities and Futures Commission and the Insurance Authority undertaking international obligations and/or participating in international co-operation pursuant to their regulatory functions;

5. construction personnel tasked to carry out off-site duties in foreign places that are essential and cannot be replaced by other means to ensure the quality, integrity and statutory

compliance of services or components to be used in government projects;

6. experts, personnel of the academic sectors or of international authorities who are engaged in research and/or provide advice in combating the COVID-19 infection to the HKSAR Government;

7. staff and personnel of public bodies and their partners for the supply of wristbands and related materials for home quarantine; and

8. personnel of public bodies and their partners, agencies, companies or organisations for the supply to Hong Kong of personal protective equipment (PPE) or materials/equipment for the production of PPEs.

CHP would launch a pilot project tomorrow, under which returnees at Hong Kong International Airport would be given bottles to place their deep throat saliva specimens for COVID-19 testing.

19.03 The HA expected the referral to public hospitals by the Port Health Division of the DH of a large number of people suspected to be infected with COVID-19 to arrive at Hong Kong via the Hong Kong International Airport every day. The HA was reported to be working on the establishment of test centres at

the AsiaWorld-Expo and the North Lantau Hospital under the instruction of the Government's Steering Committee in relation to the COVID-19 virus. Starting on March 20, people arriving Hong Kong with upper respiratory symptoms would be sent to the test centres at the AsiaWorld-Expo or the North Lantau Hospital for the viral test and to wait for the laboratory results.

CHP announced that the Enhanced Laboratory Surveillance Programme, which would provide a free testing service for COVID-19, would be further extended to cover asymptomatic persons under the Compulsory Quarantine of Persons Arriving at Hong Kong from Foreign Places Regulation (Cap. 599E).

The Public Health Laboratory Services Branch of the CHP would provide testing for 5,000 samples from the relevant persons per week. Taking reference from clinical and research statistics around the globe, the DH concurred that elderly people infected with COVID-19 usually present with a more serious clinical condition or are more prone to complications, and are thus subject to higher potential risk.

20.03 The Commerce and Economic Development Bureau announced that it approved the first two production lines

under the Local Mask Production Subsidy Scheme.

21.03 The Government announced applications from foreign domestic helpers to extend their limit of stay in Hong Kong as visitors would be flexibly considered.

The HA said it stepped up monitoring of laboratory procedures for testing COVID-19 specimens following a mix up in results.

Secretary for Education Kevin Yeung said the Government would take the necessary measures to ensure the Hong Kong Diploma of Secondary Education Examination (HKDSE) would be held in a controlled and safe environment.

Socio-Economic Policy Packages

16.03 The Government would launch the Retail Sector Subsidy Scheme under the Anti-epidemic Fund on March 23. A sum of $5.6 billion was earmarked under the fund for the scheme which is expected to benefit some 70,000 retailers.

17.03 the Government announced the details of the one-off subsidy to the transport trades under the Anti-epidemic Fund.

A sum of $1.4 billion was earmarked under the Fund to provide a one-off non-accountable subsidy, which was expected to benefit the registered owners of some 130,000 commercial vehicles.

20.03 The Government welcomed the approval of a new loan guarantee commitment of $20 billion under the Commerce and Economic Development Bureau to introduce a new Special 100 per cent Guarantee Product under the SME Financing Guarantee Scheme (SFGS) by the Finance Committee of the Legislative Council. The Government planned to roll out the new product within April.

22.03 –28.03 (582/4; 125 recoveries)**

Public Health Policies

22.03 The HA and the DH would enhance tests for people returning to Hong Kong from overseas.

Chief Executive Carrie Lam said the Government would help residential care homes for the elderly and residential care homes for people with disabilities to strengthen disease prevention. Mrs Lam noted she had earlier decided to provide one million surgical masks monthly to these institutions for use by the nursing staff, and that would now be doubled to two million a month. The Social Welfare Department would arrange for an anti-bacteria coating developed by a local university's innovation and technology team to be sprayed in these institutions to strengthen virus prevention.

LegCo Secretariat announced that all public services in the LegCo Complex, including the Public Complaints Office, Library and Archives, would be suspended from March 23. Secretariat staff would work from home, except those who provide support services to the meetings of LegCo and its Committees, maintain basic operation of the Secretariat and who are on essential duties.

23.03 The Government announced that it would ban non-Hong Kong residents coming from overseas countries or territories arriving at the airport from entering Hong Kong for 14 days starting from March 25. Non-Hong Kong residents arriving in Hong Kong from the Mainland, Macau and Taiwan who had been to overseas countries or territories in the past 14 days would also be banned from entering.

Chief Executive Carrie Lam announced that the Government plans to temporarily ban alcohol sales in bars and restaurants as one of its latest anti-epidemic measures.

Government requested the clubs on private recreational leases to immediately close all of their recreational and sports facilities, changing rooms and play rooms for young children in the clubs. The Government also appealed to other private clubs and gymnasia to

adopt the same measure to reduce the risk of the spread of the virus.

24.03 The DH said the Enhanced Laboratory Surveillance Programme that provided free COVID-19 testing would be extended to cover asymptomatic travellers arriving from the UK, other European countries and the US in phases beginning on March 25.

25.03 The Office of the Government Chief Information Officer (OGCIO) announced that it has enhanced support for people under quarantine who are using the StayHomeSafe mobile app.

The HA announced that it would set up COVID-19 triage and test centres in some of its accident and emergency (A&E) departments in hospitals from this week to alleviate pressure on public hospitals' in-patient isolation facilities.

The DH would set up a temporary specimen collection centre at the AsiaWorld-Expo on March 26 to speed up the collection of specimen from inbound travellers from overseas for conducting testing for COVID-19 and facilitate those who have difficulty in arranging family members or friends to submit their specimen.

26.03 The Government modified the quarantine measures for the second batch of people returning from Hubei and placed

them under home quarantine.

27.03 Six more production lines (total 8) were approved under the Local Mask Production Subsidy Scheme by the Commerce & Economic Development Bureau .

Country park barbecue sites and campsites of the AFCD would be closed from 6pm on March 28 for 14 days.

The Government announced new regulations to combat the spread of COVID-19, including a ban on gatherings of more than four people in a public place.

A second regulation would require restaurants only to serve half their capacity of customers. Each table needed to be separated by at least 1.5m and only four people could be seated at a table. The second regulation would come into effect at 6pm on March 28 for 14 days.

Venues such as cinemas, fitness centres, amusement game centres, bathrooms, place of amusement and place of public entertainment were required to close.

Socio-Economic Policy Packages

23.03 A $1 billion package of relief measures for the aviation industry was announced to help the industry tide over the sustained challenges due to the COVID-19 outbreak.

The Government and the Airport Authority jointly rolled out the package.

*29.03 –04.04 (863/4; 180 recoveries)***

Public Health Policies

29.03 The HA said 400 isolation beds would be available in the coming week to help accommodate the increasing number of confirmed COVID-19 cases in the city.

31.03 Chief Executive Carrie Lam said it was unsatisfactory that some patients were not sent straight to hospital as soon as they were diagnosed with COVID-19 and she hoped the second-tier isolation ward beds being made available would help alleviate the situation.

01.04 The HA said the test centre located in AsiaWorld-Expo would provide COVID-19 tests to people under home quarantine if they developed relevant symptoms.

The Secretary for Food and Health (SFH) issued directions to be effective for 14 days from 6pm:

a. The closure of karaoke establishments and the suspension of karaoke activities in catering premises and clubhouses;

b. The closure of mahjong-tin kau establishments and the suspension of mahjong-tin kau activities in catering premises and club-houses;

c. The closure of establishment (commonly known as club or nightclub) that is open late into the night, usually for drinking, and dancing or other entertainment;

d. A person must wear a mask at any time where practicable within the beauty parlour, clubhouse and massage establishment premises as set out

e. Body temperature screening on a person must be conducted before the person is allowed to enter the beauty parlour, clubhouse and massage establishment premises as set out

f. Hand sanitizers must be provided at any beauty parlour, club-house and massage establishment premises

02.04 Participants of a COVID-19 surveillance programme could make use of a door-to-door specimen collection service starting April 3 to submit their deep throat saliva specimens to the DH for coronavirus testing.

The operating hours of passenger clearance services at the Shenzhen Bay Port would be adjusted to 10am to 8pm daily from April 3 until further notice.

The Secretary for Food and Health (SFH) has

issued directions through notices in the Gazette to be effective for 14 days from 6pm on April 3, 2020, such that –

a. any premises (commonly known as bar or pub) that is exclusively or mainly used for the sale or supply of intoxicating liquors as defined in section 53(1) of the Dutiable Commodities Ordinance (Cap. 109) ("intoxicating liquors") for consumption in that premises must be closed;

b. any part of a catering business premise that is exclusively or mainly used for the sale or supply of intoxicating liquors for consumption in that part must be closed; and

c. any area in a clubhouse that is exclusively or mainly used for the sale or supply of intoxicating liquors for consumption in that area must be closed.

Contravening the above requirements would be a criminal offence. Offenders are subject to a maximum fine of $50,000 and imprisonment for six months.

03.04 The HA said it was asking local scientists if the N95 respirator masks could be decontaminated and reused to combat the shortage of medical masks amid the COVID-19 pandemic.

The Government noted that starting April 10, all

cross-boundary goods vehicle drivers entering Shenzhen via its ports would need to present the "i Shenzhen" health certification code.

They should also present proof of a negative result for a nucleic acid test conducted within the previous seven days to Shenzhen customs officers for examination before entering the city.

Sixty-five Hong Kong residents took a chartered flight arranged by the Government out of Lima to London, then a regular connecting flight with secured bookings from London to Hong Kong.

04.04 The operating hours of passenger clearance services at the Hong Kong-Zhuhai-Macao Bridge Hong Kong Port would be shortened starting April 5.

Socio-Economic Policy Packages

01.04 Support measures of the Anti-epidemic Fund would be extended to the construction industry, the Development Bureau announced. The support measures would also cover small and medium-sized enterprise (SME) consultants which are company members of professional institutions and associations. The bureau expected that the new arrangement would further benefit about 240,000 construction workers and 400 SME consultants to help cover

their extra expenses in enhancing anti-epidemic equipment amid the outbreak.

03.04 As the outbreak continued, the HKMA and the HKMCI put forward another round of five initiatives to further support SMEs in addressing cash-flow pressure:

1. The HKMA would introduce a series of measures aimed at increasing the banking sector's liquidity so that banks would have ample liquidity to support local economic activities.

2. The current level of regulatory reserves would be reduced by half to release a total of HK$200 billion of lending capacity, providing banks with more room on their balance sheets to cater for future financing needs.

3. The HKMA asked banks to consider arrangements to automatically offer extensions of loan tenor or principal repayment holidays to qualified SMEs without requiring them to make an application.

4. Preparatory work by HKMCI and banks for the special 100 per cent Loan Guarantee under the SME Financing Guarantee Scheme announced in the Budget entered an advanced stage.

5. Banks said that they would allow SME

customers in the import-export and manufacturing sectors facing cash-flow pressure due to delays in shipments to further extend the repayment period of trade financing facilities.

04.04 The Inland Revenue Department announced that it had extended tax deadlines in view of the latest COVID-19 situation.

05.04 –11.04 (1,000/4; 336 recoveries)**

Public Health Policies

06.04 The Leisure & Cultural Services Department launched a one-stop online resources centre for the public to view or participate in multi-faceted leisure and cultural activities from home.

The Government announced that it would extend the entry restriction on non-Hong Kong residents and quarantine and airport transit measures until further notice.

07.04 The DH would strengthen health quarantine and COVID-19 testing arrangements for all inbound travellers from April 8.

Under the Prevention & Control of Disease Regulation, all asymptomatic inbound travellers arriving at Hong Kong International Airport would be required to have their deep throat saliva samples taken at the Temporary Specimen Collection

Centre at AsiaWorld-Expo for COVID-19 testing.

Taking reference from the testing arrangements for Peru returnees by chartered flights, the department said that letting travellers from places with higher risk wait for test results at the Specimen Collection Centre could efficiently identify patients with the virus and help in arranging their close contacts to be sent to quarantine centres.

As 248 of the 359 imported cases recorded in the past 14 days involved people who had been to the UK, the department decided to adopt this testing arrangement for inbound travellers from the country starting April 9.

Starting April 8, the Enhanced Laboratory Surveillance Programme would also be further extended to inbound travellers who had been to Hubei Province in the past 14 days arriving through Shenzhen Bay Port and Hong Kong-Zhuhai-Macao Bridge Hong Kong Port.

08.04 The Government extended measures regulating catering business premises, scheduled premises and prohibiting group gatherings to April 23. They also include the closures of beauty parlours and massage establishments.

Patients arranged to be tested for COVID-19 by private doctors could

make use of a door-to-door specimen collection service starting April 14 to submit their deep throat saliva specimens to the DH for the test.

The Agriculture, Fisheries and Conservation Department (AFCD) announced that the country park barbecue sites and campsites would continue to be closed until April 23

09.04 Confinees at quarantine centres would be quarantined for the first 10 days then put under home quarantine for the remaining four days starting from April 11, CHP announced. Confinees would undergo COVID-19 viral tests before being discharged from quarantine centres. They will also have to wear electronic wristbands to comply with the home quarantine requirement before they are discharged.

10.04 Twenty-seven Hong Kong residents were on a flight chartered by the Chinese Embassy in the Kingdom of Morocco that would bring home Chinese citizens stranded in Morocco, the Government announced .

11.04 Asymptomatic inbound travellers arriving on flights from the US and other areas in Europe would be required to proceed to the Temporary Specimen Collection Centre at the AsiaWorld-Expo for their deep throat saliva sample collection and wait for the COVID-19 test results there from

April 13.

If they tested positive, they would be arranged for admission to hospital as soon as possible for treatment, while the close contacts who travelled with them would be sent to designated quarantine centres.

Those who tested negative can go home or to a designated place to continue completion of the 14-day compulsory quarantine.

The Executive Council would be on recess on April 14 and would resume on April 21.

Socio-Economic Policy Packages

08.04 The Government announced a $137.5 billion package of relief measures to help individuals and businesses tide over financial difficulties during the COVID-19 epidemic, including the introduction of an $80 billion Employment Support Scheme.

Announcing the new measures at a press conference this evening, Chief Executive Carrie Lam said this third round of relief is in addition to the $120 billion package announced in the Budget and the $30 billion Anti-epidemic Fund.

For the Dedicated Fund on Branding, Upgrading & Domestic Sales (BUD Fund), the cumulative funding ceilings for each enterprise to undertake projects in the Mainland;

and projects in other economies with which Hong Kong has signed Free Trade Agreements, were $2 million respectively. The Government decided to remove the two individual ceilings, so that enterprises could flexibly make use of the total funding of up to $4 million to expand to new markets.

Due to the impact of the epidemic, virtual exhibitions opened up a new avenue for business promotion. In this context, the Hong Kong Trade Development Council organized Spring Virtual Expo in April.

In tandem, the Hong Kong Export Credit Insurance Corporation (HKECIC) immediately implemented a new round of support measures for one year to strengthen support for policyholders, in particular the Small Business Policy (SBP) holders, so as to provide greater protection to small and medium-sized exporters.

09.04 The Government would enhance the BUD Fund and the SME Export Marketing Fund (EMF) within April to strengthen support for enterprises facing difficulties amid the COVID-19 outbreak.

*12.04 – 18.04 (1,023/4; 567 recoveries)***

Public Health Policies

15.04 The Government confirmed that the Hong Kong Diploma of Secondary Education (DSE) Examination could be held on April 24.

16.04 Community pharmacies offered to help refill patient prescriptions during the COVID-19 epidemic, the HA said.

17.04 The Commerce & Economic Development Bureau announced that it approved five more production lines under the Local Mask Production Subsidy Scheme (total 13).

18.04 The HA announced that its temporary COVID-19 test centre at AsiaWorld-Expo would be suspended from April 19 due to the declining number of inbound travellers.

Socio-Economic Policy Packages

14.04 The Home Affairs Department announced that the Anti-epidemic Support Scheme for Property Management Sector would be extended to cover industrial and commercial buildings.

15.04 The Home Affairs Bureau said a subsidy scheme would be launched under the Anti-epidemic Fund to provide relief to fitness centre operators to tide over the financial difficulties during the COVID-19 epidemic.

16.04 The maximum monthly rental subsidy for each recycler under the One-off Rental Support Scheme would be increased from $25,000 to $37,500, the Environmental Protection Department announced .

To help the recycling industry cope with the current economic situation and operational difficulties due to the COVID-19 epidemic, the Recycling Fund allocated $50 million in additional funds to raise the scheme's subsidy level.

The fund earmarked up to $250 million in total funding to fight the virus and help the recycling industry ride out difficult times.

17.04 The banking sector launched a scheme to alleviate the cashflow pressure faced by corporate customers in light of the economic challenges brought about by the COVID-19 outbreak.

Jointly announced by the Monetary Authority and the Banking Sector SME Lending Coordination Mechanism, the Pre-approved Principal Payment Holiday Scheme was estimated to cover more than 80% of all corporate borrowers in Hong Kong.

18.04 The second round of the Anti-epidemic Fund and other relief measures was passed by the LegCo Finance Committee.

*19.04 – 25.04 (1,038/4; 772 recoveries)***

Public Health Policies

20.04 The Government announced that starting April 22, all asymptomatic inbound travellers arriving at Hong Kong International Airport must wait for COVID-19 test results at a designated location.

The DH would arrange asymptomatic inbound travellers who need to wait for test results overnight to be temporarily accommodated in its holding centre for test result set up in the Regal Oriental Hotel.

21.04 Secretary for Food & Health Prof Sophia Chan announced that most social distancing measures to fight COVID-19 would be extended for another 14 days, requiring restaurants to serve at 50% capacity would be suspended.

AFCD announced that its barbecue sites and campsites in country parks would be closed until May 7.

22.04 The HA began using rapid tests to check for COVID-19 at its hospitals.

Results could be produced in one to two hours.

23.04 To reduce social contact in light of the COVID-19 epidemic, the Primary One Central Allocation results would be posted to parents.

A special programme would be launched on April 24 to provide free Chinese medicine outpatient rehabilitation service to discharged

COVID-19 patients, the Food & Health Bureau announced.

24.04 The Commerce & Economic Development Bureau announced that it approved the remaining seven production lines under the Local Mask Production Subsidy Scheme.

Given the approval of 13 production lines earlier, the quota of 20 production lines under the scheme was fully allocated.

Police announced its decision to prohibit two public meetings and object to a public procession intended to be held on Hong Kong Island on May 1.

Socio-Economic Policy Packages

20.04 With reference to the practice of some overseas governments in providing wage subsidies to employers and following the funding approval by the LegCo Finance Committee, the Government would launch the $81 billion Employment Support Scheme (ESS) as soon as possible.

The scheme would provide time-limited financial support to employers to retain workers who would inevitably be made redundant due to the downturn in business.

Wage subsidies provided under the ESS were calculated based on 50% of wages in a specified month subject to a wage cap of $18,000 per month

for six months.

Under the ESS, self-employed people who have contributed to the MPF from January 1, 2019 to March 31 would be granted a one-off subsidy of $7,500. Regarding job creation, the Government earmarked $6 billion to create about 30,000 time-limited jobs in public and private sectors in the coming two years for people of different skills and academic qualifications.

All borrowers of the Tertiary Student Finance Scheme would be offered an interest-free deferral of loan repayment from April 1 this year to March 31, 2022, including their loan instalments and interests.

The Development Bureau said a one-off subsidy of $7,500 would be offered to each eligible construction worker.

At the same time, a one-off subsidy would be provided to 30,000 construction-related enterprises, generally small-scaled, which cannot benefit from the first round of the Anti-epidemic Fund.

The Government would also provide a direct subsidy of $3 million to each non-profit-making organisation running the 10 projects under the Revitalising Historic Buildings Through Partnership Scheme, PMQ and the Energizing Kowloon East -

Fly the Flyover Operation.

24.04 The Government launched the second phase of the Anti-epidemic Support Scheme for Property Management Sector to extend the subsidy coverage to industrial buildings and commercial buildings.

25.04 The Government announced it would provide subsidies to local primary producers to give them immediate financial relief. For instance, it would provide a subsidy of $10,000 to each local primary producer, including owners of vegetable farms, hydroponic farms, flower farms and nurseries, marine fish culture farms, pond fish farms, fishing vessels and fish collector vessels, but excluding livestock farms.

26.04 –02.05
Public Health Policies

27.04 The Research Council chaired by the Secretary for Food & Health approved $111 million in funding to support the medical schools of the University of Hong Kong (HKU) and Chinese University (CUHK) to conduct 26 research studies on COVID-19. The research studies would last from 12 to 24 months

28.04 Secretary for Food & Health Prof Sophia Chan said exemptions from compulsory quarantine included cross-boundary students and those whose business

activities were in the interest of Hong Kong's economic development.

LCSD announced that some of its leisure venues would be reopened in phases on May 6 and May 11.

CE announced most of the 180,000 government employees would stop working from home, and all public services would revert to normal business hours, noting the number of confirmed Covid-19 cases in the city had decreased in recent weeks.

29.04 The first batch of about 300 Hong Kong residents stranded in Pakistan would take a chartered flight tentatively scheduled to leave Islamabad on the morning of April 30 and arrive in Hong Kong in the afternoon.

Socio-Economic Policy Packages

27.04 The Government announced the establishment of a LawTech Fund to help law firms and barristers' chambers procure and upgrade information technology (IT) systems and arrange lawtech training courses for their staff.

28.04 Tenants of the EcoPark, country park refreshment kiosks and the Hong Kong Wetland Park would benefit from increased rental concessions for government premises.

03.05–09.05

Public Health Policies

03.05 The Government announced the mechanism for Hong Kong enterprises with manufacturing operations in the Mainland to apply for exemption from the compulsory quarantine arrangement.

04.05 The Commerce & Economic Development Bureau announced that the subsidy quota for three mask production lines had been reassigned.

The CHP said that it could not conclude that local COVID-19 transmissions had stopped.

Chief Executive Carrie Lam said because Hong Kong had not reported a local COVID-19 case for over two weeks and imported cases were low, some anti-epidemic measures could be lifted.

07.05 The CHP said recovered COVID-19 patients or those who did not have any symptoms might be discharged from hospital 10 days after the onset of symptoms or a positive test result.

09.05 More than 8,200 applications for the Anti-epidemic Support Scheme for Property Management Sector were received, with over 3,850 approved.

Socio-Economic Policy Packages

04.05 The Social Welfare Department launched a subsidy scheme to support all the some 1,000 residential care homes for the elderly and people with disabilities to give their premises an anti-virus coating spray.

The Food & Environmental Hygiene Department announces applications for the Catering Business (Social Distancing) Subsidy Scheme, under the second round of the Anti-epidemic Fund, would start from May 5.

05.05 A scheme that provides a $100,000 one-off subsidy to licensed billiard establishments, public bowling alleys and skating rinks opened for applications.

The Office of the Communications Authority (OFCA) announced the launch of the Subsidy Scheme for Encouraging Early Deployment of 5G under the second round of the Anti-epidemic Fund.

Chief Executive Carrie Lam said that Hong Kong's needy and disadvantaged would receive masks as part of the Government's new mask distribution programme.

Secretary for Education Kevin Yeung said the Government is confident that classes can resume on May 27.

The Government would distribute free reusable face masks to all Hong Kong citizens, the Innovation & Technology Bureau announced.

06.05 The Government would launch the Subsidy Scheme for Beauty Parlours, Massage Establishments & Party Rooms under the second round of the Anti-epidemic Fund on May 11.

The Tour Service Coach Drivers (Mainly Serving Tourists) Support Scheme, under the second round of the Anti-epidemic Fund, was open for applications.

08.05 Premises could still operate other licensed businesses which were not required to be suspended if they were operating more than one licensed business before the closure, the Food & Health Bureau said.

Subsidies to local primary producers and wholesale traders operating in fresh food wholesale markets were being disbursed, the Agriculture, Fisheries & Conservation Department announced.

09.05 The CuMasks have undergone strict testing and certification processes before the product would be distributed to help people combat the COVID-19 virus, Secretary for Innovation & Technology Alfred Sit said.

Major Development

04.05 Hong Kong's economy in the first quarter of 2020 contracted 8.9% over a year earlier, the largest decline on record since 1974, the Census & Statistics Department announced.

05.05 SCMP[5]: Hong Kong employers pushed for minimum wage freeze amid economy battered by Covid-19.

SCMP[6]: Reusable masks from Hong Kong government can filter bacteria, fungi and viruses. A government source told SCMP more than 7 million of the face coverings would be ready for distribution later this month. The filtration technology developed by the Hong Kong Research Institute of Textiles and Apparel won a top European prize in 2018.

SCMP[7]: Hong Kong public hospitals began return of services cancelled because of coronavirus.

---

5   *SCMP*: www.scmp.com/news/hong-kong/hong-kong-economy/article/3082830/hong-kong-employers-push-minimum-wage-freeze-amid

6   *SCMP*: www.scmp.com/news/hong-kong/health-environment/article/3082818/coronavirus-hong-kong-based-research-institute

7   *SCMP*: www.scmp.com/news/hong-kong/health-environment/article/3082896/hong-kong-public-hospitals-begin-return-services

06.05 A recovered COVID-19 patient tested positive for the virus again, the HA announced.

07.05 SCMP[8]: From Hong Kong to Britain, governments ranked poorly for their response to Covid-19. Survey of 23 economies found 'major cracks' in self-belief across the Western world. China, Vietnam and India had impressed with their responses to Covid-19, while Hong Kong and Japan languished at the bottom.

SCMP[9]: First chartered flights in works for Hong Kong residents stuck in India.

Apple Daily[10]: The government reusable masks are doubted for Blackbox operation.

SCMP[11]: More reports of violence against women, children in Hong Kong since start of pandemic.

08.05 SCMP[12]: University of Hong Kong study found eyes were 'important route' for coronavirus, up to 100 times more infectious than Sars.

SCMP[13]: Professor Samuel Yeung-shan Wong said Canada should follow Hong Kong by supporting public mask wearing and testing all arrivals at airports for coronavirus. A study by Wong, published in Canada, said Hong Kong's aggressive contact tracing and quarantine measures also helped restrict the spread of the disease.

09.05 SCMP[14]: University of Hong Kong found out three medicals effective in repressing the virus and shorten hospital stays for patients: interferon, protease inhibitor, and ribavirin.

SCMP: Hong Kong recorded no new cases, as government adviser suggested easing border restrictions with Macau.

10.05–16.05

Public Health Policies

11.05 The DH reminded parents to maintain up to date immunisation for their children for comprehensive and timely protection against infectious diseases and not to delay vaccination due to the COVID-19 outbreak.

12.05 The CHP said saliva specimen bottles were distributed to residents of a housing estate block in Tsuen Wan where two of the locally transmitted COVID-19 cases live.

13.05 The first chartered flight to take Hong Kong residents stranded in India home was tentatively scheduled to depart New Delhi on May 17 at the earliest

15.05 The Housing Authority said it would proactively inspect the communal drainage pipes of all its public rental housing, including the pipes inside some of the units.

Socio-Economic Policy Packages

10.05 Changing rooms and shower facilities would be reopened on May 11 along with the leisure facilities of the LCSD, Secretary for Home Affairs Caspar Tsui announced.

In view of the latest COVID-19 situation, the LCSD announced that more of its venues would be reopened on May 21 and some recreation and sports programmes would resume from June 1.

11.05 The Government earmarked $135 million under the second round of the Anti-epidemic Fund to provide a cash subsidy to individual licensees in the estate agency sector.

Hongkong Post reported a smooth start on the first-day delivery of CuMask by arranging the delivery of around 97% of about 120,000 items received from the Government the preceding day.

12.05 The Government unveiled details concerning the latest arrangements for the Employment Support Scheme, which employers and self-employed people would be able to apply online for starting from May 25.

The Government announces that the disbursement of subsidies under the Club-house

---

8   *SCMP*: www.scmp.com/week-asia/politics/article/3083185/coronavirus-mainland-chinese-impressed-their-leaders-hongkongers

9   *SCMP*: www.scmp.com/news/hong-kong/society/article/3083201/coronavirus-first-chartered-flights-works-hong-kong

10 *Apple Daily*: https://hk.news.appledaily.com/local/20200507/2CHY4R7T4V4NYC3E6CAGRAMIRQ/

11 *SCMP*: www.scmp.com/news/hong-kong/health-environment/article/3079338/stuck-home-monster-more-reports-violence-against

12 *SCMP*: www.scmp.com/news/hong-kong/health-environment/article/3083394/university-hong-kong-study-finds-eyes-are

13 *SCMP*: www.scmp.com/news/world/united-states-canada/article/3083417/masks-tests-quarantine-centres-what-can-canada

14 *SCMP*: www.scmp.com/news/hong-kong/health-environment/article/3083627/coronavirus-hong-kong-records-no-new-cases-covid

Subsidy Scheme under the Anti-epidemic Fund has started.

15.05 The Scheme on Relief Grants for Interest Class Instructors Hired by Organisations Subvented by the Social Welfare Department opened for applications.

16.05 More than 5,400 applications for the Anti-epidemic Support Scheme for Property Management Sector were approved, involving subsidies of over $200 million

The Distance Business Programme under the Anti-epidemic Fund of the Government would accept applications from enterprises from 9am on May 18 until October 31.

Major Development

11.05 On.cc[15]:Hong Kong, Macau and Guangdong are researching on relieving the compulsuary quarantine arrangement through collaboration

12.05 SCMP[16]: Hongkonger without travel history confirmed as infected. The woman said she had not knowingly been in contact with any Covid-19 patients, nor been abroad

13.05 On.cc[17]: Residents of the 2 entire blocks of buildings of the 2 new local cases, after a clean period of more than 3 weeks, would be mass tested with a view to contain infection and search for origins.

SCMP[18]: Hong Kong study findings indicate novel coronavirus most likely came from Asian bat.

14.05 Two people running catering businesses were convicted of contravening the Prevention & Control of Disease (Requirements & Directions) (Business & Premises) Regulation and were fined $3,000 each.

15.05 Hong Kong's economy in the first quarter contracted sharply by 8.9% over a year earlier, after declining by 3% in the preceding quarter

Mingpao[19]: Three patients who recovered from COVID-19 donated their blood to cure other confirmed cases, while only this three out of 30 recovered people took action.

SCMP[20]: Cathay Pacific and Cathay Dragon reported combined HK$4.5 billion loss for start of 2020. Senior manager Ronald Lam called financial outlook 'very bleak'

16.05 Apple[21]: Two old-brand Hong Kong department stores were sold to Chinese capitals due to COVID-19 impacts. (Bossini, Sincere)

17.05 – 23.05

Public Health Policies

17.05 A chartered flight taking 249 Hong Kong residents stranded in India back home departed from New Delhi at around 11pm.

18.05 The Government announced that people conducting audit services or enterprises providing construction-related services on the Mainland could apply for exemption from the compulsory quarantine arrangement.

19.05 The requirement limiting group gatherings in public places to a maximum of eight people would be extended to June 4, but religious gatherings would be exempt with certain restrictions to be imposed on them.

The Government was further enhancing laboratory testing capabilities for COVID-19 and the scope of testing, Secretary for Food & Health Prof Sophia Chan said.

Secretary for Food & Health Prof Sophia Chan said the Government was using a "suppress and lift" strategy in considering the restrictions or relaxation of social distancing measures, and the Government had been using a risk-based approach.

20.05 The Government introduced statutory restrictions on group gatherings in public places with a view to reducing risks of virus transmission and claimed no political considerations have ever come into play.

15 On.cc: https://hk.on.cc/hk/bkn/cnt/news/20200511/mobile/bkn-20200511094227412-0511_00822_001.html

16 *SCMP*: www.scmp.com/news/hong-kong/health-environment/article/3083978/coronavirus-hong-kong-hits-23-days-without

17 On.cc: https://hk.on.cc/hk/bkn/cnt/news/20200513/bkn-20200513163041235-0513_00822_001.html

18 SCMP: www.scmp.com/news/hong-kong/health-environment/article/3084261/novel-coronavirus-most-likely-came-asian-bat-hong

19 *Mingpao*: https://news.mingpao.com/pns/%E6%B8%AF%E8%81%9E/article/20200515/s00002/1589482319460/30%E4%BA%BA%E5%90%88%E9%81%A9%E5%83%85%E6%8D%90%E8%A1%80%E6%BC%BF-%E7%9E%9E%E5%AE%B6%E4%BA%BA%E6%8D%90%E8%80%85-%E5%8F%AF%E6%8D%90%E6%98%AF%E5%B9%B8%E9%81%8B

20 *SCMP*: www.scmp.com/news/hong-kong/transport/article/3084514/cathay-pacific-and-cathay-dragon-report-combined-hk45

21 *Apple Daily*: https://hk.news.appledaily.com/finance/20200515/AFR2CVWQG37VCSTCZ4SUNPRA3Y/ & https://hk.news.appledaily.com/finance/20200515/2GZMWTRNJRUO2XNXUM2ZD2CKXE/

21.05 The Government announced that enterprises with an operating base relating to logistics, port or shipping business on the Mainland could apply for an exemption from the compulsory quarantine arrangement.

22.05 The Government announced a mechanism for directors of listed companies or listing applicants to apply for exemption from the compulsory quarantine arrangement.

Socio-Economic Policy Packages

17.05 The Government announced that it appointed Pricewaterhouse-Coopers Advisory Services as the central processing agent for the implementation of the Employment Support Scheme (ESS).

18.05 The subsidy scheme for the securities industry under the second round of the Anti-epidemic Fund would launch and open for applications on May 25, the Financial Services & the Treasury Bureau announced.

About $1.2 billion in subsidies were disbursed so far to about 160,000 construction workers under the second round of the Anti-epidemic Fund, the Development Bureau announced.

Subsidies for the first tranche of the Employment Support Scheme (ESS) would be calculated on the basis of the wages paid in one of the months specified by the employers from December 2019 to March 2020.

19.05 The Government announced it would receive masks from 19 production lines under the Local Mask Production Subsidy Scheme starting from late this month.

The mechanism for legal practitioners, arbitrators or mediators providing necessary professional services in the Mainland, Macau or Taiwan to apply for exemption from the compulsory quarantine arrangement was announced.

the LCSD would reopen 33 public swimming pools on May 21 from 6.30am to 10pm for three sessions daily with two breaks.

20.05 The Government considered that the $10,000 to be disbursed to residents under the Cash Payout Scheme was an appropriate amount, after having thoroughly examined their financial impact on society.

An initial implementation plan was formulated on the feasibility of class resumption for about 2,500

cross-boundary secondary students, the EDB said.

23.05 More than 6,900 applications for the Anti-epidemic Support Scheme for Property Management Sector were approved, involving subsidies of over $240 million.

Major Development

18.05 SCMP[22]: Hamster research showed effectiveness of masks 'huge' in Covid-19 battle, Hong Kong scientists said.

19.05 The seasonally adjusted unemployment rate increased to 5.2% in the period between February and April, the Census & Statistics Department announced.

24.05 – 30.05

Public Health Policies

25.05 The Government would relax social distancing measures in accordance with the "suppress and lift" strategy. Starting May 29, bathhouses, party rooms, clubs or nightclubs and karaoke establishments could resume operation.

Socio-Economic Policy Packages

25.05 The Recycling Fund disbursed over $90 million in anti-epidemic and rental support subsidies to recyclers through

the One-off Recycling Industry Anti-epidemic Scheme and the One-off Rental Support Scheme.

Members of the Commission on Children, were briefed on support measures for children and their families during the COVID-19 epidemic: support measures for children and their families, especially those with children with special needs, amid disruption of childcare services and class suspensions owing to the epidemic.

26.05 The disbursement of subsidies to approved applicants of the Subsidy Scheme for Beauty Parlours, Massage Establishments & Party Rooms began through bank transfer.

The ESS received about 72,000 applications from employers and 61,000 from self-employed people from the first day of the application period on May 25 until 6pm on May 26.

27.05 The Government would publish pieces of subsidiary legislation in the Gazette on May 29 to implement the waiver of statutory registration fees for 13 healthcare professions.

The Government provided a time-limited unemployment support

---

22 *SCMP*: www.scmp.com/news/hong-kong/health-environment/article/3084779/coronavirus-hamster-research-proof-effectiveness

scheme to provide timely and basic assistance to unemployed people, Secretary for Labour & Welfare Dr Law Chi-kwong said.

29.05 The Anti-epidemic Subsidy Scheme for the Laundry Trade opened for applications and would run until June 12 to help the trade cope with challenges brought by the current economic situation.

As of 28 May, more than 7,100 applications received for the Catering Business (Social Distancing) Subsidy Scheme set under the second round of the Anti-epidemic Fund.

Applications opened for the subsidy scheme for public light buses, local ferries and taxis under the second round of the Anti-epidemic Fund.

30.05 The Government would enhance the Anti-epidemic Support Scheme for Property Management Sector.

Major Development

25.05 Chief Executive Carrie Lam claimed that some in the community opined that the Government's decision on prohibiting group gatherings was politically driven.

Such a claim was totally unfounded. Adjustment to control measures was always based on public health considerations.

Customs arrest an online trader's director in connection with a case of supplying surgical masks in violation of the Trade Descriptions Ordinance.

26.05 SCMP[23]: China's 'Sars hero' Zhong Nan-shan urged Hong Kong to relax border controls with mainland and Macau. He also praised Hong Kong for its efforts to defeat the coronavirus, saying city had 'done beautifully'. He said mutually recognised health system between Hong Kong and the mainland could enable cross-boundary travellers to skip quarantine.

30.05 SCMP[24]: So hard to get Hong Kong's 'hidden youth' to leave home, now pandemic drives them into isolation again.

Three imported cases on the QR818 flight from Pakistan, a previous same flight also had 13 confirmed cases.

31.05–06.06

Public Health Policies

31.05 The Government announced that two special flights would be

arranged to bring Hong Kong residents stranded in Nepal back to Hong Kong.

01.06 The DH urged private doctors to be vigilant by offering COVID-19 testing for patients who come to them with symptoms.

The Government was highly concerned about a COVID-19 community cluster linked to a Lek Yuen Estate resident as it reflected some characteristics not seen before.

02.06 The Government would extend compulsory quarantine measures for people arriving in Hong Kong from both the Mainland and foreign places.

The CHP said the residential building where four newly confirmed COVID-19 patients reside would not be evacuated.

-The second batch of Hong Kong residents stranded in India would take a special flight arranged by the Government to return to Hong Kong on the morning of June 3 at the earliest.

04.06 Residents living in units 10 and 12 in Luk Chuen House in Lek Yuen Estate, Sha Tin, would be evacuated, the CHP announced.

Socio-Economic Policy Packages

02.06 The LCSD provided ex-gratia payment to personnel affected by the cancellation of programmes to relieve the impact of the pandemic.

The Labour Department announced that the SSE Agencies would be introduced under the Anti-epidemic Fund to assist them in tiding over the difficulties arising from the COVID-19 epidemic.

03.06 Financial regulators and the trade adopted measures to maintain business operations and provide necessary services while minimising the risk of infection amid the COVID-19 epidemic.

05.06 The Working Family & Student Financial Assistance Agency would start disbursing a one-off special allowance under the Anti-epidemic Fund to Working Family Allowance and Student Financial Assistance households from June 9.

-The ESS received more than 140,000 applications from employers and 170,000 from self-employed people from the first day of the application period on May 25 until 6pm on June 5.

23 *SCMP*: www.scmp.com/news/hong-kong/health-environment/article/3086021/coronavirus-chinas-sars-hero-zhong-nanshan-urges

24 *SCMP*: www.scmp.com/news/hong-kong/society/article/3086617/so-hard-get-hong-kongs-hidden-youth-leave-home-now-pandemic

Major Development

31.05 The Innovation & Technology Bureau announced that the CuMask online registration system received over 1.37 million registrations, covering more than 3.75 million registrants in total.

SCMP[25]: coronavirus pandemic exposed Hong Kong's insensitivity to its ethnic minorities.

SCMP[26]: doctors blamed Hong Kong's outdated IT systems for slowing Covid-19 response, delaying reopening of mainland border.

01.06 SCMP[27]: Hong Kong to get its own health code system for travels to Guangdong, Macau after Covid-19 border restrictions were lifted. A source said the system, meant to certify whether a traveller was free of the virus, would not contain transfer of any personal data.

SCMP[28]: Hong Kong bankers suffered sharp cuts in pay, bonuses as pandemic-driven downturn weighs on outlook, headhunters said.

02.06 Secretary for Food & Health Prof Sophia Chan said that the Government's anti-epidemic strategy was based on public health factors and not on other considerations.

04.06 The StartmeupHK Festival 2020, scheduled for July 6 to 10, would transform its in-person event into a fully virtual experience, Invest Hong Kong announced.

05.06 SCMP[29]: Hong Kong public housing estate evacuated after cluster of Covid-19 infections found. Officials have moved some residents from Luk Chuen House at Lek Yuen Estate in Sha Tin. Authorities were investigating whether the virus was spread through pipes.

SCMP[30]: kitchen exhaust fans could be behind latest Hong Kong cluster, sayid leading infectious disease expert.

06.06 Apple Daily[31]: IT, Tourism and Accounting sectors plan strike, to be figured out by mid of June.

SCMP[32]: World Health Organisation finally advised the public to wear masks in crowded places to combat coronavirus, with conclusion supported by successful cases in Asian such as Hong Kong.

*07.06–13.06 (1,110/4)***

Public Health Policies

08.06 The Government announced a mechanism for directors or executives of specified listed companies to apply for exemption from the compulsory quarantine arrangement.

09.06 The EDB announced that Secondary 3 to 5 cross-boundary students would resume classes on June 15.

10.06 LCSD would reopen more public swimming pools, gazetted beaches, libraries and museums.

Socio-Economic Policy Packages

07.06 Classes were gradually resuming after more than three months of suspension due to COVID-19. During the period, the EDB provided support and resources to equip teachers with teaching strategies for e-learning.

08.06 The Hong Kong Export Credit Insurance Corporation announced the launch of a 100% Credit Limit Top-Up Scheme.

The Government said the vetting work of the Retail Sector Subsidy Scheme under the first round of the Anti-epidemic Fund was completed.

The Government announced that more support would be provided for the travel industry by enhancing the Green Lifestyle Local Tour Incentive Scheme and extending the subsidy initiative for tourist guides.

---

25 *SCMP*: www.scmp.com/comment/opinion/article/3086531/how-coronavirus-pandemic-has-exposed-hong-kongs-insensitivity-its

26 *SCMP*: www.scmp.com/news/hong-kong/health-environment/article/3086826/coronavirus-doctors-blame-hong-kongs-outdated-it

27 *SCMP*: www.scmp.com/news/hong-kong/health-environment/article/3086827/coronavirus-hong-kong-get-its-own-health-code

28 *SCMP*: www.scmp.com/business/banking-finance/article/3086700/hong-kong-bankers-suffer-sharp-cuts-pay-bonuses-pandemic

29 *SCMP*: www.scmp.com/news/hong-kong/health-environment/article/3087526/coronavirus-new-cluster-infection-expands-elderly

30 *SCMP*: www.scmp.com/news/hong-kong/health-environment/article/3087709/coronavirus-kitchen-fans-could-be-behind-latest

31 *Apple Daily*: https://hk.news.appledaily.com/local/20200606/XGX5G2RUDL3JE545JLSMZV5NJM/

32 *SCMP*: www.scmp.com/news/china/science/article/3087824/wear-masks-crowded-places-combat-coronavirus-world-health

09.06 The Government would invest in Cathay Pacific Airways to protect Hong Kong's role as a leading international aviation hub in the region as well as the city's long-term economic development, Financial Secretary Paul Chan said.

The Fitness Centre Subsidy Scheme received more than 1,900 applications during the application period of over four weeks, of which 600 had so far been approved with $60 million disbursed.

The Food & Environmental Hygiene Department announced that over $4.3 billion in subsidies has been disbursed to the food business sector through various schemes under the Anti-epidemic Fund.

11.06 The Anti-epidemic Fund would offer a one-off subsidy to employers in the construction sector who employed casual employees on a long-term basis, the Development Bureau announced.

The Government would provide salary subsidies to employers who hire graduates and assistant professionals of the engineering, architectural, surveying, town planning and landscape sectors, the Development Bureau announced.

12.06 About 3,400 applications were approved for disbursement of subsidies totalling over $150 million under the five tourism industry support schemes in the second round of the Anti-epidemic Fund.

The application deadline for the Student Grant of $3,500 for secondary day school, primary school and kindergarten students in the 2019-20 school year was extended to June 30, the Government announced.

The Government started to disburse the first tranche of wage subsidies under the ESS to a total of 49,500 employers and self-employed people applicants.

13.06 About 9,300 applications for the Anti-epidemic Support Scheme for Property Management Sector were approved, involving subsidies of around $310 million.

Major Development

12.06 Customs urged people to stop using a type of surgical mask which had a bacterial count that exceeded the permitted limit.

14.06 – 20.06
Public Health Policies

15.06 The Centre for Food Safety said it had taken salmon samples from import and wholesale levels at different places for novel coronavirus testing as a precautionary measure.

16.06 Prof Chan explained that the number of people allowed in group gatherings in public places would be relaxed from eight to 50.

17.06 LCSD announced that it would reopen more of its facilities and venues.

18.06 The Government said it strengthened the testing for inbound travellers from Beijing in response to the latest COVID-19 situation there.

Socio-Economic Policy Packages

14.06 The Subsidy Scheme for Encouraging Early Deployment of 5G received 81 applications since its launch, of which three applications were approved with the first portion of the subsidy to be disbursed within June.

15.06 The Government announced that it received a total of 428,659 applications for the ESS, including 168,799 from employers and 259,860 from self-employed people (SEP).

16.06 The Government announced that the monthly $1,000 allowance under the Anti-epidemic Fund for outsourced cleaning and security workers of the Government and the Housing Authority would be provided for a further three months, from the previously set "no fewer than four months."

17.06 The taxi or red minibus driver subsidy under the second round of the Anti-epidemic Fund was open for applications until September 30, the Transport Department announced.

The Environment Bureau announced that a subsidy programme for graduates would be launched under the Green Employment Scheme to subsidise private companies to employ fresh graduates.

18.06 The Government announced plans to double the cash incentives for travel agents organising tours under the Green Lifestyle Local Tour Incentive Scheme so as to foster local economic revival and relaunch the tourism industry.

19.06 The Labour Department announced that the SSE Agencies would be open for applications from June 22 to July 21. The scheme would grant a $50,000 subsidy for each main license of employment agencies that provide a foreign domestic helper (FDH) placement service.

The Government announced it would offer more than 700 time-limited jobs in Executive Service Assistant and Support Service Assistant positions to increase employment opportunities.

The Home Affairs Bureau announced an additional subsidy of $80,000 from the $150 million scheme would be disbursed to 44 Arts Development Council-funded arts groups, 14 venue partners under the LCSD and 34 Arts Capacity Development Funding Scheme grantees.

20.06 About 9,900 applications for the Anti-epidemic Support Scheme for Property Management Sector were approved, involving subsidies of around $330 million, the Government announced.

Major Development

16.06 SCMP[33]: Hong Kong unemployment hit 15-year high, with 5.9 per cent out of work. Jobless rate rose for eighth month in a row, surpassing the figure from the aftermath of the global financial crisis. Labour market worsening with large parts of the city's economy still 'in the doldrums', minister said.

17.06 About 280 Hong Kong residents stranded in India would return to the city by two special flights arranged by the Government.

SCMP[34]: HSBC planned to cut as many as 35,000 jobs as part of a massive overhaul first unveiled in February. The London-based lender paused jobs cuts in March because of the 'extraordinary impact' of the coronavirus pandemic on the global economy.

20.06 SCMP[35]: China's aim to integrate Greater Bay Area comes together

with Hong Kong health care providers playing a leading role. The inclusion of Hong Kong-based health care providers in mainland's insurance network was likely to spur cross-border flow of talent in the Greater Bay Area. Availability of world-class medical services and education was crucial in attracting Hong Kong residents to live and work in the bay area.

21.06–27.06 (1,195/7)**

Public Health Policies

23.06 Travelers' health code mooted: Chief Executive Carrie Lam said the Government was actively working with Guangdong and Macau on introducing a health code which would allow more people to travel again.

24.06 Secretary for Food & Health Prof Sophia Chan said the governments of Guangdong and Hong Kong were considering the launch of a pilot scheme to relax the cross-boundary flow of people between the two places within certain limits. The mutual recognition would be done through the health code of the two places.

The Transport Department said its licensing offices would resume walk-in counter services in full from June 29.

25.06 Labs played a key role: To tackle the unprecedented COVID-19 challenge, Hong Kong has put in place a surveillance programme with more than 300,000 samples tested for COVID-19 so far.

Chief Executive Carrie Lam: From next week, a pack of 10 disposable masks would be distributed to each residential address in Hong Kong. These masks were the first batch of masks procured by the Government under the Local Mask Production Subsidy Scheme.

The Government would deliver 30 million masks for free to all residential addresses in the city through Hongkong Post starting June 30.

26.06 The Government announced that the use of Chun Yeung Estate in Fo Tan as quarantine centre would cease in end-July as the COVID-19 outbreak in Hong Kong had begun to stablise.

Socio-Economic Policy Packages

22.06 The ESS Secretariat published the list of the

first batch of employers who received wage subsidies. Most of them are micro/small/medium-sized enterprises below 50 employees.

The Anti-epidemic Fund would cover vehicle maintenance workshops by granting a one-off non-accountable subsidy of $50,000 to each eligible workshop, the Government announced.

23.06 The Government clarified that the ESS would not require employers to use the wage subsidies to subsidise at maximum $9,000 or half of the wages of each employee. The Government explained that should the employer spend all the wage subsidies on paying employees' wages and not make redundancies during the subsidy period, the secretariat would not need to claw back wage subsidies from relevant employers.

24.06 Applications for the Dishware Washing Trade Subsidy Scheme under the Anti-epidemic Fund opened, the Food & Environmental Hygiene Department announced.

The Transport Department said an additional $20,000 subsidy would be provided to kaito

---

33 *SCMP*: www.scmp.com/news/hong-kong/politics/article/3089230/hong-kong-unemployment-continues-rise-slower-rate-carrie

34 *SCMP*: www.scmp.com/business/banking-finance/article/3089380/hsbc-resume-retrenchment-plan-after-pausing-job-cuts-march

35 *SCMP*: www.scmp.com/business/companies/article/3089800/chinas-aim-integrate-greater-bay-area-comes-together-hong-kong

operators for each vessel deployed in kaito services, involving about $1.8 million.

26.06 The Innovation & Technology Commission announced an additional provision of $1 billion under the Anti-epidemic Fund for the Distance Business Programme in addition to the original $500 million.

27.06 Property sector: About 10,300 applications for the Anti-epidemic Support Scheme for Property Management Sector were approved, involving subsidies of over $340 million.

Major Development

22.06 Now[36]: It was investigated that the government CuMasks could not pass 'infiltration test' after it was washed for over 50 times.

27.06 SCMP[37]: Hong Kong mulled ban on home quarantine for domestic helpers as influx expected in coming weeks. Labour chief revealed plan to change quarantine rules for helpers as city reached two weeks without any locally transmitted cases of Covid-19 and 10,000 workers from the Philippines are expected to arrive in Hong Kong in the short term.

28.06–04.07 (1,256/7)**

Public Health Policies

30.06 Government announced that the previous flexibility arrangement to assist foreign domestic helpers and their employers would be extended with immediate effect.

The Government announced it would further relax the social distancing measures in relation to catering businesses and scheduled premises, while the limitation on group gatherings in public places would be maintained.

Socio-Economic Policy Packages

29.06 The ESS Secretariat published the list of the second batch of employers who received wage subsidies. The list covered 33,679 employers, 98% of whom are micro, small or medium-sized enterprises with fewer than 50 employees.

The Department of Justice said a COVID-19-related scheme was launched to provide speedy and cost effective online dispute resolution services to the general public and businesses.

01.07 The FinTech Anti-epidemic Scheme for Talent Development (FAST Scheme) under the second round of the Anti-epidemic Fund would be launched on July 2, the Financial Services & the Treasury Bureau announced.

Major Development

28.06 The COVID-19 pandemic brought global air traffic to a near standstill and left many Hong Kong people stranded abroad. At this critical juncture the Immigration Department assisted thousands of people who needed help getting home.

01.07 The Researcher Programme and the Postdoctoral Hub were merged to become the Research Talent Hub to nurture more innovation and technology talents, the Innovation & Technology Commission announced.

02.07 Customs was investigating a case in which surgical masks with suspected false trade descriptions were being supplied to the Government Logistics Department. Four people were arrested. The GLD announced that it immediately stopped making payments and has rescinded procurement contracts to the supplier of surgical masks bearing false trade descriptions.

05.07–11.07 (1,430/7)**

Public Health Policies

07.07 Secretary for Food & Health Prof Sophia Chan said hotels maybe used as designated places for foreign domestic helpers to undergo quarantine when they came to Hong Kong.

Public hospitals would enhance infection control measures to combat the next wave of epidemic, the HA announced.

09.07 The Government would tighten existing social distancing measures.

LCSD announced it would enhance measures on prevention and control of infection for its recreational and cultural facilities.

10.07 Secretary for Education Kevin Yeung announced that all secondary schools, primary schools and kindergartens could advance the beginning of their summer holiday to July 13.

11.07 Secretary for Food & Health Prof Sophia Chan said social gatherings pose certain health risks amid the rising number of COVID-19 cases and that those organising events must adhere to infection control measures.

36   Now: https://news.now.com/home/local/player?newsId=395306

37   *SCMP*: www.scmp.com/news/hong-kong/health-environment/article/3090853/coronavirus-hong-kong-mulls-ban-home-quarantine

Socio-Economic Policy Packages

06.07 The ESS Secretariat publishes the list of the third batch of employers who received wage subsidies.

The Government announced that the Cash Payout Scheme dispersed payment to 3.15 million people who registered electronically through banks on or before June 30.

07.07 The ESS Secretariat announced that the fifth batch of wage subsidies totaling $4.2 billion and covering more than 190,000 employees would be disbursed. Together with the first four batches of wage subsidies that were disbursed, the wage subsidies in all five batches amount to about $29.6 billion, covering nearly 110,000 employers and more than 1.3 million employees.

About 1.24 million people who registered electronically with banks by June 30 received the $10,000 cash payout, bringing the cumulative total of recipients to over 4.3 million.

08.07 The Government increased the rental concessions for eligible tenants of its premises to alleviate the pressure arising from the pandemic on businesses, Secretary for Commerce & Economic Development Edward Yau said.

In light of the gradual resumption of convention and exhibition activities in July, the Government would launch the Convention & Exhibition Industry Subsidy Scheme under the Anti-epidemic Fund with a commitment of $1.02 billion.

10.07 The Government would grant another $6,000 ex-gratia payment under the Anti-epidemic Fund to prospective tenants who accepted advance allocation offers for Fai Ming Estate in Fanling and Chun Yeung Estate in Fo Tan.

The Government launched a subsidy scheme to provide relief to gold and silver traders affected by the COVID-19 pandemic.

11.07 About 10,500 applications for the Anti-epidemic Support Scheme for Property Management Sector were approved, involving subsidies of over $370 million.

Major Development

09.07 SCM[38]: United Airlines and American Airlines cancelled recently resumed services to Hong Kong. Foreign aircrew refusing to fly to Hong Kong over mandatory Covid-19 testing concerns, throwing flight operations into chaos

11.07 Commercial Radio 881[39]: Previous HKU researcher claimed China held back information of COVID-19, who has been threatened and gone to US.

SCMP[40]: Cathay Pacific averted financial collapse with distress call to tap the HK$4 trillion war chest of Hong Kong's financial tsar. The Hong Kong government wanted to dress up the bailout dubbed Project Apollo as a "short-term investment" amid political scrutiny. Bailout size grew during negotiations to restore confidence among creditors and investors in the airline's survival.

*12.07 –18.07 (1,775/12)***

Public Health Policies

12.07 The HA would boost the supply of isolation beds to accommodate the increasing number of confirmed COVID-19 patients. HA had around 1,150 first-tier isolation beds for admission of confirmed (COVID-19) cases.

13.07 Chief Executive Carrie Lam announced the Government would tighten social distancing measures and mandate that people wear masks on public transport from midnight on July 15.

LCSD announced that its leisure and cultural facilities would be closed from July 15 until further notice.

14.07 EDB announced its decision to further tighten up measures in all schools.

The Social Welfare Department's units which provide direct services to the public, including social security field units, would continue with their normal services. But all aided childcare centres, day care centres or units for the elderly, sheltered workshops, integrated vocational rehabilitation services centres, integrated vocational training centres and day activity centres would suspend

---

38 *SCMP*: www.scmp.com/news/hong-kong/transport/article/3092420/coronavirus-united-airlines-stops-resumed-hong-kong

39 雷霆881: www.881903.com/news/local/2346532/%E6%B8%AF%E5%A4%A7%E5%89%8D%E7%A0%94%E7%A9%B6%E5%93%A1%E6%8C%87%E4%B8%AD%E5%9C%8B%E9%9A%B1%E7%9E%9E%E7%96%AB%E6%83%85-%E5%8F%97%E7%94%9F%E5%91%BD%E5%A8%81%E8%84%85%E9%80%83%E5%88%B0%E7%BE%8E%E5%9C%8B

40 *SCMP*: www.scmp.com/business/banking-finance/article/3092678/cathay-pacific-averts-financial-collapse-distress-call-tap

their service delivery from July 15.

The Home Affairs Department announced that all community halls and centres, except when being used as temporary night heat shelters, would be closed until further notice.

The Environmental Protection Department's public facilities would stop services. Visitor and education programmes at Community Green Stations would be cancelled.

The Fire & Ambulance Services Education Centre & Museum under the Fire Services Department would also be closed and all public education programmes would be cancelled.

The Government made use of the Anti-epidemic Fund to conduct large scale COVID-19 testing for designated high-risk groups in the community on a voluntary basis, and expanded Hong Kong's overall testing capacity.

15.07 The HA announced that it was expanding its standard of screening patients for COVID-19 upon their admission to public hospitals, which allowed doctors to execute clinical judgment on whether they think patients should be in the high-risk group according to the history taken from the patient.

The CHP said it would target people in high-risk groups when conducting COVID-19 tests. Priority was given to people experiencing coronavirus symptoms and those living in buildings with more than one unit with unlinked cases.

16.07 The Government announced that designated staff canteens and catering businesses providing meals for staff members to eat in would be exempted from the restrictions on dine-in services starting tonight.

The Transport Department on July 17 would commence registration for taxi drivers to make appointments for one-off COVID-19 testing.

17.07 The Government announced that its free COVID-19 testing services were not for private use and explained that the objective was to encourage people with symptoms to take the test as soon as possible.

The Government called on restaurant operators to register online for a scheme that provides free COVID-19 testing for catering business workers.

18.07 The Government announced it had gazetted specifications to impose conditions on travellers who visited specific high-risk places

within 14 days before arriving in Hong Kong to reduce the number of imported cases.

The Food & Environmental Hygiene Department said that 12 public markets in Kowloon would close earlier for deep cleaning and disinfection in the coming days.

Socio-Economic Policy Packages

12.07 Secretary for Justice Teresa Cheng posted a blog article and concluded that 'The pandemic has caused an unprecedented impact on Hong Kong's economy... We have been closely monitoring the situation in the legal and dispute resolution sector to provide timely support'.

14.07 The ESS Secretariat published the list of the fourth batch of employers who received wage subsidies.

15.07 The Government announced that the subsidy scheme for vehicle maintenance workshops under the Anti-epidemic Fund would open for applications from July 16.

16.07 The application deadline for the Scheme on Relief Grants for Interest Class Instructors Hired by Organisations Subvented by the Social Welfare Department was extended.

17.07 The ESS Secretariat announced that the sixth batch of wage subsidies totalling $4.7 billion and covering about 200,000 employees would be disbursed.

18.07 More than 10,500 applications under the Anti-epidemic Support Scheme for Property Management Sector were approved, involving subsidies of over $410 million.

The Anti-epidemic Subsidy Scheme for the Laundry Trade received over 1,400 applications, of which around 1,000 applications were approved, involving subsidies of about $60 million.

Major Development

12.07 SCMP[41]: University of Hong Kong dismissed allegations from former employee that Beijing covered up outbreak. Yan Limeng, formerly of HKU's school of public health, said the university had failed to act on her findings in late December of human-to-human transmission. University brushed off her allegations as hearsay, said her Fox News interview did not tally with its facts and had no scientific basis.

13.07 The chance of contracting COVID-19 from infected blood is very low, the HA said in response

---

41   *SCMP*: www.scmp.com/news/hong-kong/health-environment/article/3092868/coronavirus-university-hong-kong-dismisses

to an incident where a person confirmed to have the virus donated blood last week.

14.07 The CHP said it was worried about a surge in locally transmitted COVID-19 cases with unknown sources of infection. They were having difficulty tracking down the source of infection connected to half of the 48 newly-confirmed patients.

The HA was investigating how two patients at Princess Margaret Hospital and Queen Elizabeth Hospital contracted COVID-19.

SCMP: Hong Kong third wave: learn from Covid-19 social-distancing mistakes and overhaul quarantine exemption policy, health experts told officials. Four leading public health figures commented on government's coronavirus strategy, urging officials to prepare more isolation and quarantine facilities. Testing, quarantine exemptions and total lift of eight-person maximum at restaurant tables were key failures, said Chinese University's Dr David Hui.

15.07 SCMP[42]: 64-year-old could be first prosecuted for violating new public transport mask rules amid Covid-19 spike. The man allegedly became agitated and produced a wooden pole when MTR staff demanded he wear a mask. Separately, police were hunting for a man caught beating a McDonald's employee on video after being asked to don a mask in the restaurant.

16.07 SCMP[43]: HKU school head chided former worker for tarring reputation of ex-colleagues on American TV over alleged research cover-up. Professor Keiji Fukuda from HKU's School of Public Health issued internal memo to staff, expressing concern over allegations and impact on 'highly respected members'.

SCMP[44]: Hong Kong third wave: Covid-19 infections soar to record high of 67, more than half from unknown source. Ticket issued to owner of dim sum place for breaching evening dine-in ban, representing first legal

action under sweeping measures.

17.07 The CHP reported 58 additional COVID-19 cases, of which 50 were locally transmitted including three linked to an elderly care home, while eight were imported.

The Civil Service Bureau reminded bureaus and departments that they should handle the work arrangements for their staff with flexibility while maintaining the provision of public services amid the COVID-19 pandemic.

18.07 SCMP[45]: Number of people confirmed with Covid-19 in Hong Kong surpassed the 1,755 recorded for severe acute respiratory syndrome in 2003. Infection of three health workers at Tuen Mun Eye Centre sparked Covid-19 cluster fears as city marks grim milestone.

*19.07–25.07 (2,503/19)***

Public Health Policies

19.07 SCMP[46]: Carrie Lam revealed major upgrade of quarantine, isolation facilities for Covid-19 fight

as city reported daily high of 108 confirmed infections, of which 83 were locally transmitted and 25 imported. City's leader also announced work-from-home arrangements for civil servants (starting July 20), extension of compulsory mask wearing to public spaces inside.

The Government was looking into using Asia World-Expo as a community isolation facility to combat the COVID-19 pandemic.

20.07 Government anticipated that classes of all schools, including international schools and kindergartens, would not commence earlier than August 17.

The directions under the Prevention & Control of Disease (Requirements & Directions) (Business & Premises) Regulation (Cap 599F) to extend existing social distancing measures were gazetted, from July 22 to 28.

The Home Affairs Department and the Association of Property Management Companies launched Community Testing of

42 *SCMP*: www.scmp.com/news/hong-kong/health-environment/article/3093270/hong-kong-third-wave-64-year-old-becomes-first

43 *SCMP*: www.scmp.com/news/hong-kong/health-environment/article/3093342/coronavirus-hku-school-head-chides-former-worker

44 *SCMP*: www.scmp.com/news/hong-kong/health-environment/article/3093409/hong-kong-third-wave-about-50-new-cases

45 *SCMP*: www.scmp.com/news/hong-kong/health-environment/article/3093745/hong-kong-third-wave-fears-fresh-covid-19-cluster

46 *SCMP*: www.scmp.com/news/hong-kong/health-environment/article/3093795/hong-kong-third-wave-more-100-confirmed-and

COVID-19 for Frontline Property Management Workers to arrange a free virus testing service for frontline workers.

21.07 The DH reminded citizens that some of its non-urgent services have been adjusted or suspended.

The Food & Environmental Hygiene Department started to distribute face masks and hand sanitisers to market and hawker bazaar operators, and placed hand sanitisers at communal areas for market patrons.

The LCSD strongly urged members of the public not to go swimming or sunbathing at closed beaches.

The Immigration Department would implement a new arrangement on applications for foreign domestic helper visas.

22.07 The Government announced it would further enhance anti-epidemic measures, mandating people to wear masks not only on public transport but at all indoor public places.

The CHP urged the public to stay at home as far as possible to prevent the spread of COVID-19 in the community.

23.07 Government said it converted Lei Yue Mun Park & Holiday Village into a community isolation facility.

The Government announced that aside from those providing emergency services and essential public services, all other government employees would continue to work from home until August 2.

24.07 The CHP urged the public to stay at home as the surge in COVID-19 cases continues.

As some new COVID-19 cases were found to be related to Hung Hom and To Kwa Wan markets, the Food & Environmental Hygiene Department said it immediately cleaned and disinfected areas used by patients.

25.07 The Food & Environmental Hygiene Department would arrange for the 12 public markets on Hong Kong Island and in the New Territories to be closed earlier at 7pm for deep cleaning and disinfection from July 26 to 28.

The HA announced that specimen bottles would be available at 22 of its general out-patient clinics from July 27 for members of the public to collect their deep throat saliva samples for virus testing.

Socio-Economic Policy Packages

19.07 Chief Executive instructed the Home Affairs Department to arrange provision of food packs for the elderly.

20.07 A subsidy programme for graduates under the Green Employment Scheme received dozens of applications covering around 120 jobs, representing more than half of the jobs under the programme, the Environment Bureau said.

21.07 The ESS Secretariat published the list of the fifth batch of employers who received wage subsidies.

24.07 the Law Tech Fund application period deadline would be extended to September 6 to allow eligible law firms and chambers more time to prepare their applications. Around 400 applications were received so far.

The Home Affairs Department said it gave more than 5,000 food packs to the elderly living in Kowloon East public housing estates with confirmed COVID-19 cases.

25.07 More than 10,600 applications under the Anti-epidemic Support Scheme for Property Management Sector were approved, involving subsidies of over $440 million.

Major Development

19.07 The Government clarified that the existing exemption arrangement under the compulsory quarantine regime was essential to maintain the necessary operation of society and the economy and to ensure an uninterrupted supply of daily necessities.

Chief Executive Carrie Lam said it was not realistic for Hong Kong to adopt citywide COVID-19 testing.

20.07 The CHP announced that an investigation would be carried out after the COVID-19 test results concerning two people were mixed up.

SCMP[47]: Hong Kong third wave: authorities weighed lockdown after 73 new Covid-19 cases reported. Authorities turned to unprecedented measures, including requiring people to wear masks indoors at public venues, possibly starting this week.

21.07 In response to a media report that a lawyer was preliminarily tested positive for COVID-19 after visiting people in custody, the Correctional Services Department said the people concerned were currently asymptomatic.

The Government clarified the rumour that it might impose a so-called lockdown in the coming few days in view of the COVID-19 outbreak was unfounded.

The Government strongly condemned the selfish and illegal acts of

---

47   *SCMP*: www.scmp.com/news/hong-kong/health-environment/article/3093866/hong-kong-third-wave-infectious-disease-experts

disorderly people who gathered inside a mall in Yuen Long, gravely increasing the risk of spreading COVID-19.

SCMP[48]: Experts pointed to policy loopholes in handling returning domestic helpers and stopover sea or aircrew, as SCMP found significant proportion among imported cases involve such groups. They also singled out public complacency as another factor, stressing that government measures could only do so much.

SCMP[49]: Hong Kong's third wave of Covid-19 killed two more elderly patients as public hospitals warned they could run out of first-tier isolation beds. Personal carer who visited more than 10 homes for the elderly and accompanied residents on hospital consultations was among those infected.

22.07 SCMP[50]: 'Mainland Chinese health authorities have offered Covid-19

help, with city likely to accept'. Official agencies among the mainland health organisations willing to provide medical equipment, expertise and testing support, source said.

24.07 The Exchange Fund recorded an investment loss of $10.6 billion in the first half of the year, the Monetary Authority announced.

25.07 Secretary for Commerce & Economic Development Edward Yau participated in the first-ever Virtual Ministers Responsible for Trade Meeting of Asia-Pacific Economic Cooperation 2020.

RTHK[51]: Shenzhen and Zhuhai suspended the mutual recognition of quarantine with Hong Kong.

HKCNews[52]: Under pandemic, about 60% of the countries postponed the election, and 40% unchanged. Most countries held election after the

COVID-19 cases dropped down. Professor David Hui of Respiratory Medicine in CUHK suggested that government could make decision at the end of August.

26.07 –01.08 (3,395/33)**

Public Health Policies

26.07 The Government announced that crew change arrangements for passenger vessels and goods vessels without a cargo operation in Hong Kong would be suspended from July 29 until the local epidemic situation was contained.

The Transport Department announced that from July 27, the voluntary and free of charge COVID-19 testing service would be extended from taxi drivers to public light bus drivers.

The Government said the tightening of measures for sea and air crew would take effect on July 29.

27.07 Chief Secretary Matthew Cheung announced that the Government would further tighten social distancing measures and extend the mask-wearing requirement to cover all outdoor public places from midnight on July 29 until August 4.

The Home Affairs Department would launch a programme to test public housing estate residents in Tsz Wan Shan for COVID-19 given the relatively severe epidemic situation there.

The EDB announced that schools would continue to suspend all on-campus activities from July 29 to August 16.

The CHP called on employers to adopt work from home arrangements to prevent a community-wide COVID-19 outbreak.

The HA explained that with the number of COVID-19 cases increasing daily, those severely ill were considered top

48 *SCMP*: www.scmp.com/news/hong-kong/health-environment/article/3093978/hong-kong-third-wave-how-did-citys-scariest-surge

49 *SCMP*: www.scmp.com/news/hong-kong/health-environment/article/3094030/hong-kong-third-wave-covid-19-bed-situation

50 *SCMP*: www.scmp.com/news/hong-kong/health-environment/article/3094173/hong-kong-third-wave-health-authorities-mainland

51 RTHK: https://news.rthk.hk/rthk/ch/component/k2/1539830-20200725.htm

52 HKCNews: www.hkcnews.com/article/32297/2020%E7%AB%8B%E6%B3%95%E6%9C%83%E9%81%B8
%E8%88%89-%E5%A4%96%E5%9C%8B%E9%81%B8%E8%88%89-%E7%BE%8E%E5%9C%8B%E7%
B4%84%E7%BF%B0%E9%9C%8D%E6%99%AE%E9%87%91%E6%96%AF%E5%A4%A7%E5%AD%
B8%EF%BC%88the_johns_hopkins_university%EF%BC%89-32297/%E5%A4%9A%E5%9C%8B%E5%9
C%A8%E7%96%AB%E6%83%85%E5%9B%9E%E8%90%BD%E8%BE%A6%E9%81%B8%E8%88%89-
%E8%A8%B1%E6%A8%B9%E6%98%8C%EF%BC%9A%E6%B8%AF%E5%BA%9C%E5%8F%AF%E6%9C%88
%E5%BA%95%E6%89%8D%E6%B1%BA%E5%AE%9A%E7%AB%8B%E6%9C%83%E5%AE%89%E6%8E%92?f
bclid=IwAR3ri-gN_RiN361Efx8nOAlUug0uVY-s5hbJm0LexkX1hS9nIsM7XX1evzw

priority when it came to admitting patients to the hospital.

The New Territories South Animal Management Centre would be launched on July 28 as another quarantine facility for pets related to COVID-19 cases, the Agriculture, Fisheries & Conservation Department announced.

28.07 Chief Executive Carrie Lam called on the public to follow strictly the social distancing measures and stay at home as far as possible in view of the COVID-19 epidemic.

29.07 As some new COVID-19 cases were found to be related to Tung Yick Market in Yuen Long, the Food & Environmental Hygiene Department said it would close the market an hour earlier on July 30 for deep cleaning and disinfection.

30.07 The Government allowed the resumption of daytime dine-in services from 5am to 5.59pm from July 31, having noted the difficulties the previous arrangement caused those not working from home.

The Government announced that aside from those providing emergency services and essential public services,

all other government employees should continue to work from home until August 9.

The HA said the Asia-World-Expo community treatment facility with 500 beds was expected to open on August 1, further boosting the authority's bed capacity.

01.08 The Food & Environmental Hygiene Department announced that it has further enhanced anti-epidemic measures in its markets and would clean and disinfect all public markets.

The HA's COVID-19 community treatment facility at AsiaWorld-Expo, which provided 500 beds, started operation.

The CHP urged the public to avoid family gatherings due to a rise in COVID-19 family clusters.

Under the Community Testing of COVID-19 for Frontline Property Management Workers, 11,500 tests were completed, the Home Affairs Department announced.

The Home Affairs Department would cease opening the 19 community halls or community centres in 18 districts for members of the public to take their own meal to have lunch from August 2.

Socio-Economic Policy Packages

27.07 As of July 26, more than $4.8 billion were disbursed to about 490,000 construction workers and 19,000 construction-related enterprises via two rounds of the Anti-epidemic Fund, the Development Bureau said.

28.07 The Housing Authority announced that it would provide a two-month rent waiver for public rental housing tenants along with a 9.66% rent increase that would take effect September 1.

29.07 The ESS Secretariat published the list of the sixth batch of employers who received wage subsidies, covering about 11,600 applicants and subsidies totalling about $4.7 billion. (Seventh batch of about 17,300 successful employer applicants to be started next week, with subsidies totalling about $6.4 billion covering around 283,000 employees.)

30.07 The Development Bureau further extended the application deadline for Batch VI of the Revitalising Historic Buildings Through Partnership Scheme to September 3.

Major Development

26.07 HKU[53]: Team of Professor Yuen Kwok-yung of

Department of Microbiology in HKU found compounds from existing medicals to restrain the virus replication.

Apple Daily[54]: HA rejected the imported "Mainland help" and emphasized that there were not enough beds and about one hundred patients were waiting to be hospitalized.

27.07 Three people were prosecuted on July 27 for failing to wear a mask while in markets, contravening (Cap 599I) under the Prevention & Control of Disease (Wearing of Mask) Regulation.

Leading medical experts Yuen Kwok-yung and David Hui have said the government's policy of exempting 33 types of inbound travellers from the 14-day mandatory quarantine was the "biggest loophole" in battling the new wave of coronavirus. But the government hit back and said it was a "misunderstanding," defending the arrangements by arguing they were necessary to ensure the "normal operation" of the city. The health minister has now said that the government is to tighten its quarantine policy on sea and air crew, while the CHP – which earlier failed to identify the

53 HKU: https://fightcovid19.hku.hk/zh/%E8%A2%81%E5%9C%8B%E5%8B%87%E5%9C%98%E9%9A%8A%E7%99%BC%E7%8F%BE%E5%A4%9A%E7%A8%AE%E8%97%A5%E7%89%A9%E4%B8%AD%E7%9A%84%E5%8C%96%E5%90%88%E7%89%A9%E5%8F%AF%E6%8A%91%E5%88%B6%E6%96%B0%E5%86%A0%E7%97%85/
54 *Apple Daily*: https://hk.appledaily.com/local/20200726/J6MTMACAZEUARLELDKN7PA6L7Q/

source of the current outbreak – vowed to carry out "serious follow-up." [55]

Mingpao[56]: When asked about whether he would apologize to the health experts, Under Secretary for Food and Health Dr CHUI Tak-yi did not response but only claimed that he would respect the experts' opinions and would not cease reviewing the development of the pandemic. Expert Adviser David Hui commented that the responsibility of expert adviser was to stop up a loophole and prevent the fourth wave from happening. On whether the HKSAR government should apologize or not, Hui believed that 'it doesn't matter and there is no need to do so'.

28.07 SCMP[57]: coronavirus might have stopped mutating, making it more infectious, study found. Polytechnic University team studied samples taken from different clusters since late June and found no genetic difference. Either the virus ceased to mutate, or the cases all contracted the virus at the same place in a short period of time.

29.07 Hong Kong's economy in the second quarter of 2020 contracted 9% over a year earlier, slightly lower than the 9.1% decrease in the first quarter, the Census & Statistics Department announced.

The HA said it is using all available resources to admit more COVID-19 patients, in the situation that people who had recently been notified that they were positive for the virus have to wait before they could be hospitalized.

The COVID-19 Community Testing Scheme in Tsz Wan Shan, launched by the Home Affairs Department and the Tung Wah Group of Hospitals, collected 4,150 sets of registration forms and specimens.

SCMP[58]: FedEx pilots wanted US company to suspend flights to Hong Kong, said Covid-19 measures present 'unacceptable risk'.

Online opposition to the ban on daytime dine-in services as employees who could not work from home struggled having meals outside.

30.07 Expanded by the Lei Yue Mun community isolation facility with 350 beds and the AsiaWorld-Expo community treatment facility with 500 beds, the bed capacity that the HA could handle is about 1,500, capacity increased by 50%.

On.cc[59]: Association of Hong Kong Nursing Staff collected over 120,000 countersigns to oppose the freezing salary announced by the HA and to ask for subsidies from the "Anti-Epidemic Fund" by the government.

SCMP[60]: Officials scrapped coronavirus-related ban on eating in restaurants after just 24 hours.

SCMP[61]: Hong Kong needs citywide coronavirus testing, Zhong Nanshan said. Dine-in ban was 'crucial' to contain third wave but compulsory tests across the population was also needed.

HKU[62]: HKU Professor Malik Peiris found through investigating the virus that there were at least four sources of virus, and only one type of virus caused large scale infection, which was imported. Government should be cautious on exemption list.

31.07 Customs seizes 434 boxes of surgical

55   Hong Kong Free Press: https://hongkongfp.com/2020/07/28/covid-19-surge-hong-kong-admits-quarantine-exemptions-may-be-to-blame-as-city-sees-106-new-infections/

56   *Mingpao*: https://news.mingpao.com/pns/%E8%A6%81%E8%81%9E/article/20200727/s00001/1595788838967/%E6%B8%AF%E5%BA%9C%E4%B8%8A%E5%91%A8%E7%A8%B1%E3%80%8C%E5%85%8D%E6%AA%A2E8%80%85%E6%98%AF%E7%96%AB%E6%BA%90%E3%80%8D%E5%B1%AC%E8%AA%A4%E8%A7%A3-%E8%A2%AB%E5%95%8F%E9%81%93%E6%AD%89-%E5%BE%90%E5%BE%B7%E7%BE%A9-%E5%B0%8A%E9%87%8D%E5%B0%88%E5%AE%B6%E6%84%8F%E8%A6%8B

57   *SCMP*: www.scmp.com/news/hong-kong/health-environment/article/3095062/hong-kong-third-wave-coronavirus-may-have-stopped

58   *SCMP*: www.scmp.com/news/hong-kong/transport/article/3095094/hong-kong-third-wave-fedex-pilots-want-us-company-suspend

59   On cc：https://hk.on.cc/hk/bkn/cnt/news/20200730/bkn-20200730101041408-0730_00822_001.html

60   *SCMP*: www.scmp.com/news/hong-kong/health-environment/article/3095283/hong-kong-third-wave-government-changes-mind

61   *SCMP*: www.scmp.com/news/china/society/article/3095277/hong-kong-needs-citywide-covid-19-testing-chinas-sars-hero-zhong

62   HKU: https://fightcovid19.hku.hk/zh/%e7%97%85%e6%af%92%e5%ad%b8%e6%ac%8a%e5%a8%81%e8%a3%b4%e5%81%89%e5%a3%ab%ef%bc%9a%e7%ac%ac%e4%b8%89%e6%b3%a2%e7%96%ab%e6%83%85%e7%97%85%e6%af%92%e5%9f%ba%e5%9b%a0%e5%b9%be%e4%b9%8e%e5%ae%8c%e5%85%a8/

masks which had a bacterial count suspected of exceeding the limit.

HKU[63]: Professor Yuen Kwok-yung of microbiology suggested the government should target to reduce cross infection, by providing take-aways and places for dining.

01.08 SCMP[64]: free Covid-19 tests for residents as mainland Chinese clinical teams head to city. Sixty lab technicians from public hospitals in Guangdong province would be picked for Hong Kong stint.

Seven members of the Mainland nucleic acid test support team arrived Hong Kong to support anti-epidemic work.

Commercial Radio 881[65]: Dr Chuang Shuk Kwan: only knew Mainland clinical teams to come from news, but the Department of Public Health might have known.

Chief Executive's Office expressed regret on individual misleading media reports[66]: She said clearly that she had not discussed the postponement of the election with any of the government expert advisers.

Apple Daily[67]: Loopholes in exemption policies caused the third wave, but the government emphasizes on citizens to reduce social activities.

02.08–08.08 (4,008/47)**
Public Health Policies

03.08 The Transport Department announced that its voluntary and free of charge COVID-19 testing service for taxi and public light bus drivers (PLB) would be extended starting August 4.

04.08 Prof Yuen Kwok-yung inspected Hung Hom and To Kwa Wan markets in view of recent COVID-19 cases related to these facilities.

The CHP expressed concern about the possible spread of COVID-19 at two different markets.

05.08 The CHP said it is tracing about 28 foreign domestic helpers in relation to a confirmed case announced on August 4.

The HA announced that it was investigating the connection between two COVID-19 cases at Pamela Youde Nethersole Eastern Hospital.

The Government urged members of the public to ensure that they could meet Guangdong Province's updated prevention and control measures when travelling there. The negative test result would be valid within 24 hours from the report's issue time.

Virus testing arrangement: The Government decided to procure testing services from three providers by direct procurement with funding from the Anti-epidemic Fund so as to roll out large-scale testing as soon as possible to safeguard public health.

06.08 The Government announced that aside from those providing emergency services and essential public services, all other government employees would continue to work from home until August 16.

The Home Affairs Department announced that the COVID-19 Community Testing Scheme would be extended to four districts, involving 46 buildings and about 86,000 residents.

The CHP expressed concern over a possible COVID-19 outbreak in hostels used by foreign domestic helpers.

The Government announced measures to reduce the health risks faced by foreign domestic helpers staying in boarding facilities of employment agencies and reduce the risk of COVID-19 transmission in the community.

07.08 As a new COVID-19 case was found to be related to Tai Po Hui Market, the Food & Environmental Hygiene Department said it would close the market an hour earlier on August 7 for deep cleaning and disinfection.

The Government distributed 28 million disposable adult masks to about 2.8 million residential addresses in Hong Kong in the past month, with each household receiving 10 masks.

63 HKU: https://fightcovid19.hku.hk/zh/%E8%A2%81%E5%9C%8B%E5%8B%87%EF%BC%9A%E6%94%BF%E5%B
A%9C%E8%A6%81%E6%9C%89%E9%87%9D%E5%B0%8D%E6%80%A7%E6%8E%AA%E6%96%BD%E9%98
%BB%E6%AD%A2%E9%A3%9F%E8%82%86%E4%BA%A4%E5%8F%89%E6%84%9F%E6%9F%93/

64 *SCMP*: www.scmp.com/news/hong-kong/health-environment/article/3095646/hong-kong-third-wave-mainland-clinical-teams

65 雷霆881：www.881903.com/news/local/2350125/%E5%BC%B5%E7%AB%B9%E5%90%9B%E7%9C%8B%E6%96
%B0%E8%81%9E%E6%89%8D%E5%BE%97%E7%9F%A5%E4%B8%AD%E5%A4%AE%E6%B4%BE%E5%93%
A1%E4%BE%86%E6%B8%AF%E5%B1%95%E9%96%8B%E5%AF%A6%E9%A9%97%E5%AE%A4%E5%B7%A
5%E4%BD%9C

66 CE's Office: www.info.gov.hk/gia/general/202008/01/P2020080100845.htm

67 *Apple Daily*: https://hk.feature.appledaily.com/wars/article/1_61235562?appId=598aee533b729200504d1f2e

Chief Executive Carrie Lam announced the Government would introduce a universal and voluntary COVID-19 testing programme with the support of the central government.

The Government said that a Mainland medical laboratory team, which would help run the universal community COVID-19 testing programme, would be able to operate in Hong Kong under a qualification exemption.

The Government said the Mainland nucleic acid test support team commenced work to assist in enhancing virus testing capacity, establishing a temporary hospital as well as expanding the scale of community treatment facilities.

The Government announced that it would continue to impose conditions on travellers who visited specific high-risk places within 14 days before arriving in Hong Kong and simplify relevant conditions.

08.08 The Food & Environmental Hygiene Department announced that it would arrange for 12 public markets to be closed earlier at 7pm for deep cleaning and disinfection from August 9 to 11.

The Labour Department, Police and the Food & Environmental Hygiene Department conducted mobile broadcasts in popular gathering places of foreign domestic helpers to urge them to comply with anti-epidemic measures.

Socio-Economic Policy Packages

03.08 The Government said its decision to postpone the 2020 LegCo General Election for a year on public health grounds was reasonable, legal and in the public interest, in response to the statement by HKBA.

Major Development

02.08 The HA apologised for inappropriately sending a woman who was not infected with COVID-19 to the Asia-World-Expo community treatment facility.

SCMP[68]: Hong Kong's City University began testing animals for coronavirus amid owners' concerns. So far, two dogs and four cats tested positive for the coronavirus.

Apple Daily[69]: Online sources showed that Beijing Genomics Institute was recruiting nurses from Mainland to Hong Kong for operation of tests. But there is no such recruitment information on the official website.

SCMP[70]: officials to prioritise next round of testing for Covid-19 as first experts from mainland China arrived to help with fight.

SCMP[71]: Hong Kong cash handout: the new immigrants struggling to ride out the Covid-19 crisis without HK$10,000 government payment. Non-permanent residents were still waiting to be given the nod to apply for the cash support.

03.08 Mingpao[72]: National Health Commission sent 60-people "nucleic acid testing support team" who stay for a month and 6-people "cabin hospital support team" with practical experience who stay for half a year.

HKU[73]: Professor Yuen Kwok-yung suggested the possibility of universal testing.

04.08 SCMP[74]: Hong Kong jobs crisis sparked rise in serious emotional and mental health problems, experts warned.

05.08 The Research Council chaired by the Secretary for Food & Health approved a further

68   *SCMP*: www.scmp.com/news/hong-kong/education/article/3095667/cityu-lab-begins-testing-animals-covid-19-hong-kong

69   *Apple Daily*: https://hk.appledaily.com/local/20200802/OHLNKE2WNOX2JAXFQFFXAJVBN4/

70   *SCMP*: www.scmp.com/news/hong-kong/health-environment/article/3095690/hong-kong-third-wave-prioritise-high-risk-groups

71   *SCMP*: www.scmp.com/news/hong-kong/society/article/3095715/hong-kong-cash-handout-new-immigrants-struggling-ride-out

72   *Mingpao*: https://news.mingpao.com/pns/%E8%A6%81%E8%81%9E/article/20200803/s00001/1596392374987/%E6%AA%A2%E6%B8%AC%E9%9A%8A%E6%8A%B5%E6%B8%AF-%E5%8A%A9%E5%BB%BA%E5%AF%A6%E9%A9%97%E5%AE%A4%E5%A4%A7%E7%AF%A9%E6%9F%A5-%E4%BA%9E%E5%8D%9A%E5%BB%BA%E6%96%B0%E7%A4%BE%E5%8D%80%E6%B2%BB%E7%99%82%E8%A8%AD%E6%96%BD-%E3%80%8C%E6%96%B9%E8%89%99%E9%9A%8A%E3%80%8D%E7%A8%B1%E6%8C%87%E5%B0%8E%E9%81%8B%E4%BD%9C%E4%B8%8D%E6%B2%BB%E7%97%85

73   HKU: https://fightcovid19.hku.hk/zh/%e8%a2%81%e5%9c%8b%e5%8b%87%e8%aa%8d%e7%82%ba%e8%a6%81%e6%80%9d%e8%80%83%e5%85%a8%e6%b0%91%e6%aa%a2%e6%b8%ac%e7%9a%84%e5%8f%af%e8%a1%8c%e6%80%a7/

74   *SCMP*: www.scmp.com/news/hong-kong/health-environment/article/3095837/covid-19-time-bomb-hong-kong-jobs-crisis-sparks

$59 million in funding to support local universities to conduct research studies on COVID-19 under the Health & Medical Research Fund.

Police condemned netizens for spreading fake news that the Commissioner of Police was infected with COVID-19 and called the rumour totally groundless and fictitious.

The Agriculture, Fisheries & Conservation Department said a pet cat and a pet dog belonging to two close contacts of confirmed COVID-19 cases tested positive for the virus.

The Government condemned the acts of some non-establishment camp district council members and people who held demonstrations outside the hotel where the Mainland nucleic acid test support team was staying in.

06.08 SCMP[75]: restaurant, retail and hotel bosses tried to reinvent themselves digitally as pandemic keeps visitors away. Anxiety set in for thousands made jobless, or told to stay home on reduced pay or no pay. Hard-hit sectors got creative, with city tours designed for Hongkongers, staycation deals.

09.08 – 15.08 (4,008/47)**

Public Health Policies

09.08 The Labour Department launched a free, one-off COVID-19 testing service for all foreign domestic helpers staying in boarding facilities of employment agencies.

The LCSD said it stepped up patrols in its venues on August 8 and 9 to urge people to comply with anti-epidemic regulations.

Major Development

09.08 The HA said the chance that a 70-year-old patient at Kwong Wah Hospital, who preliminarily tested positive for COVID-19 after two negative tests, got infected with the virus at the hospital was low.

Mingpao[76]: A private laboratory that helped the government undertake the high-risk group testing pointed out that they found a higher rate of positive than the government public laboratory and warned that the problematic collection process might have caused false negative.

Mingpao[77]: Professor Yuen Kwok-yung listed three major loopholes in the third-wave containment measures, that was, slow testing process, long period in waiting for hospitalization and loose end in measures such as exemption.

10.08 Apple Daily[78]: The latest study by team of Professor Yuen Kwok-yung showed that the third wave outbreak was hardly connected to the first two waves. There was still unknown connection between the third wave and the imported cases, and the virus had gene mutation in Hong Kong. Experts thought it was crucial to tighten exemption, or the universal testing would be useless.

16.08 – 22.08 (4,658/76)**

Public Health Policies

17.08 Services at the Lei Yue Mun community isolation facility were temporarily suspended to facilitate upgrade works there, the HA announced.

18.08 Chief Executive Carrie Lam said the COVID-19 epidemic situation was still very severe in Hong Kong and that it was not the time to relax social distancing measures.

19.08 The Agriculture, Fisheries & Conservation Department announced it had started to provide free COVID-19 testing services to all Hong Kong mobile fishermen and their deckhands on board vessels operating in Mainland waters.

20.08 The HA would distribute specimen packs and collect deep throat saliva specimens at 22 general outpatient clinics for another three months.

The Government announced that its departments would resume

---

75 *SCMP*: www.scmp.com/news/hong-kong/hong-kong-economy/article/3096150/hong-kong-tourism-distress-restaurant-retail-and

76 *Mingpao*: https://news.mingpao.com/pns/%E6%B8%AF%E8%81%9E/article/20200809/s00002/1596909
712636/%E9%86%AB%E8%AD%B7%E5%8A%A9%E6%8E%A1%E6%A8%A3-%E9%99%BD%E6%
80%A7%E6%AF%94%E7%8E%87%E8%B6%85%E6%94%BF%E5%BA%9C%E9%A9%97%E9%AB-
%98%E5%8D%B1%E7%BE%A4%E7%B5%84-%E5%8C%96%E9%A9%97%E6%89%80%E6%86%82%E5%85%A
8%E6%B0%91%E6%AA%A2%E6%B8%AC%E6%8E%A1%E6%A8%A3%E4%B8%8D%E7%95%B6%E6%90%8D
%E6%88%90%E6%95%88

77 *Mingpao*: https://news.mingpao.com/pns/%E6%B8%AF%E8%81%9E/article/20200809/s00002/1596909713032/%E8%
A2%81%E5%9C%8B%E5%8B%87%E5%88%97%E4%B8%89%E5%A4%A7%E9%8C%AF%E8%AA%A4-%E6%A
A%A2%E6%B8%AC%E6%85%A2%E9%80%81%E9%99%A2%E6%85%A2%E6%8E%AA%E6%96%BD%E6%94
%BE%E9%AC%86

78 *Apple Daily*: https://hk.appledaily.com/local/20200810/UFEGJSFRRI3ZS2WG6AKXOENFII/

basic public services in a safe and orderly manner from August 24 to meet the needs of the public and enterprises.

The Food & Environmental Hygiene Department launched a one-off free COVID-19 testing service for supermarket workers, catering business staff at eligible clubhouses as well as licensed hawkers.

21.08 The Government would launch the Universal Community Testing Programme on September 1 to provide a one-off free testing service for members of the public.

Socio-Economic Policy Packages

18.08 Chief Executive Carrie Lam announced the Government would launch a new round of Anti-epidemic Fund to help sectors affected by COVID-19.

The Innovation & Technology Commission introduced measures to enhance the Distance Business Programme.

The Government announced that the second tranche of the ESS would invite applications from August 31 to September 13.

19.08 The Monetary Authority announced that the countercyclical macroprudential measures for mortgage loans on non-residential properties would be relaxed from August 20.

More than 11,000 applications were approved so far under the Subsidy Scheme for Beauty Parlours, Massage Establishments and Party Rooms, involving about $560 million in subsidies.

The ESS processing agent was verifying whether employers who had received the first tranche of wage subsidies have complied with the scheme's terms.

20.08 The ESS Secretariat published the list of the eighth batch of employers who received wage subsidies.

21.08 More than 430 time-limited Support Service Assistant positions offered by various government bureaus and departments were open for application.

The Food & Environmental Hygiene Department said it would enhance the Catering Business (Social Distancing) Subsidy Scheme to help those who were eligible but had not submitted applications for the first tranche of the subsidy.

Major Development

16.08 Secretary for Justice Teresa Cheng: Now that the postponement of the election and the constitutional lacuna were addressed, we must fight the COVID-19 pandemic in solidarity and focus on our economic development and improving people's livelihoods.

21.08 The Government welcomed the arrival of a Mainland nucleic acid test support team.

23.08 – 29.08 (4,787/86)**

Public Health Policies

23.08 The Government would on August 24 begin registration for foreign domestic helpers whose previous employment contracts expired or were terminated and were waiting to join new employers to book a COVID-19 test.

24.08 The Environmental Protection Department announced that it had arranged COVID-19 testing on August 25 and 26 for about 500 frontline staff who had frequent contact with the public.

25.08 The Government said it would relax several social distancing measures on August 28.

The Electrical & Mechanical Services Department announced it would arrange free and voluntary COVID-19 testing for lift and escalator trade practitioners from August 26.

The Government said that the medical and healthcare sectors responded positively to the Universal Community Testing Programme, with more than 5,000 personnel enrolled to participate in it so far.

The Government said the terminal operators of Kwai Tsing Container Ter-

minals had returned over 90% or more than 7,100 of the distributed bottles with specimens to the DH for COVID-19 testing.

26.08 The Government said all private laboratories providing testing services for the Government must take part in and pass the CHP's External Quality Assessment Programme for COVID-19 testing.

Apple Daily : BGI (one of the contracted private laboratories) produced high sensitivity self-testing suit leading to 3,700 false positive cases in Sweden. It could mistakenly identify 54 types of respiratory diseases and present cross reaction.

27.08 The Government would recruit experienced and well-trained personnel to conduct COVID-19 tests for the Universal Community Testing Programme.

The Food & Environmental Hygiene Department provided updated guidelines on the provision of dine-in services to licensees and operators of food premises in light of the latest COVID-19 public health risk assessment.

For the prevention and control of COVID-19, all secondary and primary students would learn from home with the support of schools once the new academic year starts on September 1, the EDB said.

The Tourism Commission announced that it would launch a free and voluntary COVID-19 testing scheme for registered frontline hotel staff on August 28.

28.08 Secretary for the Civil Service Patrick Nip announced that 141 specimen collection centres would operate in 18 districts under the Universal Community Testing Programme.

The taxi industry would launch the Anti-epidemic Name Tag for Taxi Drivers Scheme to encourage taxi drivers to participate in the Universal Community Testing Programme, the Transport Department said.

Socio-Economic Policy Packages

23.08 The Government introduced a penalty clause in the second tranche of the Employment Support Scheme to boost deterrence against employers from significantly laying off employees.

Major Development

24.08 The CHP said the overall COVID-19 caseload trend was decreasing and the Universal Community Testing Programme, to be launched on September 1, would help identify silent carriers.

Apple Daily[80]: Alfred Sit, Secretary for Innovation and Technology, expressed on 24 August that Health Code would not be used to track citizen's locations or limit the entrance to public places.

25.08 The Universal Community Testing Programme would help the Government consider measures to return Hong Kong's economy to normal as soon as possible, Chief Executive Carrie Lam said.

Chief Executive Carrie Lam: A key task that required our concerted efforts and everyone's active participation is the Universal Community Testing Programme which aimed to identify asymptomatic patients in the community to further curb the epidemic.

28.08 Chief Executive Carrie Lam attended a ceremony at Sun Yat Sen Memorial Park Sports Centre to welcome the arrival of the Mainland nucleic acid test support team.

29.08 The Government said the Universal Community Testing Programme was one of the important measures in fighting the COVID-19 epidemic and should not be compared with the 2020 LegCo General Election.

*30.08 –05.09 (4,858/94)***

Public Health Policies

30.08 As at 6pm on August 30, more than 420,000 people registered for the Universal Community Testing Programme that would begin on September 1.

31.08 Secretary for Education Kevin Yeung announced that schools would resume face-to-face lessons on a half-day basis in two phases from September 23.

The Transport & Housing Bureau woiuld provide regular COVID-19 tests for frontline workers at Kwai Tsing Container Terminals starting September 1.

01.09 Chief Executive Carrie Lam and principal officials took part in the Universal Community Testing Programme on its launch day on September 1 at the Central Government Offices testing centre.

The Government would increase the booking quota for the Universal Community Testing Programme at all centres from September 3.

The Universal Community Testing Programme was launched, with all 141 community testing centres operating smoothly as a whole and about 126,000 people attending the centres for specimen taking.

02.09 The Government announced it would further relax social distancing measures on September 4.

A total of about 798,000 people had made appointments to take part in the Universal Community Testing Programme.

03.09 The Social Welfare Department announced that aided childcare centre and special childcare centre services provided by non-governmental organisations would resume in phases.

04.09 The Universal Community Testing Programme will be extended for four days to September 11.

The Government announced that it submitted the expression of interest to participate in the COVID-19 vaccine Global Access (COVAX) Facility as part of Hong Kong's two-pronged strategy for vaccine procurement.

A total of about 953,000 people made appointments to take part in the Universal Community Testing Programme.

05.09 A total of about 1,058,000 people made appointments to take part in the Universal Community Testing Programme.

Socio-Economic Policy Packages

01.09 The Government announced that the second tranche of the ESS

---

80 *Apple Daily*: https://hk.appledaily.com/local/20200824/UDP5YN7YPVFD3HQYRSZMKFTVMI/

received about 83,000 applications from employers and over 6,000 from self-employed people as of 6pm on September 1.

02.09 The application period for principal moratorium for the 80% Guarantee Product and the 90% Guarantee Product under the SME Financing Guarantee Scheme was extended to March 31, 2021, HKMC Insurance announced.

Over $6 billion in subsidies was approved in the Retail Sector Subsidy Scheme and the Subsidy Scheme for Beauty Parlours, Massage Establishments & Party Rooms..

04.09 Due to the severe blow to various sectors brought about by the COVID-19 pandemic, the Home Affairs Bureau said it would provide more than 2,500 time-limited jobs under the Anti-epidemic Fund's Job Creation Scheme.

Major Development

30.08 The Government expressed regret over false information on the internet and social media about the Universal Community Testing Programme and said the programme would help identify asymptomatic COVID-19 patients in the community.

31.08 The HA expressed support for the Universal Community Testing Programme.

Singtao[81]: Alfred Sit explained that Health Code would only be deployed after outbreak stabilized and that there would be quota for Health Code for the early stage trial; information was needed for transferring the code to the destination city, for example Macau and Mainland cities.

01.09 The value of total retail sales in July, provisionally estimated at $26.5 billion, fell 23.1% year-on-year, the Census & Statistics Department announced.

03.09 The Government welcomed the arrival of the third batch of Mainland nucleic acid test support team members.

09.09 HKU[82]: The State Key Laboratory for Emerging Infectious Diseases of the University of Hong Kong (the SKL) has partnered with Xiamen University and Wantai Biopharmaceutical company to rapidly develop a vaccine candidate against COVID-19. The vaccine candidate has been approved by China's National Medical Products Administration (NMPA) for clinical trial in humans.

*06.09–12.09 (4,938/100)***

Public Health Policies

09.09 Secretary for Food & Health Prof Sophia Chan announced that the China Certification & Inspection Group (CCIC) was the fourth private contracted laboratories providing testing services for the Government.

The government announced that the Universal Community Testing Programme would be extended for three days to September 14.

11.09 The Government relaxed social distancing measures, with the maximum number of people allowed to be seated together at one table at catering business premises increased from two to four.

Some leisure venues were reopened in phases.

*13.09–19.09 (5,009/103)***

Public Health Policies

14.09 SCMP[83]: the Universal Community Testing Programme ended with 42 carriers found among 1.78 million people

Some museums, performance venues and public libraries would reopen gradually.

15.09 The government fully resumed normal public services.

Secretary for Food & Health Prof Sophia Chan said surveillance of the community's COVID-19 situation would be increased.

16.09 The Hospital Authority announced that the number of general outpatient clinics distributing specimen collection packs will be increased from 22 to 31 starting 18 Sept.

18.09 The Government extended the dine-in hours allowed at catering business premises to midnight.

Secretary for Food & Health Prof Sophia Chan said the fourth wave of COVID-19 might be more severe than the third, adding that target group testing would be regularised.

Prof Chan made the remarks at a press conference that the Government was taking a two-pronged approach in procuring vaccines.

Socio-Economic Policy Packages

14.09 The second adult-sized CuMask were distributed to eligible citizens for free.

81   *Singtao*: https://std.stheadline.com/daily/article/2271930/日報-港聞-薛永恒-疫情穩定才推健康碼

82   HKU: www.hku.hk/press/news_detail_21583.html

83   *SCMP*: www.scmp.com/video/coronavirus/3101541/hong-kongs-covid-19-mass-testing-ends-least-42-carriers-found-among-178

The Government announced that the second tranche of ESS received a total of 184,723 applications

15.09 The government announced the third round of Anti-epidemic Fund, with a new assistance package totalling HKD 24 billion.

16.09 The Government announced that the Rating (Exemption) Order 2020 (Amendment) Order 2020 would be gazetted and take effect on September 18 to implement a further rates relief to non-domestic tenements for the third and fourth quarters of 2020-21.

The ESS Secretariat notified the first batch of 20,000 successful employer applicants of the results for the scheme's second tranche with subsidies totalling $7.2 billion.

Major Development

14.09 HKU[84]: Professor Ben Cowling, Head of Division of Epidemiology and Biostatistics, addressed a letter to the late Professor Anthony Hedley from HKU's School of Public Health. He expressed that public health policies should be based on scientific evidence.

*20.09 – 26.09 (5,009/105)***

Public Health Policies

23.09 The Government announced the social distancing measures currently in place would be largely maintained until October 1 and performances with a live audience might resume from that date.

24.09 The Government gazetted the latest specifications to impose conditions on travellers who visited the United Kingdom within 14 days before arriving in Hong Kong to reduce the number of imported COVID-19 cases, including UK to specified high-risk places from Oct 1.

The Hospital Authority announced that the number of general outpatient clinics distributing specimen collection packs would be increased from 31 to 46 starting 28 Sept.

25.09 Chief Executive Carrie Lam said with the epidemic situation stabilising gradually in Hong Kong, the government will strive to restart discussions with relevant authorities to enable members of the public to resume travel as soon as possible.

The Food & Environmental Hygiene Department announced it would continue to arrange voluntary free COVID-19 testing services for targeted groups to safeguard public health.

Socio-Economic Policy Packages

21.09 The Housing Authority's Commercial Properties Committee approved the extension of rent concessions for eligible non-domestic tenants or licensees for another six months from October 1.

Chief Secretary Matthew Cheung chaired the first meeting of the fourth-term Commission on Poverty, in which the extension of six Community Care Fund programmes was endorsed.

22.09 The Government said applications for the second tranche of the Employment Support Scheme from the two supermarket chains, Wellcome and PARKnSHOP, were approved. The two chains would receive wage subsidies of $184.5 million and $161.96 million to maintain a paid headcount of 10,149 and 8,215.

23.09 The extension of existing waivers or concessions of government fees and charges implemented in 2019 and the implementation of new waivers would be gazet-

ted by the Government on 25 Sept. The estimated revenue forgone to the Government arising from the measures amounted to $2.048 billion.

The Employment Support Scheme Secretariat notified the second batch of over 82,500 successful employer applicants of the results for the scheme's second tranche with subsidies totalling $11.5 billion to cover a committed headcount of over 480,000 paid employees.

24.09 A 100% venue rental subsidy would be provided for organisers of exhibitions and international conventions held at the Hong Kong Convention & Exhibition Centre and AsiaWorld-Expo, the Government announced.

25.09 The Anti-epidemic Subsidy Scheme for the Laundry Trade under the Anti-epidemic Fund concluded with $85 million in subsidies approved, the Environment Bureau said.

The Financial Industry Recruitment Scheme for Tomorrow under the second round of the Anti-epidemic Fund would open for applications on September 30, the Financial Services & the Treasury Bureau announced. $180 million was set for the scheme to help create 1,500 new jobs in the

---

84   HKU: https://fightcovid19.hku.hk/ben-cowling-public-health-policies-should-be-based-on-scientific-evidence/

financial services industry to employ local people and further the industry's development.

Major Development

21.09 HKU[85]: Ben Cowling warned of the fourth wave of infections sooner than expected. He said the fourth wave could result from leftover infections from the third wave instead of from imported cases.

23.09 The overall situation concerning the face-to-face class resumption of Secondary and Primary 1, 5 and 6 as well as Kindergarten 3 was smooth in general, the Education Bureau says.

27.09–03.10 (5,109/105)**

Public Health Policies

29.09 Relaxation of the boundary controls between Hong Kong and the Mainland might proceed in a gradual manner with due consideration given to the public health risks posed by COVID-19, Chief Executive Carrie Lam said.

The Government announced that the requirements and restrictions applicable to catering and scheduled premises would be largely maintained until 8 Oct and rules on team sports and religious gatherings will be eased.

The Labour Department announced the free COVID-19 testing service for foreign domestic helpers waiting to join their new employers would be extended to 15 Oct.

30.09 The Transport Department today announced that free, voluntary COVID-19 tests would be arranged for taxi and public light bus drivers starting 3 Oct.

Socio-Economic Policy Packages

28.09 Further to the first and second rounds of the Anti-epidemic Fund, the Government said it would continue to support the tourism industry to help tide it over this challenging time, benefitting about 23,400 people.

29.09 The Government invited contactless payment service providers to indicate interest and submit service package information for promotion purposes under the subsidy scheme for promotion of contactless payment in public markets. The Government would provide a one-off subsidy to stall tenants of markets and cooked food stalls at a flat rate of $5,000 per stall.

30.09 The Club-house Subsidy Scheme was open for applications until 30 Oct.

04.10–10.10 (5,176/105)**

Public Health Policies

05.10 SCMP[86]: Experts warned that fourth wave infection in Hong Kong was looming.

06.10 The Government announced that the social distancing measures would be maintained until 15 Oct and rules on team sports held at public skating rinks would be eased.

08.10 The Hospital Authority announced that the distribution hours for specimen collection packs at 46 general outpatient clinics would be extended from October 9 to tie in with the Government's epidemic control strategy.

09.10 In view of the recent confirmed COVID-19 cases involving Thai people, the Home Affairs Department and Lok Sin Tong would jointly arrange a voluntary free testing service for them in Kowloon City.

The Government announced that it would set up temporary testing centres in locations related to recent community outbreak clusters in view of the worsening COVID-19 epidemic situation, four districts, namely Wan Chai, Kwai Tsing, Kowloon City and Yau Tsim Mong.

Socio-Economic Policy Packages

05.10 The Education Bureau issued letters or circular memorandum to all kindergartens, private primary and secondary day schools as well as tutorial schools to inform them of the details of a one-off grant under the Anti-epidemic Fund ranging from $30,000 to $80,000 each.

06.10 The Social Welfare Department launched the second round of a special grant to assist child care centres to tide over financial difficulties arising from the prolonged service suspension.

08.10 The Food & Environmental Hygiene Department announced that the subsidy schemes for commercial bathhouse licence holders and places of public entertainment licence holders will open from 9 Oct.

The Education Bureau would provide one-off relief grants for catering service suppliers for schools and post-secondary education institutions

---

85   HKU: https://fightcovid19.hku.hk/ben-cowling-warns-of-the-fourth-wave-of-infections-sooner-than-expected/

86   *SCMP*: www.scmp.com/news/hong-kong/health-environment/article/3104111/coronavirus-when-will-hong-kongs-fourth-wave

as well as interest class providers and school bus services. The additional expenditure was estimated to be $248.9 million.

09.10 The Scheme on Relief Grants for Interest Class Instructors Hired by Organisations Subvented by the Social Welfare Department (Phase 2) opened for applications, providing a one-off relief grant of $5,000 to interest class instructors.

Eligible cinemas, places of amusement and sports coaches could apply for one-off grants under the third round of the Anti-epidemic Fund from 9 Oct, the Government announced.

Fresh rounds of the Amusement Game Centres Subsidy Scheme and the Mahjong/Tin Kau Licence Holder Subsidy Scheme under the Anti-epidemic Fund opened for applications on 9 Oct.

The Catering Business Subsidy Scheme under the third-round of the Anti-epidemic Fund would invite applications from 13 Oct to 12 Nov, which provided subsidies ranging from $ 50,000 to 250,000 to eligible applicants. It would benefit about 17,000 catering outlets. So far, over $ 3.2 billion was disbursed.

Major Development

06.10 Secretary for Food & Health Prof Sophia Chan today attended a virtual meeting of the World Health Organiza-tion (WHO) Regional Committee for the Western Pacific.

07.10 The 8th Hong Kong Games was post-poned for a year due to the COVID-19 epidemic situation, the Leisure & Cultural Services Department announces.

08.10 Director of Health Dr Constance Chan said the increasing trend in the number of local COVID-19 cases with an unknown source of infec-tion was worrying.

09.10 Secretary for De-velopment Michael Wong and Under Secretary for Food & Health Dr Chui Tak-yi inspected the newly completed com-munity treatment facility expansion at AsiaWorld-Expo, adding nearly 1,000 beds.

*11.10 – 17.10 (5,238/105)***

Public Health Policies

11.10 The Government said the temporary test-ing centres in Wan Chai and Kwai Tsing collected specimens from 1,844 people for COVID-19 nucleic acid testing.

12.10 The Government said the temporary test-ing centres in Wan Chai, Kwai Tsing, Kowloon City and Yau Tsim Mong dis-tricts collected specimens from 4,938 people for COVID-19 nucleic acid testing.

13.10 The Government announced the social distancing measures cur-rently in place would be maintained until 22 Oct.

The Food & Environmen-tal Hygiene Department met representatives of catering businesses to discuss strengthening anti-epidemic measures in catering premises to minimise the COVID-19 transmission risk.

14.10 The Government said the temporary test-ing centres in Wan Chai, Kwai Tsing, Kowloon City and Yau Tsim Mong district collected speci-mens from 8,676 people for COVID-19 nucleic acid testing as of 8pm.

15.10 Hong Kong reached a milestone agreement with Singa-pore to establish a travel bubble with a view to re-viving air travel between the two places in a safe and progressive way.

The Government decided to extend the operation period of the temporary testing centre in Yau Tsim Mong to 18 Oct after reviewing all four testing centres' usage and public demand for the testing service.

16.10 The Government would gazette the latest conditions on travellers who visited France and Russia within 14 days before arriving in Hong Kong.

The Food & Environmen-tal Hygiene Department launched a voluntary on-line declaration scheme on air changes in catering premises.

The Food & Environ-mental Hygiene Depart-ment announced that it arranged for a testing agency to deliver speci-men bottles at bar areas to encourage voluntary COVID-19 testing.

The Government said the temporary testing centres in Wan Chai, Kwai Tsing, Kowloon City and Yau Tsim Mong districts collected specimens from 14,824 people for COVID-19 testing as of 8pm on 16 Oct.

17.10 The Food & Environmental Hygiene Department and Police stepped up inspections and take enforcement ac-tion at catering business premises including bars and upstairs restaurants in Wan Chai District.

Yau Tsim Mong Tem-porary Testing Centre collected specimens from 711 people for COVID-19 nucleic acid tests, bring-ing the number of speci-mens collected at all four temporary testing centres to 15,535.

Socio-Economic Policy Packages

14.10 The Leisure & Cul-tural Services Department provided a new round of ex-gratia payment to personnel affected by the cancellation of programmes scheduled to be held in its venues or facilities due to the COVID-19 epidemic.

The Housing Author-ity would pass on the

enhanced rates concession for the third and fourth quarters to its non-domestic tenants and licensees, with a cap of $5,000 per quarter for each rateable property.

Major Development

12.10 Princess Margaret Hospital apologised for an incident involving the handling of specimens.

13.10 The Cultural Centre's Auditoria Building and Concert Hall were temporarily closed from 13 Oct as a musician who performed at the Concert Hall preliminarily tested positive for COVID-19.

HKU[87]: HKU researchers find Covid-19 treatment with ulcer drug, offering a new and readily available therapeutic option.

Stand News[88]: A letter to Professor Yuen Kwok-yung urged that a well-respected medical experts should not be used as political tool.

14.10 HKU[89]: HKU microbiologist Prof Yuen proposed mandatory testing for people with respiratory symptoms. He also called for the use of contactless payment methods to minimise cross infections.

15.10 Under Secretary for Food & Health Dr Chui

Tak-yi urged private doctors to arrange COVID-19 testing for those who have symptoms to help detect cases.

18.10 – 24.10 (5,290/105)**

Public Health Policies

18.10 The Government said the Yau Tsim Mong Temporary Testing Centre collected specimens from 1,267 people for COVID-19 nucleic acid tests, bringing the number of specimens collected at all four temporary testing centres to 16,802.

20.10 The Government announced it would relax several social distancing measures on 23 Oct, including lifting the restrictions on the number of people allowed at wedding ceremonies and indoor meeting from 20 to 50.

The Social Welfare Department announced that the fourth round of free COVID-19 testing services would be arranged for staff of residential care homes for the elderly and persons with disabilities and nursing homes from 21 Oct.

22.10 The Labour Department announced the free COVID-19 testing

service would continue to be provided for foreign domestic helpers waiting to join their new employers from 27 Oct to November 21.

Socio-Economic Policy Packages

19.10 The Fitness Centre Subsidy Scheme under the third round of the Anti-epidemic Fund opened for applications, providing a one-off subsidy of $50,000 to each eligible fitness centre.

21.10 The second round of the Subsidy Scheme for Beauty Parlours, Massage Establishments & Party Rooms under the Anti-epidemic Fund would accept applications from 23 Oct to 1 Nov.

Up until 21 Oct, the Employment Support Scheme had approved wage subsidies to a total of about 135,000 employers under the second tranche, with subsidies totalling almost $37 billion and a total committed headcount of paid employees of about 1.56 million.

23.10 The Pyrotechnics & Special Effects Operators Subsidy Scheme under the Anti-epidemic Fund was open for application until 13 Nov, a one-off

$7,500 subsidy.

The Distance Business Programme received 27,785 funding applications from enterprises, the Innovation & Technology Commission announced. As of 22 Oct, 17,252 applicants had received the funding totalling up to $970 million.

Major Development

19.10 The second-term Human Resources Planning Commission convened its second meeting to brief members on the key findings of a study on the COVID-19 pandemic's impact on the Asia-Pacific (APAC) region's labour market.

The Department of Health apologised for the inappropriate quarantine arrangement made for a COVID-19 case involving a man who arrived in Hong Kong from India.

SCMP[90]: Pandemic took 'deep toll' on Hongkongers' mental health, former justice minister said. He called for increased public vigilance against symptoms of mental health problems amid the pandemic

20.10 Apple Daily[91]: While the Hong Kong government considered imposing manda-

87   HKU: https://fightcovid19.hku.hk/hku-researchers-find-covid-19-treatment-with-ulcer-drug/

88   *Stand News*: www.thestandnews.com/society/致袁教授的信-勿讓萬人敬仰的醫學專家被利用作政治工具/

89   HKU: https://fightcovid19.hku.hk/hku-microbiologist-suggests-mandatory-testing-for-sick-people-and-using-contactless-payment-methods/

90   *SCMP*: www.scmp.com/news/hong-kong/health-environment/article/3105959/covid-19-time-bomb-pandemic-takes-deep-toll

91   *Apple Daily*: https://hk.appledaily.com/news/20201020/JF3KNCHZ5BAJLCYGSJV5HQ2LUE/

tory COVID-19 testing on patients with mild symptoms and residents of buildings with positive cases, medical experts warned that compulsory testing could backfire.

SCMP[92]: Cathay Pacific would 'axe 6,000 staff and Dragon brand' in bid to stay afloat, with most cuts aimed at Hong Kong workforce. It would also axe its Cathay Dragon sister airline brand. It reduced the lay-offs from about 8,000 to 5,000 after government intervention.

21.10 The Government required Cathay Pacific Airways to fully consider the potential impact on Hong Kong's status as an international aviation hub when restructuring its business, Financial Secretary Paul Chan said.

Chief Executive Carrie Lam said the government's commitment to medical research is clearly evident in the Government's efforts to combat COVID-19. To date, the government had already allocated nearly US$35 million in support of some 50 COVID-19 research studies.

Apple Daily[93]: The Hong Kong Laboratory Accreditation Scheme (HOKLAS) include wide ranges of accreditation, for example, food, Chinese medicine, chemistry, building materials. It also covers the qualification of testers and protection of privacy.

Apple Daily[94]: Five virus testing laboratories were found not accreditated by HOKLAS. The five labs conducted over 27,3000 tests, estimated to cost over $101 million.

23.10 SCMP[95]: Hong Kong was battling a potentially deadly superbug:136 cases of fungal infection Candida auris so far this year, compared to 20 in whole of 2019. This could be due to indirect impacts from Covid-19 as isolation wards were being used up.

25.10 – 31.10 (5,324/105)**

Public Health Policies

26.10 The Transport Department announced that free, voluntary COVID-19 tests would be arranged for taxi and public light bus drivers from 27 Oct to 9 Nov.

27.10 The Government announced social distancing measures would be further relaxed from October 30 for seven days, including raising the maximum number of people allowed to be seated together at one table from four to six in restaurants and bars and allowing dine-in services until 2am.

The government announced to add Belgium to high-risk list.

The Leisure & Cultural Services Department announced that all gazetted beaches under the department would reopen on 3 Nov.

30.10 Sixty-three projects had been approved under the Public Sector Trial Scheme to combat the COVID-19 epidemic with total funding of over $102 million, the Innovation & Technology Commission announced.

Socio-Economic Policy Packages

30.10 The Sports Premises Subsidy Scheme under the third round of the Anti-epidemic Fund was opened for applications, which would provide a one-off subsidy of $30,000 to each eligible sports premises.

Major Development

25.10 Chief Executive Carrie Lam described the epidemic situation in Hong Kong as generally stable.

27.10 HKU[96]: Prof. Yuen Kwok-yung called on to test patients with mild symptoms, which could reduce hidden community spread.

28.10 Chief Executive Carrie Lam received the seasonal influenza vaccination and urged citizens to get vaccinated early to prepare for the winter influenza surge.

Customs announced it detected the largest-ever counterfeit face mask case on 28 Oct, when it seized about 100,000 masks in a special operation. It was estimated the market value reached about $3 million and were intended to be transshipped overseas via Hong Kong.

30.10 The Government announced it recorded a $279.8 billion deficit for the six months ending 30 Sept. Expenditure for the period was $427.8 billion and revenue was $148 billion. Fiscal reserves stood at $880.5 billion at the end of September.

01.11 – 07.11

Public Health Policies

02.11 The Social Welfare Department launched a new round of the Anti-virus Coating Spray

92   *SCMP*: www.scmp.com/news/hong-kong/transport/article/3106279/cathay-pacific-axe-6000-staff-and-close-dragon-brand-bid

93   *Apple Daily*: https://hk.appledaily.com/local/20201021/PJZ55ABA4NFE3BZINYKG2ABPAI/

94   *Apple Daily*: https://hk.appledaily.com/local/20201021/CMG3XWGKVBBUDHJ7JBRZZJZMNA/

95   *SCMP*: www.scmp.com/news/hong-kong/health-environment/article/3106874/hong-kong-battling-potentially-deadly-superbug

96   HKU: https://fightcovid19.hku.hk/zh/袁國勇呼籲盡量檢測有病徵者/

Subsidy to support about 1,100 residential care homes for the elderly and the disabled.

03.11 The Government was setting up four longer-term COVID-19 community testing centres at Quarry Bay Community Hall, Henry G Leong Yaumatei Community Centre, Lek Yuen Community Hall and Yuen Long Town East Community Hall.

The Government announced the social distancing measures currently in place would be maintained until 12 Nov.

The Government announced to add Turkey on the high-risk list.

The Hospital Authority announced that time slots for distribution of specimen collection packs would be increased at 46 general outpatient clinics for more convenient COVID-19 testing.

Free COVID-19 testing for teachers and staff in kindergartens and primary, secondary and special schools would be arranged from November 9, the Education Bureau announced.

04.11 The Food & Environmental Hygiene Department announced it would contact bar and pub operators to arrange voluntary free COVID-19 testing for their staff.

The Government launched a 24-month special measure through the second round of the Anti-epidemic Fund to in-

spect the external drainage systems of about 20,000 private buildings, Secretary for Development Michael Wong said.

The government had been following up proactively on the exemption from compulsory quarantine for Hong Kong residents in Guangdong and Macau, Chief Secretary Matthew Cheung said.

The Government would arrange a testing agency to distribute and collect specimen bottles in Mui Wo and Tai Wai for three consecutive days from November 5 for people to undergo COVID-19 testing.

Socio-Economic Policy Packages

02.11 As of noon 2 Nov, the Distance Business Programme had received 38,572 funding applications, among which it had processed 20,772 applications and approved 18,025 of them with total funding of around $1.02 billion.

The Housing Authority extended for another six months the time-limited arrangement allowing banks and financial institutions to offer a mortgage principal moratorium plan to Subsidised Sale Flats Scheme mortgagors.

Major Development

03.11 The Government reminded employers not to dismiss foreign domestic helpers who have contracted COVID-19.

08.11 – 14.11
Public Health Policies

08.11 The Government arranged a testing agency to distribute and collect deep throat saliva specimen bottles in Tai Po for three consecutive days from 8 Nov.

The Leisure & Cultural Services Department stepped up patrols of public beaches to call on users to comply with regulations on the limit on the number of people in group gatherings and the mask-wearing requirement.

COVID-19 in Macao:
A Brief Review of the Macao Government's Anti-epidemic Measures

Li Lue

The measures taken by the Macau government to fight the pandemic display the characteristics of "QPRS": Quick, Precise, Ruthless, and Strong. 'Quick' refers to the speed of setting up a response mechanism, starting medical check and quarantine, and effecting public dissemination. 'Precise' refers to the precision of the control and supply chain measures for essential items such as masks. 'Ruthless' refers to the decisive cancelation of all large-scale events, quarantines of all Wuhan visitors, closure of casinos, schools and government agencies. 'Strong' refers to the strength of the economic assistance to residents and business. Macao has thus successively contained Covid-19 pandemic.

Foreword

Macao is a tourist city, with nearly 40 million tourists in 2019, and nearly 7 million tourists in January-February 2019 alone. In addition, Macao has close contacts with surrounding areas, and the number of arrivals and departures in 2019 reached 194 million. Therefore, when the new crown epidemic occurred in 2020, Macao's risks and pressures were enormous. Fortunately, the government's response measures are timely and effective. Until May 20, 2020, there were only 45 confirmed cases, with zero death, zero health care–associated infection (HAI or HCAI), zero community infection, and all have been healed and discharged[1].

Looking back on the experience of Macao in the fight against the epidemic, it can be divided into two phases. The first phase is from January 1 to March 14. From January 1st, the response measures were taken, to the first confirmed case on January 22[2], and then new response measures were continuously added and the response was strengthened. Leading up to the tenth case confirmed on February 4, there were 10 confirmed cases in 14 days, including 8 imported cases and 2 related cases. After February 4, there were 40 days with no more case.

From March 15 to present is the second stage of the fight against the epidemic. As the overseas epidemic worsened, many Macao residents living overseas returned to Macao. By April 8th, there were an increase of 35 imported cases in 24 days, making Macao a total of 45 cases. Since April 8, there has been no more new case, and all cases were discharged from the hospital by May 19. Only on June 26, 2020 there came one more case.

Recalling the anti-epidemic measures of the Macao SAR Government, it can be summarized as the following characteristics: "QPRS", quick, precise and ruthless, and plus the economic aid measures are "strong".

---

1   Most of the statistics data comes from the webpages of Statistics and Census Service, Government of Macao Special Administrative Region: www.dsec.gov.mo/en-US/

2   Most of the epidemic data comes from the special webpage against epidemics: www.ssm.gov.mo/apps1/PreventCOVID-19/en.aspx#clg17458

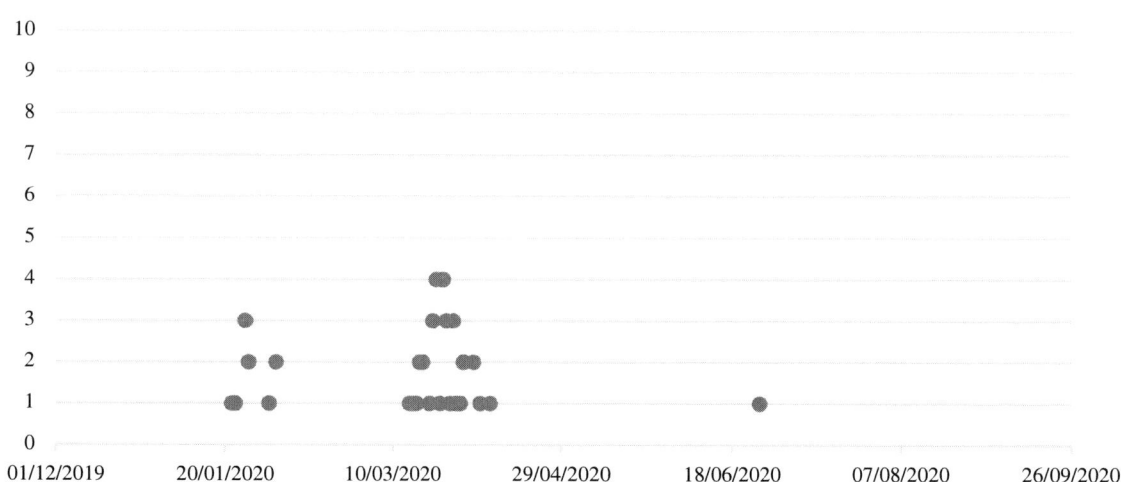

Figure 6.1 Confirmed new cases of Covid-19 in Macao

Table 6.1 Main monitoring

Country or Regions	updated on	Cumulative cases	No. of cases	Serious cases	Cured	deadly cases	Cumulative number of suspected cases (confirmed cases not included)	
							Not confirmed	To be confirmed
Macao Situation – China	31/08/2020	46	0	1	46	0	4191	0

Quick

Quick Start of Quarantine Measures

Macao received a notice from the National Health Commission on unexplained viral pneumonia in Wuhan on December 31, 2019[3]. The SAR government immediately conducted body temperature screening at the Macao International Airport for passengers from Wuhan on the next day, January 1, 2020. The government also increased the number of personnel to strengthen the health and quarantine measures at all ports, especially airports. From January 2, 2020, passengers from Wuhan flights were required to complete a health declaration form. From January 4, 2020, the temperature screening for all drivers and passengers was expanded to all ports[4].

---

3   Macao SAR Government Portal. Retrieved June 2, 2020 from www.gov.mo/zh-hant/news/312621/
4   Same as above.

**Table 6.2 Information about confirmed diagnosed patients
with novel coronavirus (Covid-19) in Macau SAR[5]**

| Case Number | Patient brief details | | | Diagnosis date | Patient Condition |
	Region or Country	Sex	Age		
No. 1	Wuhan	F	52	22/01/2020	Recovered and discharged
No. 2	Wuhan	M	66	23/01/2020	Recovered and discharged
No. 3	Wuhan	F	57	26/01/2020	Recovered and discharged
No. 4	Wuhan	F	39	26/01/2020	Recovered and discharged
No. 5	Wuhan	F	21	26/01/2020	Recovered and discharged
No. 6	Wuhan	M	15	27/01/2020	Recovered and discharged
No. 7	Wuhan	F	67	27/01/2020	Recovered and discharged
No. 8	Macao	F	64	02/02/2020	Recovered and discharged
No. 9	Macao	F	29	04/02/2020	Recovered and discharged
No. 10	Macao	M	56	04/02/2020	Recovered and discharged
No. 11	Korea	F	26	15/03/2020	Recovered and discharged
No. 12	Spain	M	47	16/03/2020	Recovered and discharged
No. 13	Macao	F	20	17/03/2020	Recovered and discharged
No. 14	Indonesia	F	42	18/03/2020	Recovered and discharged
No. 15	Philippines	M	31	18/03/2020	Recovered and discharged
No. 16	Macao	F	19	19/03/2020	Recovered and discharged
No. 17	Indonesia	M	11	19/03/2020	Recovered and discharged
No. 18	Macao	F	50	21/03/2020	Recovered and discharged
No. 19	Macao	M	19	22/03/2020	Recovered and discharged
No. 20	Macao	M	20	22/03/2020	Recovered and discharged
No. 21	Macao	F	19	22/03/2020	Recovered and discharged
No. 22	Macao	M	44	23/03/2020	Recovered and discharged
No. 23	Macao	M	12	23/03/2020	Recovered and discharged
No. 24	Macao	M	21	23/03/2020	Recovered and discharged
No. 25	Indonesia	M	41	23/03/2020	Recovered and discharged
No. 26	Macao	F	17	24/03/2020	Recovered and discharged
No. 27	Macao	M	28	25/03/2020	Recovered and discharged
No. 28	Macao	M	18	25/03/2020	Recovered and discharged
No. 29	Macao	F	15	25/03/2020	Recovered and discharged
No. 30	Australia	M	52	25/03/2020	Recovered and discharged
No. 31	Macao	M	27	26/03/2020	Recovered and discharged
No. 32	Philippines	M	31	26/03/2020	Recovered and discharged
No. 33	Philippines	F	37	26/03/2020	Recovered and discharged
No. 34	Macao	M	43	27/03/2020	Recovered and discharged
No. 35	Macao	M	19	28/03/2020	Recovered and discharged
No. 36	Macao	M	21	28/03/2020	Recovered and discharged
No. 37	Macao	M	32	28/03/2020	Recovered and discharged
No. 38	Macao	M	44	29/03/2020	Recovered and discharged
No. 39	Macao	F	9	30/03/2020	Recovered and discharged
No. 40	Macao	F	47	31/03/2020	Recovered and discharged
No. 41	Macao	M	20	31/03/2020	Recovered and discharged
No. 42	Macao	M	58	03/04/2020	Recovered and discharged
No. 43	Macao	F	53	03/04/2020	Recovered and discharged
No. 44	Macao	M	52	05/04/2020	Recovered and discharged
No. 45	Macao	M	32	08/04/2020	Recovered and discharged
No. 46	Macao	M	57	26/06/2020	Recovered and discharged

Note: Content in the above table is updated after 16:00 daily.

5   Same as above.

Set Up a Response Mechanism Quickly

On January 5, 2020, the SAR government established the "Macao's Inter-departmental Taskforce on Pneumonia of Unknown Cause" to respond to the epidemic and raise the early warning level to level III (heavier)[6].

Since Macao is dominated by the gambling industry, the prevention and control measures for infectious diseases in casinos was implemented right away from January 6, 2020, to detect body temperature for people entering casinos[7].

With the development of the epidemic, new measures have been continuously introduced. With the increase of the domestic epidemic and the emergence of overseas epidemics, he Novel Coronavirus Response and Coordination Centre (NCRCC) was established by the government on January 21, 2020[8]. The Centre is directly under the supervision of the Chief Executive and the Secretary for Social Affairs and Culture is the Centre's vice chairperson. The Centre is responsible for the overall planning, guidance and coordination of public and private entities on the prevention, control and treatment of novel coronavirus epidemics.

With the first diagnosis of pneumonia in Macao on January 22, 2020, in a 52-year-old female tourist from Wuhan, the public sector implemented measures to deal with novel coronaviruses, including to monitor the body temperature, provide hand sanitizer and masks for coughers in the government building. All frontline staff were required to wear masks.[9]

From January 23, 2020, health declarations were implemented in every port, either in paper or in electronic form. Passengers could scan the QR code posted on every port using their mobile phones or enter the website https://service.ssm.gov.mo/ hdeclaration / and fill in personal health information. After completion, the health declaration certificate would be displayed in their mobile phones. Passengers must show their health declaration certificate to the officers when passing the customs[10].

Publish Information Fast

On January 23, 2020, the NCRCC released a special webpage for information release, as well as some social media. The Information Bureau also launched the Telegram group of the novel coronavirus epidemic channel on January 26, 2020.[11]

---

6 Macao SAR Government Portal. Retrieved June 2, 2020 from www.gov.mo/zh-hant/news/312833/

7 Macao SAR Government Portal. Retrieved June 2, 2020 from www.gov.mo/zh-hant/news/312929/

8 www.gov.mo/zh-hant/news/314619/

9 www.gov.mo/zh-hant/news/314825/

10 www.gov.mo/zh-hant/news/315005/

11 www.gov.mo/zh-hant/news/315233/

Precise

Precise Control of the Customs

Because the outbreak of Covid-19 in the mainland was concentrated in Wuhan in the beginning, the initial prevention and control measurement of Macao was also directed at Wuhan. For example, from January 1, 2020, the temperature of passengers from Wuhan was screened at Macao International Airport. From January 2, all passengers from Wuhan were required to fill out health declaration form[12].

With the first case diagnosed on January 22, the second case on January 23, and three more cases on January 26, all of them from Wuhan, from January 27, 2020 all travelers from Hubei and travelers who have been to Hubei within 14 days were required to present a health certificate that is free of novel coronavirus infection[13].

With the rapid development of the Korean epidemic, on February 24, 2020, the Macao government announced that people who had visited South Korea within 14 days before arriving in Macao should go to the Workers Stadium or the checkpoint at Bei'an Pier in Taipa for medical examination. On February 26, 2020, all people who have visited South Korea within 14 days before entry, including Macao residents, passengers and foreign employees, are required to conduct 14-day medical observations at designated locations in accordance with the requirements of the health authorities after entry[14].

With the development of overseas epidemic situation, the Macao SAR Government announced on February 29, 2020 that all immigrants who have been to Italy or Iran within 14 days before entering Macao must undergo medical observation at the designated location for 14[15]. Then on March 8, it was announced that all immigrants who had been to Germany, France, Spain, or Japan within 14 days before entry must undergo medical examination[16]. On March 12, it was announced that all immigrants who had been to Norway within 14 days before entry must undergo medical examination[17]. It was announced on March 14 that all students returning to Macao from overseas, including students who return to Macao regardless of education stage, must undergo a 14-day medical observation[18].

With the continuous confirmation of imported cases after March 15th, it was announced on March 17th that all persons who have visited countries or regions outside China within 14 days prior to entry must follow the requirements of the Health Bureau and accept 14 days of medical observation at designated locations after entry[19]. The next day, it announced an almost-closed- customs-ban on all non-local residents, except residents of the Mainland of China, Hong Kong and Taiwan and holders of identification cards for foreign employees who enter the Macao Special Administrative Region[20]. On March 19, all foreign employee are prohibited from entering Macao, except whom from mainland China, Hong Kong and Taiwan. On March 25, all residents of the Mainland, Hong Kong and Taiwan

---

12 www.gov.mo/zh-hant/news/312621/

13 www.gov.mo/zh-hant/news/315240/

14 www.gov.mo/zh-hant/news/320064/

15 https://news.gov.mo/detail/en/N20BcSVHAA?2

16 www.gov.mo/zh-hant/news/322218/

17 https://news.gov.mo/detail/zh-hant/N20CKha831?3

18 www.gov.mo/zh-hant/news/323213/

19 www.gov.mo/zh-hant/news/323430/

20 www.gov.mo/zh-hant/news/323457/

who have visited a foreign country within 14 days before entry are prohibited from entering Macao. All persons who have visited the Hong Kong or Taiwan within 14 days prior to entry must be subject to 14 days of medical observation at designated locations as required by the health authorities[21].

As can be seen from the above, with the development of the external epidemic situation, the SAR government has gradually implemented increasingly stringent immigration control measures, effectively restricting imported cases.

Precise Collection of Information

After receiving the notification from the National Health Commission for the first time on December 31, 2019, Macao SAR government maintained close contact with it and also monitored the epidemic situation in the Mainland closely. From January 13th to 14th, 2020, according to the arrangement of the National Health Commission, the SAR Government sent three representatives to Wuhan to investigate the local situation and exchange information with representatives from the mainland to understand the local unexplained pneumonia epidemic situation, patient diagnosis, treatment and prevention[22].

On January 21, 2020, the government established a novel coronavirus infection response coordination center, operating 24 hours, and set up a hotline 2870-0800 to serve the public[23].

On January 22, 2020, Chief Executive Ho Iat Seng met with Academician Zhong Nanshan, the head of the Expert Group of the National Health and Welfare Commission[24]. He pointed out that Macao's population is highly concentrated, and there are many Casino hotels. Macao should cooperate with Guangdong to prevent the "super spreaders" and control the spread of the epidemic. At the same time, Macao also needed to strengthen the protective measures of hospitals and medical staff to ensure safety. In addition, on a press conference of high-level panel of experts from the National Health Commission about the new coronavirus pneumonia on January 20, 2020, both Dr. Yuen Kwok-yun and Academician Zhong Nanshan clearly proposed the role of masks in preventing the new coronavirus. The Macao government changed the general policy of wearing masks only when needed, began to call on the public to wear surgical masks in public, and launched a plan to supply masks to Macao residents on January 23, 2020[25].

Precise Information Dissemination for Residents

From the beginning, many special lectures were held for the medical, tourism, and education sectors to introduce measures and precautions for the prevention and control of the epidemic[26].

Beginning on January 26, the Higher Education Bureau followed up the situation of Macao students studying in Wuhan, suggesting them staying at home for self-isolation for 14 days after returning to Macao, and paying attention to physical conditions. If you feel unwell, you should see a doctor immediately. The government urges Macao residents on vacation in the Mainland to return to

---

21   www.gov.mo/zh-hant/news/324556/
22   www.ssm.gov.mo/apps1/PreventCOVID-19/ch.aspx#clg17458
23   www.gov.mo/zh-hant/news/314619/
24   www.gov.mo/zh-hant/news/314871/
25   www.gov.mo/zh-hant/news/315010/
26   https://news.gov.mo/detail/zh-hant/N20AZ52ujH?0

Macao as soon as possible, and calls for staying at home for 14 days of self-isolation; civil servants must fill out a health declaration form before going to work. In response to the development of novel coronavirus epidemics, the start date of basic education and higher education has been continuously delayed to avoid crowds. For students studying overseas, the Higher Education Bureau can assist them in purchasing masks after registration. The Social Work Bureau has set up a psychological support hotline 28261126 for Macao residents or people in Macao when they need help. The hotline (2870 0800) for enquiries on epidemic matters has been increased to 12 lines, and a team has been set up to follow up on handling rumors.

Precisely Resolve Citizens' Concerns: Ensure the Supply of Masks

Because of the experience of SARS in 2003, the government released the information as early as January 8, 2020 that the Macao market has enough masks to supply so the public needed not worry too much[27]. At that time the government still believed that the public did not need to wear masks at all times[28]. On January 13, 2020, the government emphasized again that the supply of masks is sufficient and the public needed not worry too much. The government would ensure that the stock and supply of masks in Macao was stable[29]. On January 23, the Health Bureau launched a plan to ensure the supply of masks to Macao residents[30]. Residents can hold permanent / non-permanent resident ID cards or foreign employee identification cards to buy 10 masks for MOP$8, in 56 registered pharmacies in Macao. A repeat purchase can be made after 10 days. Moreover, since many shops are closed for holidays during the Spring Festival, residents can go to 8 health centers and 2 health stations under the Health Bureau to purchase masks for the mask plan.

Ruthless

Cancel All Large-scale Chinese New Year Events

On January 23, 2020, the government announced the cancellation of all large-scale public events during the Spring Festival, and urged the public to reduce their outings during the Spring Festival, and hope that the cultural activities and spring tea held by various societies can be cancelled or postponed to avoid crowding and to reduce risk[31].

On January 25, 2020, the Novel Coronavirus Infection Response Coordination Center called on theaters and large-scale performances to be suspended, and citizens should wear masks on buses[32].

27　www.gov.mo/zh-hant/news/313187/

28　Same as above.

29　www.gov.mo/zh-hant/news/313811/

30　www.gov.mo/zh-hant/news/315010/

31　www.gov.mo/zh-hant/news/314986/

32　www.gov.mo/zh-hant/news/315188/

Restrict and Isolate Wuhan Passengers

Starting at 0:00 on January 27, all non-local Macao residents from Hubei Province and non-local Macao residents who have been to Hubei Province within 14 days before entering Macao must present a non-infected certificate of novel coronavirus issued by a legal medical institution[33]. The staff of the Health Bureau will verify the relevant certificate in accordance with the law. If necessary, they will confirm with the medical institution that issued the certificate. Those who cannot produce or fail to verify the relevant certificate will be refused entry into Macao.

In addition, all people who have visited Hubei Province within 14 days before entering Macao are restricted from entering casinos.

Starting at 9 a.m. on January 27, the SAR government contacted about 1,113 tourists from Hubei. Among them, more than 700 people were in Macao hotels. If there were no suspected symptoms, they were advised either they leave Macao, or if they chose to stay in Macao, they were admitted to the Hac-Sa Youth Hostel and the Urban Council Hac-Sa Training Center for compulsory isolation[34].

Restrict access to the casino

From January 27, all people who have visited Hubei Province within 14 days before entering Macao are restricted from entering any casino[35].

Government Civil Servants Exempt from work and Only Keep Emergency Services

After the Spring Festival, civil servants were exempted from going to work. The first order to stay home was only for two days[36], and then it extended to March 1 after weekly assessment. The government fully worked normally and resumed services on Match 2[37].

Delayed Start of School

With the first and second confirmed cases on January 22 and 23, it was announced on the 24th that the Chinese New Year holiday for all students would be extended to February 10[38]. Afterwards, with the development of the epidemic, it continued to be exteended. Classes were resumed gradually after the epidemic situation got stable, the higher education was resumed gradually after April 1, and non-tertiary education was resumed in separate stages on May 4[39].

---

33 www.gov.mo/zh-hant/news/315240/
34 www.gov.mo/zh-hant/news/315246/
35 www.gov.mo/zh-hant/news/315279/
36 www.macaodaily.com/html/2020-01/29/content_1412516.htm
37 www.gov.mo/zh-hant/news/317401/
38 https://news.rthk.hk/rthk/ch/component/k2/1504700-20200124.htm
39 www.exmoo.com/article/146924.html

Close Down Casinos

After evaluation, the government decided to suspend business for 15 days at 41 casinos, cinemas, theaters, bars, internet cafes, discos and dance halls across Macao starting at 0:00 on February 5. In addition, after discussions with gaming companies, the six major gaming companies promised not to require employees to take unpaid leave to reflect their responsibility to society and work together to fight the epidemic.

Strong

On February 13, 2020, the SAR Government Launched a Number of Economic Assistance Measures with Great Efforts

The total amount is about 40 billion Patacas, based on the population of 650,000 in Macao, equivalent to 61,000 Patacas per person[40]. The purpose is to "stabilize the economy and secure employment". The plan included five major directions. (1) Reductions and exemptions of Taxes and fees to reduce the burden on businesses and residents; (2) SME (Small and Medium Enterprises) assistance and interest subsidies to support the survival of enterprises; (3) Measures to strengthen people's livelihood and to support vulnerable families; (4) Improve skills training, implement work-for-relief, and protect the wage earners; (5) Launch electronic consumer cards to accelerate the recovery of people's livelihood and the economy.

(1) Reductions and exemptions of Taxes and fees to reduce the burden on businesses and residents[41]

Adjust the supplementary income tax, and deduct a cap of MOP 300,000 for the supplementary income tax in 2019. The benefit will cover commercial enterprises including SMEs, totally around 2,970 companies.

Adjust the occupation tax, refund 70% of the 2018 occupation tax paid, and the maximum amount of tax refund is MOP 20,000, benefiting 170,000 local employees.

The fixed deduction for the increase in the taxable income of the occupation tax in 2020 will be increased from the current 25% to 30%, benefiting 180,000 local employees.

Exempt all housing taxes levied on Macao residents' residences in 2019, benefiting 180,000 homes; at the same time, 25% of the housing tax on commercial premises will also be exempted, benefiting 25,000 commercial premises.

Exempt the 5% six-month tourism tax on tourist service places such as hotels, bars, fitness rooms and karaoke, benefiting 854 places.

Refund the license tax for all business vehicles.

In addition, the administrative license fees and stamp duties levied by various administrative departments and entities are exempted or refunded in 2020.

---

40 www.gov.mo/zh-hant/news/318253/
41 www.gov.mo/zh-hant/news/318146/

(2) Promote the assistance of small and medium-sized enterprises and interest subsidies to support the survival of enterprises

The temporary "SME Loan Interest Subsidy Program" was launched for SMEs that received bank loans due to a shortage of funds caused by the epidemic. The government provides 4% subsidy interest with a maximum loan amount of 2 million and a maximum of 3 years.

Launched a special "SME Assistance Program" for SMEs operating for less than 2 years, providing interest-free assistance loans with a ceiling of 600,000 patacas and a maximum repayment period of 8 years.

(3) Measures Strengthen people's livelihood and to support vulnerable families

In this year's medical subsidy program, an extra 600 MOP medical voucher is temporarily issued to each permanent resident of the SAR in response to the continuing need to fight the epidemic.

Subsidize all the water and electricity bills of Macao residents for 3 months.

Two more months of assistance will be paid to vulnerable families with financial assistance from the Social Work Bureau.

(4) Improve skills training, implement work-for-relief, and protect wage earners

When the epidemic is under control, the government would improve the professional skills training of local employees to match the government's increased infrastructure investment, and there are a large number of types of jobs in demand.

(5) Launching electronic consumer cards to accelerate the recovery of the people's livelihood and the economy

After the epidemic has eased, the SAR Government will issue electronic consumer vouchers with a value of 3,000 patacas to Macao residents. The consumption vouchers must be deducted from consumption in Macao's catering, retail, and grocery stores and are valid for a period of three months.

On March 28, 2020, the SAR Government Established a Special Fund for 10 Billion Anti-epidemic Assistance[42], and Announced the Details of the Second Round of Epidemic Economic Aid Measures on April 8, 2020[43].

The second round of economic assistance measures includes: direct financial assistance to qualified local employees, specifically based on the calculation of 25% of the median monthly working income (20,000 patacas) of Macao residents in 2019, and a three-off payment, that is, 15,000 patacas. One-time assistance for freelancers and interest subsidies for bank loans; based on the scale of the company's operations and the number of employees. Unemployment training and on-the-job training are available to all workers. From August to December of this year, an additional consumption subsidy (MOP 5,000) was issued to all Macao residents, together with the first phase of a total of MOP 8,000.

---

42   www.gov.mo/zh-hant/news/325491/
43   www.gov.mo/zh-hant/news/326766/

Summary

According to a public welfare online questionnaire survey conducted by the Macao Poll Research Association,[44] nearly 90% of the interviewed residents expressed satisfaction with the overall performance of the SAR government in responding to the epidemic (very / quite satisfied: 87.7%), and believed that the best thing the government did was "supply masks" (88.8%), followed by casino closure (77.7%), quick response (74.2%), public transport passengers must wear a mask (74.0%), reduce population flow (73.5%). In addition, the interviewed residents paid high attention to the relevant information released by the government (84.0% always pay attention or often pay attention), almost all said that the information on the epidemic situation or response measures issued by the government was helpful (97.5%). It can be seen that the government has been affirmed by most residents in different aspects such as epidemic prevention work and information distribution.

The Women's Federation of Macao launched a survey in late February, 2020[45], using an online questionnaire. It successfully collected thousands of valid questionnaires for analysis. The survey results showed a high level of satisfaction with the SAR government's anti-epidemic performance, with an overall score of 8.4 (out of 10). Nearly 85% of the interviewees believed that measures such as assisting in the sale of masks on behalf of the community would bring great help to the public and further reduce the impact of the epidemic on society.

According to a survey by the Doctoral Think Tank Committee of the Macao Youth Patriotic Education Association[46], the top five "anti-epidemic" measures that the interviewees were most satisfied with were the "Protection of Masks for the Provision of Macao Citizens Program" (88.5%), and "Immigration Measures" (82%), "Abolition of all large-scale activities during the Spring Festival" (81.4%), "Isolation Measures for Passengers from Hubei" (78.1%) and "All colleges, non-higher education institutions and private supplementary teaching aid center will delay the start of classes, and the subsidized nursery will suspend services "(76.5%).

In short, due to the quick, accurate and ruthless government prevention and control measures, Macao has achieved zero death, zero community infection, zero health care–associated infection（HAI or HCAI）, and zero community infection. Only one case of serious illness has been treated and all cases have been cured and discharged. The subsidy measures are strong, so most residents are satisfied with the performance of the SAR government in fighting the epidemic.

---

44   www.e-research-solutions.com/news/post/5e61ec5a94849e0015132017

45   www.macaodaily.com/html/2020-03/30/content_1424466.htm

46   http://tyzx.people.cn/BIG5/n1/2020/0214/c372375-31586268.html

MACAO

Li Lue
01.01–05.09 Total 46 cases / 0 deaths

01.01 – 04.01

Public Health Policies[1]

01.01 The Government of the Macao Special Administrative Region (SAR) kept in close contact with the National Health Commission of the People's Republic of China regarding the latest developments concerning a cluster of pneumonia cases in Wuhan, Hubei Province.

At the Macao International Airport, body temperature screening was implemented to passengers on flights departing from Wuhan. More manpower was deployed to various cross-boundary checkpoints, especially the airport, to reinforce health inspection and quarantine efforts.

02.01 In order to strengthen surveillance of the health status of travelers, all passengers on flights departing from Wuhan were required to fill out a health declaration form. This measure would be ongoing.

The Government held a meeting to brief representatives of the local casino gaming sector on guidelines and measures for the prevention in Macao of an outbreak of disease.

04.01 Body temperature screening was in place in all Macao-bound carriageways. Under the assistance of the officers of the Public Security Police Force, the Health Bureau conducted temperature screening to drivers and travelers who entered Macao via land-based checkpoints such as the Border Gate, Hong Kong-Zhuhai-Macao Bridge Border, Zhuhai-Macao Cross Border Industrial Zone and Cotai Frontier Post (Lotus Border).

05.01 – 11.01

Public Health Policies

05.01 Macao issued on Sunday (5 January) a Level III alert in response to the Wuhan pneumonia outbreak. The alert level meant the risk of public emergency was at moderate level, indicating public health factors – of either environmental or technological origin – requiring firm follow-up action by the local authorities.

the Macao Customs Service further deployed temperature-monitoring equipment at checkpoint facilities, and work in concert with the Municipal Affairs Bureau to combat illegal import of animal-based foodstuffs;

the Municipal Affairs Bureau stepped up effort regarding inspection and quarantine work; combine its effort with that of the Customs Service in order to strengthen efforts to prevent illegal importation and sale of animals; and strengthen hygiene maintenance in public spaces;

the Macao Government Tourism Office remained in close contact with the tourism sector, including disseminating the latest guidelines related with this matter and assisting the Health Bureau with provision – where required – of training for employees in the tourism sector;

The Gaming Inspection and Coordination Bureau and the Health Bureau continued to provide assistance to casinos for installation of temperature-monitoring equipment at venue entrances of their properties. Some casinos already installed such equipment to detect whether either any employees or any patrons might have fever;

the Government Information Bureau issued in a timely manner latest news regarding the viral outbreak and information about measures for members of the public to take especially in the travelling during Lunar New Year holidays;

the Civil Aviation Authority continued to assist the Health Bureau to monitor the respective body temperature of inbound tourists at the airport; strengthen anti-epidemic drills; and optimize where necessary relevant procedures in dealing with any outbreak of disease.

09.01 The SAR Government received a notice from the National Health Commission of the People's Republic of China explaining that preliminary investigations had identified the pathogen involved in the Wuhan outbreak as a newly-categorized coronavirus.

---

1   Most of the information comes from the special webpage against epidemics of the Macau SAR Government: www.ssm.gov.mo/apps1/PreventCOVID-19/ch.aspx#clg17458

The SAR Government formed a body called the Inter-departmental Taskforce on Pneumonia of Unknown Cause, in order to manage the local response to the Wuhan outbreak.

Any questions from the public on this topic while they were in Macao could be directed to the Health Bureau on +853 2870 0800. Alternatively, the public could visit the Bureau's website: www. ssm.gov.mo/csr to seek further information.

12.01 – 18.01
Public Health Policies

13.01 The Macao Government dispatched a team of officials to Wuhan, Hubei Province, in order for them to learn more about the latest developments regarding a pneumonia outbreak in that mainland city, particularly appropriate treatment for infected patients, and measures to prevent or if necessary control the spread of the identified coronavirus. The team of three officials visited Wuhan between 13 and 14 January. The National Health Commission of the People's Republic of China arranged the visit.

16.01 On Wednesday (16 January) Macao's Inter-departmental Taskforce on Pneumonia of Unknown Cause held a meeting to review the city's disease-control

preparations for the Lunar New Year holidays.

Response measures discussed included: issuance of guidelines for mainland students and workers that were currently based in Macao; organisation of explanatory and promotional seminars for social service institutions, schools and associations; enhancement of temperature-monitoring screening at maritime terminals and land-based checkpoints; the close monitoring of the local stocks of protective face masks; continuing provision of technical support for casinos for installation of temperature-monitoring facilities; and the strengthening of disease prevention and control measures during large-scale public events.

The Government held a press conference to provide the latest scientific findings regarding the Wuhan pneumonia outbreak. A government team was sent to Wuhan to learn more about the latest developments there.

19.01 – 25.01 (2)
Public Health Policies

21.01 Other inbound air passengers flying from the Mainland were subject to temperature checks before entering Macao.

The Government set up a "Novel Coronavirus Response and Coordina-

tion Centre" to oversee Macao's overall response effort regarding the viral pneumonia outbreak reported from Wuhan, Hebei Province. The Centre was created under an Executive Order and was directly under the supervision of the Chief Executive. The announcement of the Centre's establishment was made during a press conference in the afternoon. The Secretary for Social Affairs and Culture, Ms Ao Ieong U, who was the Centre's vice chairperson, gave the information at the press conference. The Centre adapted its strategies – as circumstances require – regarding the prevention, or if necessary, the control of the spread of the coronavirus. The Centre operated 24 hours per day. Its telephone hotline was 2870 0800.

22.01 Macao Government Tourism Office (MGTO) enhanced preventive measures in response to latest situation of Novel Coronavirus

23.01 The Guaranteed Mask Supply for Macao Residents Scheme was launched. People holding permanent or non-permanent resident identity card or non-resident worker's identification card (commonly known as the "blue card") could register and purchase masks at 56 contracted pharmacies in Macao. Each individual could purchase 10 masks every

10 days.

Health declaration was enforced in various ports of entry. Declaration could be made by paper-based or electronic means. Incoming travelers might scan the QR code displayed at the border checkpoints, or browse https://service. ssm.gov.mo/hdeclaration/ to fill out their health information. When this was done, a health declaration certificate would be generated for presentation at immigration clearance.

Macao's five Government Secretaries respectively held meetings today with representatives of community groups, in a bid to utilise the latter's community work and social networks to complement the Government's disease-control efforts.

The Chief Executive, Mr Ho Iat Seng, today announced cancellation of all Government-organised large-scale events. Mr Ho also called on local organisations to cancel their cultural events, and postpone any planned spring-gathering receptions.

24.01 In response to the current outbreak of the new coronavirus, all public libraries of the Cultural Affairs Bureau were closed from 2pm on 24 January, and all cultural venues were closed from 25 January. The reopening date of the cultural venues would be announced in due course.

Social Welfare Bureau advised parents not to bring their children back to nurseries after Chinese New Year

Ten Higher Education Institutions of Macao suspended classes till 11 February

Sports Bureau facilities were temporarily closed from 4 pm today

The DSEJ announced closure of facilities.

The plan to protect the supply of masks for Macao residents started at 6 pm on January 23. Citizens could register for purchase at 56 agreed pharmacies in Macao with permanent/non-permanent resident ID or identification card for non-resident employees. Each person could purchase 10 masks each time. , Repeat purchase after 10 days.

26.01 – 01.02 (7)

Public Health Policies

26.01 DSEJ strongly called on the teachers and students who were spending Chinese New Year in mainland China to return to Macao as early as possible.

27.01 Visitors from Hubei Province and visitors who have been to Hubei Province within the past 14 days were required to present a valid health certificate certifying that they were free from

COVID-19 to enter Macao. The Chief Executive issued an Executive Order banning from Macao casino premises anyone who had been to Hubei Province within 14 days of their arrival in Macao.

Meanwhile, the Government contacted individually – as of 9am on Monday – those 1,113 tourists visiting from Hubei Province who were still in Macao. Some 700 from that aggregate were reached via the hotels at which they were staying. They were tested for infection and if given the all-clear, offered the option of either leaving Macao or relocating – either to Pousada de Juventude de Hac-Sa or a training facility managed by the Municipal Affairs Bureau.

28.01 Civil servants were exempted from work from 30 to 31 January in accordance with the Chief Executive Writ of Instruction. During this period, Integrated Services Centre in China Plaza, Macao Government Services Centre in Islands and Northern District Public Services Centre were temporarily closed to the public.

30.01 Hong Kong Maritime Department suspended ferry services between Kowloon and Tuen Mun, to Macau and Taipa from the early morning of January 30 until further notice. The

ferries between Sheung Wan and HK airports, to Macau's outer ports and Taipa maintain service, but the density of vessels would be reduced according to actual needs.

Date of class resumption of all tertiary and non-tertiary education institutions and tutorial certres in Macao were postponed until further announcement.

The arrangements for class resumption would be announced one week before the resumption.

Socio-Economic Policy Packages

29.01 DSEJ cooperated with schools to make appropriate arrangements for students to study at home during class suspension.

31.01 The Government waived – for a period of three months – rents otherwise payable on public properties used by local businesses, in order to strengthen support for local small and medium-sized enterprises (SMEs) during the ongoing fight against the local incidence of a novel coronavirus.

The Government brought forward the date for distributing funds from the Wealth Partaking Scheme. The procedure began from April and was designed to ease economic pressure on Macao people.

02.02 – 08.02 (10)

Public Health Policies

02.02 The SAR Government announced that on the premise of ensuring emergency and basic services to the public, it continued to exempt civil servants from going to work from 3rd February (Monday) to 7th February (Friday).

04.02 The Government decided to suspend casino operations – and operation of other entertainment facilities.

The 15-day suspension also covered the following facilities: cinemas, theatres, indoor playgrounds, game centres, Internet cafes, billiard rooms, bowling alleys, steam baths, massage parlours, beauty salons, fitness centres, health clubs, karaoke premises, bars, nightclubs, discotheques, and dance halls.

07.02 The SAR Government announced that on the premise of ensuring emergency and basic services to the public, it continued to exempt civil servants from going to work from 8 February to 16 February.

The SAR government calls on all sectors of society to avoid or reduce unnecessary crowd gathering and outing activities to reduce the chance of disease transmission.

Socio-Economic Policy Packages

A new round of protection of the supply of masks was launched on February 2. The original Macao resident ID card or "blue card"wasrequired to purchase

03.02 UM professional team works with government to provide psychological counselling during epidemic period.

09.02 – 15.02 (10)

Public Health Policies

12.02 The Joint Admission Examination for Macao Four Higher Education Institutions (JAE) was rescheduled to 16-19 April.

Socio-Economic Policy Packages

The third round of the plan to guarantee the supply of masks to Macao citizens started on Feb 12.

13.02 The SAR Government adopted a series of economic assistance measures to ease the economic pressure on residents and all walks of life. The purpose was to plan the economic response and mitigation measures for Macao to "stabilize the economy and secure employment", including five major directions. 1) Tax and fee reductions and exemptions to reduce the burden on enterprises and residents; Interest subsidies to support the survival of enterprises; 3) Strengthen people's livelihood measures to support vulnerable families; 4) Improve skills training,

implement work-for-relief, and protect the wages of wage earners; 5) Launch electronic consumer coupons to accelerate the recovery of people's livelihood economy

16.02 – 22.02 (10)

Public Health Policies

16.02 Establishment of electronic system for personal health declaration

17.02 Casinos were permitted to resume operations after the stroke of midnight on Thursday (20 February), under Executive Order 39/2020 published today in the Macao SAR Gazette.

Macao non-resident workers who had been to the mainland in the 14 days prior to their intended arrival in Macao, would only be permitted to enter Macao once they have completed a 14-day period of medical observation in certain places in Zhuhai, Guangdong Province, and have obtained a certificate – issued by Zhuhai health authorities – confirming they were not infected by COVID-19. The new measure became effective after the stroke of midnight on Thursday (20 February), according to Executive Order 40/2020 published today in the Macao SAR Gazette.

Public departments resumed essential public services today. In the period to fight against Covid-19 outbreak, mem-

bers of the public entering public departments were required to check body temperature and submit a Personal Health Declaration if necessary.

20.01 Medical examination stations were set up at border checkpoints to carry out medical examination on arriving travelers from countries/areas with potential risk or high incidence of COVID-19, as well as local residents with multiple border crossings between Macao and Zhuhai in a single day.

Socio-Economic Policy Packages

18.02 Specialized Subsidy Scheme for Prevention and Response to Major Infectious Diseases was Open for Application

The 4th round of the plan to guarantee the supply of masks to Macao citizens started on Feb 22.

23.02 – 29.02 (10)

Public Health Policies

24.02 Individuals who have been to South Korea within the past 14 days prior to their entry into Macao must submit to medical examination at Workers Stadium or Taipa Ferry Terminal in Pac On.

26.02 Individuals, including Macao residents, travelers and non-resident workers, who have been to South Korea within the past 14 days prior to their entry into Macao must, at the discretion

of the health authorities, undergo medical observation for 14 days at designated venue.

27.02 The Education and Youth Affairs Bureau (DSEJ) set out the conditions for class resumption of non-tertiary education schools after it had communicated with relevant departments like the Health Bureau, education groups and school representatives as well as listened to their opinions on the class resumption plan. According to the opinions provided by the Health Bureau on class resumption, the DSEJ initially planned that when there were no new confirmed cases of novel coronavirus found in Macao and Guangdong Province for 14 consecutive days, and both Zhuhai and Zhongshan City announced that they resumed classes, the DSEJ would then announce class resumption for non-tertiary education schools 14 days in advance.

29.02 All arrivals who have been to Italy or Iran within the past 14 days prior to their entry into Macao must, at the discretion of the health authorities, undergo medical observation for 14 days at designated venue.

GGCT issues Level 2 Travel Alert for Italy

Socio-Economic Policy Packages

28.02 Public services resume normal next week

The 4th round of the plan to guarantee the supply of masks to Macao residents started tomorrow on Feb 25.

01.03 – 07.03 (10)

Public Health Policies

07.03 The Government chartered flight departed this morning from Macau International Airport to Hubei Province to bring Macao residents home.

Socio-Economic Policy Packages

The 5th round of the plan to guarantee the supply of masks to Macao residents started on March 3.

08.03 – 14.03 (10)

Public Health Policies

08.03 All arrivals who had travelled to Germany, France, Spain or Japan within the past 14 days prior to their entry into Macao must submit to medical examination.

10.03 All arrivals who had travelled to Germany, France, Spain or Japan within the past 14 days prior to their entry into Macao must, at the discretion of the health authorities, must undergo medical observation for 14 days at designated venue.

11.03 GGCT issued Level 2 Travel Alert for Germany, France, Spain and Japan

12.03 All arrivals who had travelled to Norway within the past 14 days prior to their entry into

Macao must submit to medical examination.

14.03 All students, regardless of their education level, returning from abroad must undergo medical observation for 14 days.

Socio-Economic Policy Packages

11.03 DSEJ formulated a plan for class resumption of non-tertiary education schools.

It was expected that classes would be resumed no later than 20th April.

DSEJ would strive to allow Form 6 students to go back to school at their will on 30th March.

The 6th round of the plan to guarantee the supply of masks to Macao residents started on March 13.

15.03 – 21.03 (18)

Public Health Policies

15.03 The Tourism Crisis Management Office (GGCT) issued a Level 2 Travel Alert to the following destinations:

- Europe:
- Austria, Belgium, Czech Republic, Denmark, Estonia, Finland, Greece, Hungary, Iceland, Latvia, Principality of Liechtenstein, Lithuania, Luxembourg, Malta, the Netherlands, Norway, Poland, Portugal, Slovakia, Slovenia, Sweden, Switzerland, United Kingdom;
- Americas:

- United States of America;
- Registration Notice for Macao Residents currently studying in Europe and those currently travelling in Europe

17.03 All arrivals who have been to countries/ areas outside China within the past 14 days prior to their entry into Macao must, at the discretion of the health authorities, undergo medical observation for 14 days at designated venue.

18.03 All non-Macao residents were prohibited from entering Macao, except residents of mainland China, of Hong Kong and of Taiwan, as well as holders of non-resident worker's identification card.

19.03 Macao-registered non-resident workers from overseas countries were prohibited from re-entering Macao, except those who at the same time were residents either of mainland China, Hong Kong or Taiwan.

GGCT issues Level 2 Travel Alert for All Overseas countries/ territories

Class resumption for non-tertiary education schools were postponed until further notice

20.03 A 30-day grace period ended today regarding the deadline for Macao casinos do reopen following a 15-day mandatory suspension – from 4 February to 19 Febru-

ary inclusive – to limit the spread in Macao of a novel coronavirus and its associated COVID-19 infection.

Socio-Economic Policy Packages

16.03 In order to promote consumption and revitalize the economy, the SAR Government introduced the "Consumption Subsidy Program" through Administrative Regulation No. 6/2020. Those who completed the registration during the period would be paid a subsidy of MOP 3,000.

The "Skills Upgrading and Employment Training Program" launched by the Bureau of Labor Affairs in the form of "Training with Subsidy" was launched on March 16. The program focused on successful employment of participants, and aims to provide practical relief for participants who had difficulties in employment and life through training and matching employment.

In the first round, 15 training courses would be held, involving 7 construction areas. It covers electrician, painting, plastering, carpentry, welding, truck crane and assistant construction supervisor and other projects, providing a total of 300 quota.

18.03 Non-resident workers and non-Macao residents were required to pay 5600 patacas for their stay in Golden Crown China Hotel to conduct the 14-day medical observation. The charge was the same rate as the first designated hotel for medical observation.

22.03 – 28.03 (37)

Public Health Policies

25.03 All residents of mainland China, Hong Kong and Taiwan who had visited a foreign country within 14 days prior to arriving Macao were prohibited from entering Macao.

All individuals who had been to Hong Kong Special Administrative Region or the region of Taiwan within 14 days prior to their entry into Macao must, at the discretion of the health authorities, undergo medical observation for 14 days at designated venue.

Socio-Economic Policy Packages

The 7th round of the plan to guarantee the supply of masks to Macao residents started on March 23

29.03 – 04.04 (43)

Socio-Economic Policy Packages

29.03 Macao Government provided 10-billion-pataca community-support fund amid COVID-19

The 8th round of the plan to guarantee the supply of masks to Macao residents started on April 2

05.04 – 11.04 (45)

Socio-Economic Policy Packages

08.04 The Government proposed a six-pronged approach to use of a 10-billion-pataca fund that aimed to boost financial support to the community and helped it ride out adversities linked to the COVID-19 pandemic.

The plan, part of the city's second round of financial relief countering the economic effects of COVID-19, proposed to offer additional support to a variety of groups, i.e. local employees, businesses, self-employed individuals, and the general public.

12.04 – 18.04

Socio-Economic Policy Packages

The 9th round of the plan to guarantee the supply of masks to Macao residents started on April 12

Electronic consumer cards were issued from April 14. Residents could pick up the card at the appointed place at the appointed time. A total of 150 card collection service points including government departments and banks were ready.

Registration for the second round of subsidized training by the Bureau of Labor Affairs from April 15

The Finance Bureau announced that it would issue 2018 occupational tax rebates in mid-May.

The percentage would be raised from 60% to 70%, and the cap would be raised from $14,000 to $20,000.

On April 17, the Urban Services Department announced that it would continue to launch 60 key municipal projects in May, providing more than 700 jobs to support SMEs

19.04 – 25.04

Public Health Policies

20.04 2020 Policy Address stresses post-COVID-19 economic recovery

Mr Ho delivered the Policy Address for the Fiscal Year 2020, titled "Forging Ahead Towards New Horizons".

The Government expected 2020 would see a deficit in the public budget, the first such occasion since the establishment of the Macao Special Administrative Region (SAR). Mr Ho said the Government had committed itself to spending over 50 billion patacas in response to the COVID-19 pandemic. The overall direction of the public policies would be: fighting the pandemic, safeguarding employment, stabilising the economy, caring for local people's livelihoods, implementing reform, and facilitating development.

Socio-Economic Policy Packages

19.04 DSEJ determined that non-tertiary

education schools would resume classes from May onwards: Senior secondary education: 4th May (Monday); Junior secondary education: 11th May (Monday); Primary, infant and special education: To be announced according to the epidemic situation

The first phase of UM's SME business training course received overwhelming response, the second phase was open for registration from April 21.

The 10th Round of the Plan to Guarantee the Supply of Masks to Macau Residents started on April 22.

In order to meet the needs of first-time children enrolling in school interviews on May 2 and to cooperate with the development of enrollment work, with the assistance of the Health Bureau, the Education and Youth Bureau distributed 6 child masks to approximately 6,400 children in the central registration system. Cooperating with the Macau Women's Federation, through its 5 collection points located in each district, parents of children who attend school interviews could receive masks.

Education and Youth Affairs Bureau announced the "Non-Higher Education School Staff and Cross-border Students Nucleic Acid Testing Program" on April 25.

26.04 – 02.05

Socio-Economic Policy Packages

"Training with subsidies" gradually increased courses and places, and the third round was scheduled to accept applications in May.

The 11th Round of the Plan to Guarantee the Supply of Masks to Macau Residents started on May 2

03.05 – 09.05

Public Health Policies

There were no new confirmed cases in Macao for 28 consecutive days. The "Nucleic Acid Testing Program for Macao Residents Living Cross-border" started on May 7.

Socio-Economic Policy Packages

The third phase of the UM's SME business training course opened for registration from May 5.

10.05 – 16.05

Public Health Policies

"Macau Health Code" and "Guangdong Health Code" Mutual Recognition System was activated at 10:00 on May 10.

Starting from 06:00 on May 11, holders of non-resident worker's identification card who were residents of the Mainland China were allowed to enter Macao when they cumulatively satisfied the following conditions:

(i) Possessing a Zhuhai's household registration or holding a residence permit in Zhuhai;

(ii) Holding a certificate of negative result of or a certificate of specimen collection for nucleic acid test issued by a qualified institution recognized by the health authorities or by Zhuhai within the past seven (7) days;

(iii) The Macao Health Code being displayed was in green.

(Chief Executive's Dispatch no. 120/2020)

The Education and Youth Bureau announced arrangements for the resumption of primary school education, tuition clubs and continuing education institutions to provide comprehensive services on May 11.

Socio-Economic Policy Packages

Administrative Regulation No. 15/2020 "Temporary Preferential Measures to Reduce the Negative Impact of the Novel Coronavirus Pneumonia on Various Industries" was announced and implemented on May 11.

The Cultural Industry Development Fund launched a special funding plan to help companies develop markets after the epidemic on May 12.

The 12th Round of the Plan to Guarantee the Supply of Masks to Macau Residents started on May 12

17.05 – 23.05

Public Health Policies

Individuals travelling from Macao to Zhuhai, should hold a certificate of specimen collection for nucleic acid test, which was issued by a testing institution recognized by Macao or Zhuhai; the certificate should only take effect 24 hours after sampling and valid for a period of 7 days from the effective date.

Socio-Economic Policy Packages

The 13th round of the plan to guarantee the supply of masks to Macao residents began on May 22. In response to class resumption arrangements, children aged 5 to 8 could purchase 10 masks for children

The Urban Services Department announced on May 22 that it would continue to implement food-for-work, and would launch 46 municipal construction projects in June and July to beautify the community environment, improve recreational facilities, improve the quality of urban greening and park landscapes, etc. It was expected to provide about 880 employment positions to help ensure the employment of local workers.

24.05 – 30.05

Public Health Policies

Macao residents aged either 65 or above, those aged either 18 or under, holders of Macao's disability assessment card and Macao's medical assistance card for special patients might choose to undergo the nucleic acid test either at premises in the Pac On Ferry Terminal, or at Conde S. Januário Hospital (Level C2 – former site of Child Assessment Centre) when they booked the test online.

Classes of Primary 4 to 6 resumed on May 25.

Socio-Economic Policy Packages

The "Assistance Payment Plan for Employees, Freelancers and Business Operators" (Administrative Regulation No. 19/2020) of the Ten Billion Anti-epidemic Assistance Fund Plan took effect on May 30.

Relevant assistance payments would be issued by bank transfer or mailed crossed cheques from mid-June this year, and beneficiaries did not need to apply. The entire aid plan was expected to be basically completed in early July. Assistance payments included the following three situations:

1. Eligible employees would receive 15,000 patacas (MOP, the same below).

2. Freelancers and business operators who did

not employ employees could receive 15,000 patacas; freelancers in specific industries could receive 10,000 patacas.

3. Freelancers and business operators who hired employees could receive 50,000 to 200,000 patacas.

31.05 – 06.06
Public Health Policies

Classes of Primary 1 to 3 resumed on June 1.

Socio-Economic Policy Packages

In response to the novel coronavirus epidemic, the Macau Special Administrative Region government launched the "Special Medical Subsidy Scheme" to provide eligible Macau residents with an additional medical subsidy of 600 patacas, which was launched on June 1.

The fourteenth round of the plan to guarantee the supply of masks to Macao residents started on June 1. In response to the resumption of classes, children aged 5 to 8 could purchase 10 child masks

The government launched the "Macau Heart Departure" electronic discount platform, originally planned for tourists, which was opened to local citizens on June 5.

07.06 – 13.06
Socio-Economic Policy Packages

The 15th round of guaranteeing the supply of masks to Macao residents started on June 11.

14.06 – 20.06
Public Health Policies

Zhuhai-Macao Joint Prevention and Control Working Group received notification from the Zhuhai authorities, starting 08:00 of June 16, Macao residents with official, commercial or other specific reasons, after assessment and approval by the Macao SAR Government, could be granted a medical quarantine waiver for crossing the Zhuhai-Macao border. 1,000 exemptions were issued per day for Macao residents with official or commercial purposes (valid for 7 days), the Zhuhai Government would confirm the list the Macao SAR Government approved.

All individuals who had been to Beijing within 14 days prior to their entry into Macao must, at the discretion of the health authorities, undergo medical observation for 14 days at a designated venue.

Socio-Economic Policy Packages

The 10 billion anti-epidemic aid fund plan was released from June 16.

The "SME Bank Loan Interest Subsidy Program" was launched for three months and injected nearly MOP 4.3 billion into small and medium enterprises as of June 16.

21.06 – 27.06 (46)
Public Health Policies

Without prejudice to Chief Executive's Dispatch no. 120/2020, starting from 06:00 on June 22, holders of non-resident worker's identification card who were residents of the Mainland China were allowed to enter Macao when they cumulatively satisfy the following conditions:

(i) Have habitual residence in Zhuhai, confirmed by institutions recognized by Zhuhai;

(ii) Holding a certificate of negative result of or a certificate of specimen collection for nucleic acid test issued by a qualified institution recognized by the health authorities or by Zhuhai within the past seven (7) days;

(iii) The Macao Health Code being displayed was in green.

(Chief Executive's Dispatch no. 135/2020)

Starting from June 27, the daily quota for Macao residents with official or commercial reasons applying for quarantine exemption for crossing

the Zhuhai-Macao border were increased from 1,000 to 3,000.

Socio-Economic Policy Packages

The 16th round of guaranteeing the supply of masks to Macao residents started on June 21.

In order to alleviate the employment needs of local residents, the Labor Affairs Bureau continued to hold job matching meetings to help residents who were willing to find employment to enter the workplace as soon as possible. During the period from June 8 to 22, the bureau have provided 6 job matching meetings for the trainees who completed the training programs of professional drivers, car-delivery and electricians, carpenters, hotel front office operations, hotel housekeeping operations, retail logistics and warehouse clerk to conduct job matching and interviews with companies.

28.06 – 04.07
Public Health Policies

Starting from 12:00 of June 29, Macao residents pursuing an education in Taiwan region might, by registering on the website of the Higher Education Bureau, apply for exemption of obtaining a nucleic acid certificate from medical institutions in Taiwan region before boarding a flight to Macao.

Socio-Economic Policy Packages

The 17th round of guaranteeing the supply of masks to Macao residents started on July 1.

05.07 – 11.07

Public Health Policies

Starting from 08:00 on July 6, 2020, a daily quota of 3,000 places were released for application of quarantine exemption by Macao residents with official, business or special reasons. The quarantine waiver was valid for 7 days. Applications were first assessed by the Macao SAR Government before submitted to Zhuhai City for final approval. Macao residents with official, business or special reasons granted the exemption waiver could, within 14 days after entering Zhuhai, travel within the nine Greater Bay Area (GBA) cities in Guangdong Province, namely Guangzhou, Shenzhen, Zhuhai, Foshan, Huizhou, Dongguan, Zhongshan, Jiangmen and Zhaoqing.

Socio-Economic Policy Packages

The 18th round of guaranteeing the supply of masks to Macao residents started on July 11.

12.07 – 18.07

Public Health Policies

Starting from 12:00 on July 13, all passengers travelling from Hong Kong to Macao trough Hong Kong-Zhuhai-Macao Bridge shuttle buses (golden buses) were required to present a certificate of negative result for COVID-19 nucleic acid test issued within the past 7 days.

Starting from 18:00 on July 13, all arrivals from Hong Kong were required to present a certificate of negative result for COVID-19 nucleic acid test issued within the past 7 days; those who failed to show the document Macau entry could be denied entry. Meanwhile, the measure of 14-day medical observation at the designated place for all arrivals from Hong Kong remained in force.

With effect from 18:00 of July 13, 2020, the measure for individuals who had been to Beijing within the past 14 days prior to their entry into Macao, which required them to undergo medical observation for 14 days at the designated venue at the discretion of the health authorities, have been lifted.

With effect from 18:00 of July 13, 2020, the measures for non-Macao residents from Hubei Province, Mainland China as well as non-Macao residents who had been to Hubei Province, Mainland China within the past 14 days prior to their entry into the Macao Special Administrative Region, which required them to present a medical certificate of no infection with COVID-19 issued by a legal, medical institution, have been lifted.

Starting from 00:00 on July 14, 2020, the restrictions on individuals who had visited Hubei Province of Mainland China within 14 days prior to their entry into the Macao Special Administrative Region from entering the casinos as defined in article 2 of Law no. 16/2001 "Legal Framework for the Operations of Casino Games of Fortune", was lifted.

Starting from 06:00 on July 14, 2020, all ferry and air passengers departing from Macao were required to present a certificate of a negative result for COVID-19 nucleic acid test issued within the past 7 days. The certificate could be consulted on the Macao Health Code system.

Starting from 00:00 on July 15, 2020, all individuals entering hotel establishments and guesthouses were required to receive temperature check and present a Macao Health Code (green code), while individuals entering casinos were further required to submit a valid certificate of a negative result for COVID-19 nucleic acid test. Those who failed to comply with the requirements would be prohibited from entering the premises.

The Macao Novel Coronavirus Response and Coordination Centre received notification from the Zhuhai Command Centre for COVID-19 Prevention and Control, after communication and consultation between the governments of Guangdong Province and Macao, starting from 06:00 on July 15, 2020, persons entering Guangdong Province via the Guangdong-Macao border checkpoints were no longer required to undergo 14 days of centralized medical observation (except confirmed or suspected COVID-19 patients, close contacts, persons with fever or respiratory symptoms, and those who had a foreign or other outbound travel history within 14 days prior to visiting Guangdong). Those entering Guangdong Province from Macao were only allowed to remain in nine cities, namely Guangzhou, Shenzhen, Zhuhai, Foshan, Huizhou, Dongguan, Zhongshan, Jiangmen and Zhaoqing.

19.07 – 25.07

Public Health Policies

Starting from 06:00 on July 19, 2020, special measures to limit the entry of non-resident workers who wer residents of the Mainland China, which were adopted in pursuant to Chief Executive's Dispatch no. 40/2020, no. 120/2020 and no. 135/2020, were lifted. In accordance with the announcement of the Health Bureau, the above individuals must hold a valid certificate of negative result for COVID-19 nucleic acid test and present a Macao Health Code in green to enter into Macao.

700 daily quotas (valid for seven days) were provided for non-official vehicles with Guangdong-Macao double license plate to cross the border; drivers and passengers were required to present a negative COVID-19 test certificate valid for seven days, a green colour Yuekang (Guangdong Health) Code and relevant travel documents during customs clearance. The circulation scope of the vehicles was determined with reference to the scope of activity of people entering via the Zhuhai-Macao border checkpoints.

Socio-Economic Policy Packages

The 19th round of guaranteeing the supply of masks to Macao residents started on July 22.

26.07 – 01.08

Public Health Policies

Starting from 06:00 on July 29, 2020, the 14-day medical observation exemption granted to Macau residents for entering Guangdong Province via the Guangdong-Ma-

cao border checkpoints was extended from the 9 GBA cities to the whole province.

Socio-Economic Policy Packages

The second round consumer card would be used from August 1st, and each resident would receive 5,000 patacas.

The 20th round of guaranteeing the supply of masks to Macao residents would start on July 31. For the convenience of the public, the authorities adjusted the mask sales period to the 30th, that was, the 20th round of the plan was from July 31st to August 29th. During this period, each person buys 30 masks at a time, and the price remains at 0.8 patacas each. A total of 24 patacas.

02.08 – 08.08

Public Health Policies

04.08 With effect from 06:00 on 4th August 2020, all arrivals from Hong Kong must hold a certificate of negative result for COVID-19 nucleic acid test issued within the past 72 hours; meanwhile, the measure requiring individuals who have been to Hong Kong within the past 14 days prior to arriving in Macao to undergo medical observation for 14 days at a place designated by the health authorities remains in force. Crew members of cargo vessels

sailing between Macao and Hong Kong would be managed in a closed loop upon landing in Macao in order to minimize the risk of community transmission.

With effect from 06:00 on 4th August 2020, all individuals who have been to Dalian or Urumqi within the past 14 days prior to their entry into Macao must, at the discretion of the health authorities, undergo medical observation for 14 days at designated venue.

Starting from 06:00 on 4th August 2020, 1400 daily quotas (valid for seven days) were provided for non-official vehicles with Guangdong-Macao double license plate to cross the border, with the access area extended from the 9 GBA cities to all cities of the Guangdong Province. Issues relating to immigration clearance and border checkpoints for vehicles continued to be administered in accordance with the "Notice of Zhuhai Command Centre for COVID-19 Prevention and Control Regarding the Progressive Facilitation of Clearance Procedures for Vehicles with Guangdong-Macao Double License Plate at Zhuhai-Macao Border Checkpoints" effectuated at 06:00 on 24th July 2020.

07.08 With effect from 06:00 on 7th August 2020, all arrivals from

Hong Kong must hold a certificate of negative result for COVID-19 nucleic acid test performed within the past 24 hours; meanwhile, the measure requiring individuals who have been to Hong Kong within the past 14 days prior to arriving in Macao to undergo medical observation for 14 days at a place designated by the health authorities remains in force.

09.08 – 15.08

Public Health Policies

12.08 As informed by the Hong Kong and Macao Affairs Office of the State Council: Starting 00:00 of 12th August 2020, all travelers from Macao, if they had not been to any countries and regions outside the mainland China (including Hong Kong and Taiwan) in the past 14 days prior to their arrival in the mainland China, holding a certificate or a health code containing negative result for COVID-19 nucleic acid test within 7 days were allowed to enter the mainland China without a 14-day medical observation.

16.08 – 22.08

Public Health Policies

21.08 With effect from 06:00 of 21st August 2020, individuals who have been to Nantang township in Lufeng, Shanwei City of Guangdong Province within the past 14 days prior to their entry into Macao must, at the discretion of the health authorities, undergo medical observation for 14 days at designated venue.

With effect from 06:00 of 21st August 2020, the measure for individuals who had been to Dalian within the past 14 days prior to their entry into Macao, which required them to undergo medical observation for 14 days at designated venue at the discretion of the health authorities, was lifted.

30.08 – 05.09 (46/0)

Public Health Policies

31.08 With effect from 00:00 of 31st August 2020, the measure for individuals who had been to Nantang township in Lufeng, Shanwei City of Guangdong Province within the past 14 days prior to their entry into Macao, which required them to undergo medical observation for 14 days at designated venue at the discretion of the health authorities, was lifted.

Socio-Economic Policy Packages

The 21st round of guaranteeing mask supply to Macau residents started on August 30. The sale period was 30 days, that was, from August 30 to September 28. During this period, each person could purchase 30 masks at a time for a total of 24 Macau yuan.

COVID-19 in New Zealand:
SCIENTIFIC ADVICE AND POLITICAL REALITIES

Robert Gregory

Mā pango, mā whero, ka oti te mahi — leaders and people work together to get the work done (Māori proverb).

New Zealand is commonly regarded as one of the "success" stories in the Covid-19 pandemic. Several weeks after the first few cases emerged in the country in February, 2020, the Labour-led coalition government headed by Prime Minister Jacinda Ardern launched a full national lockdown, lasting a month. In doing so it was acting on a strongly consensual body of epidemiological advice proffered by the Director-General of Health, Dr Ashley Bloomfield. The lockdown soon flattened the incidence curve, before largely eliminating the virus within the country. However, in August another significant and threatening outbreak occurred, in the country's largest city, Auckland. This impelled the government to impose partial and differential lockdowns in that region and throughout the country. The government was mindful of the economic and political consequences of its "go hard, go early" approach, and of the August outbreak, especially as a general election was scheduled for September 2020, later postponed by one month.

Introduction

New Zealand is an island nation, surrounded by vast expanses of ocean, thus rendering it relatively easy to seal itself off from the global spread of Covid-19. But, as has been the case in most other countries, no New Zealand government had previously had to cope with such a one in one hundred year public health crisis. Its emerging responses have necessarily been pragmatic, politically sensitive — 2020 being an election year — and in many ways piecemeal, though well informed by expert epidemiological knowledge from home and abroad. For students of public policymaking theory, the way governments have variously responded to this crisis could revive the old debate between those of incrementalist or rationalist persuasions. In New Zealand, it has also provided an exemplary case of technocratic decision-making in a liberal democracy, which — as elsewhere — highlights the relationship between science and politics.

Early Days

At the end of 2019 New Zealanders had begun to become aware of the disease then emerging out of Wuhan in China. However, there was no widespread alarm, and many believed that news media reports had been overplaying the potential risks of the disease spreading, let alone to New Zealand — once described as "the last bus stop on the planet." Moreover, the World Health Organisation (WHO) had not yet declared a Covid-19 pandemic.

Nevertheless, acting on the precautionary principle, the coalition government led by Prime Minister Jacinda Ardern, on 3 February 2020 barred entry into the country of foreign travellers who had departed from China, allowing only New Zealand citizens and permanent residents to return to New Zealand. Foreigners who had departed China and had spent at least 14 days in another country were allowed to enter New Zealand. (This was extended on 24 February by an additional eight days.) This decision prevented the return to New Zealand of many high fee-paying university students from China, who had enrolled in New Zealand university courses or who were returning to resume their studies. The government argued that its decision would not necessarily stand for the full year, depending on how serious the Covid-19 problem turned out to be. In the meantime, all returning New Zealanders were required to self-isolate for 14 days after entering the country, and to undergo Covid-19 tests during that period.

The Emerging Crisis

The first case of the disease was officially reported in New Zealand on 28 February. It was a woman in her 60s who had recently visited Iran before returning to Auckland. Earlier that month the Ministry of Health (MoH) had established a National Health Coordination Centre, and Covid-19 had been registered under the Health Act 1956 as an "Infectious and Notifiable Disease". The ministry had also put in place a Healthline freephone number for calls relating to Covid-19, to help deal with growing levels of public anxiety.

During March, the government responded to the pandemic through a series of steps — described by Ardern as among the "widest ranging and toughest border restrictions of any country in the world" — intended to insulate New Zealand from incursions of the virus from overseas, and to inhibit any spread within the country. The Prime Minister cancelled a national remembrance service in Christchurch for the 51 people killed on 15 March 2019 by a terrorist attack on two city mosques. A Pacific culture festival about to be held in Auckland was also cancelled. Travellers from the Pacific Islands were not required to self-isolate on entering New Zealand unless they were symptomatic. Travel from New Zealand to the Pacific Islands was barred for people showing symptoms of Covid-19 or who were close contacts of coronavirus patients. Cruise ships, which were regular and frequent arrivals at various New Zealand ports, were stopped from docking until 30 June, a prohibition that remains in force at the time of writing (late August) and will certainly not be lifted in the foreseeable future.

In mid-March the government banned public gatherings of more than 500 people, and announced that any foreign tourists who defied self-quarantining restrictions would be deported. Shortly after, the Ministry of Foreign Affairs and Trade (MFAT) exhorted all New Zealanders travelling abroad to return home, while Ardern announced that the New Zealand and Australian governments were cancelling the annual ANZAC Day (25 April) services scheduled to be held at Gallipoli in Turkey. There followed a ban on all indoor gatherings of more than 100 people, though workplaces, schools, supermarkets and public transport were exempted.

By 17 March, there were 166 new cases of Covid-19 in New Zealand, 95 (57%) of whom had recovered, while five people — all elderly — had had died from the disease. (Recovery is defined in New Zealand as being symptom-free for at least 10 days since having symptoms, and being symptom-free for the past 48 hours.)

The government's strategy was to "flatten the [infection rate] curve". Testing and contact tracing was well underway, with around 40,000 tests having been conducted throughout the country. Within two days, the government closed the borders to everyone except New Zealand citizens and permanent residents, a ban which now included Pacific Islanders, apart from those coming in for "essential" purposes, such as healthcare work. The requirement that returning New Zealanders — many of whom were brought home on international repatriation flights organised by the government — had to self-isolate for 14 days after entry into the country was later changed to mandatory self or group isolation in a managed isolation quarantine (MIQ) facility. These facilities were mainly hotels commandeered by the government in several of the major cities, particularly Auckland. All those quarantined were to be tested on the third and twelfth days of their isolation, a procedure deemed to be the most effective in detecting positive cases.[1]

---

1 www.health.govt.nz/our-work/diseases-and-conditions/covid-19-novel-coronavirus/covid-19-current-situation/covid-19-border-controls

The National Lockdown: From "Flattening the Curve" to Elimination

On 21 March Ardern announced the introduction of a country-wide alert level system, as a central feature of the strategy to control the spread of the disease. The four-level system ranged from 1, deemed appropriate for the lowest risk of infection, to 4, for the highest risk. At this time the level had been set at 2, with people over 70 years old and those with pre-existing immune system problems being encouraged to stay home. There were 255 Covid-19 cases in the country, with 103 (40%) recoveries. Two days later the government raised the alert level across the whole country from 2 to 3, and closed all schools. It declared an interim state of national emergency (extended after 31 March for a further two weeks).

After two days' notice, New Zealand went into a full level 4 lockdown at 11.59pm on 25 March. This was the main manifestation of the government's "Go hard, go early" approach to combatting the virus. By then there were 392 cases, with 113 (29%) recoveries, with new cases having increased by an average of 31 per day during the previous seven days. Five elderly people, most related to clusters of the disease in rest homes — had succumbed to Covid-19.

On 25 March a national state of emergency, separate from the lockdown, was imposed by the Minister of Civil Defence, lasting until 14 April. All people were required to stay in their "bubbles", that is, to have no physical contact with those outside their own living arrangements, and to keep at least two metres apart in public spaces. "Non-essential" services, such as public swimming pools, bars, cafes, restaurants and playgrounds were closed, but supermarkets, fuel stations and health services remained open, with strict physical distancing and hand sanitisation. Face masks in public or in organisations providing "essential" services were not mandated, however, but customer-facing businesses like supermarkets began to install transparent partitions between their check-out staff and customers. Late in March, the New Zealand Police provided an online form for people to report lockdown breaches and illegally operating businesses.

Figure 7.1 Case numbers I — Official Ministry of Health data

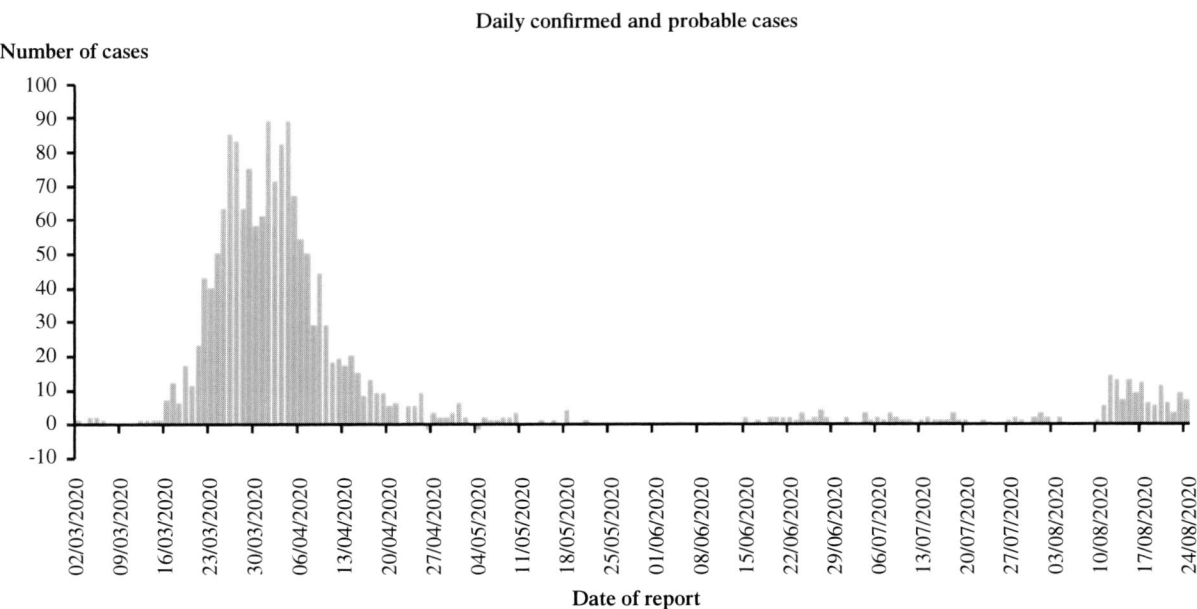

Daily confirmed and probable cases

Figure 7.2 Case numbers II — Official Ministry of Health data

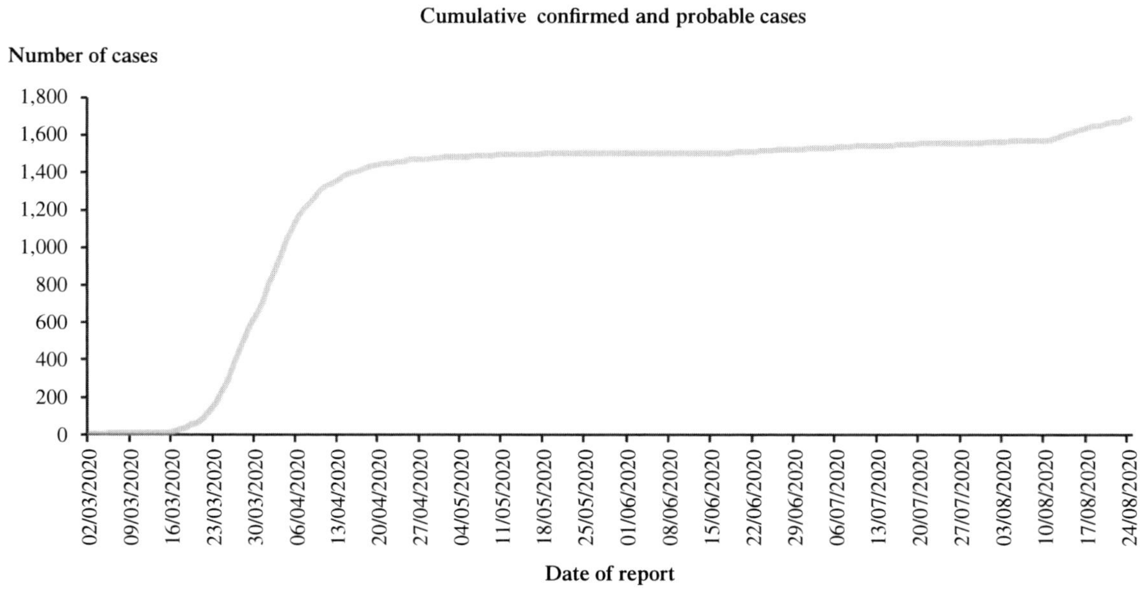

Cumulative confirmed and probable cases

Statistical modelling which had informed the government's decision to shift to level 4 had shown that if the virus had been allowed to spread largely unchecked — as in a strategy of "herd immunity" — then about 80,000 people within New Zealand would probably have died, and that the country's health systems would have been overwhelmed.[2] There would not have been nearly enough Intensive Care Units (ICUs), and respirators to cope. The government decided that it could not accept such a potential outcome, and had a pressing responsibility to do whatever was necessary to avoid it.

There was a strong consensus among the country's epidemiologists that this was the correct course of action. However, in April a group of six academics, with backgrounds collectively in health, law and economics, and led by an epidemiologist, publicly presented their "Plan B". This argued that the lockdown was unwarranted, and caused more harm to the country's wellbeing, social fabric and economy than did Covid-19. They complained that they were being kept out of the government's decision-making, and had been "shut down" in the news media.[3] The leader argued that the government should give up its elimination strategy because it was not realistic, and that Sweden's "more relaxed" approach should have been followed. The idea of a vaccine was said to be "a fantasy".[4] There was also some forceful questioning of the assumptions underpinning the modelling that had been used by the MoH in forecasting the probable mortality rate of Covid-19 in New Zealand.[5]

---

2   www.health.govt.nz/news-media/media-releases/covid-19-modelling-provides-clear-warning-consequences-not-acting-swiftly-and-decisively, www.stuff.co.nz/national/health/coronavirus/120954076/coronavirus-nz-could-have-had-200-new-covid19-cases-on-thursday-without-lockdown-modelling-shows

3   www.rnz.co.nz/national/programmes/mediawatch/audio/2018743518/covid-19-contrarians-claim-they-re-being-censored

4   www.newshub.co.nz/home/new-zealand/2020/08/coronavirus-covid-19-vaccine-a-fantasy-controversial-epidemiologist-simon-thornley.html

5   www.tailrisk.co.nz/documents/Corona.pdf?fbclid=IwAR0P_K-_SUogvodgspA-GgXHeRvQHWGGv1oKgpEq9GPwXb6nZrS7nxxVKsY

Figure 7.3 Impact of lockdown — Te Punaha Matatini, University of Auckland

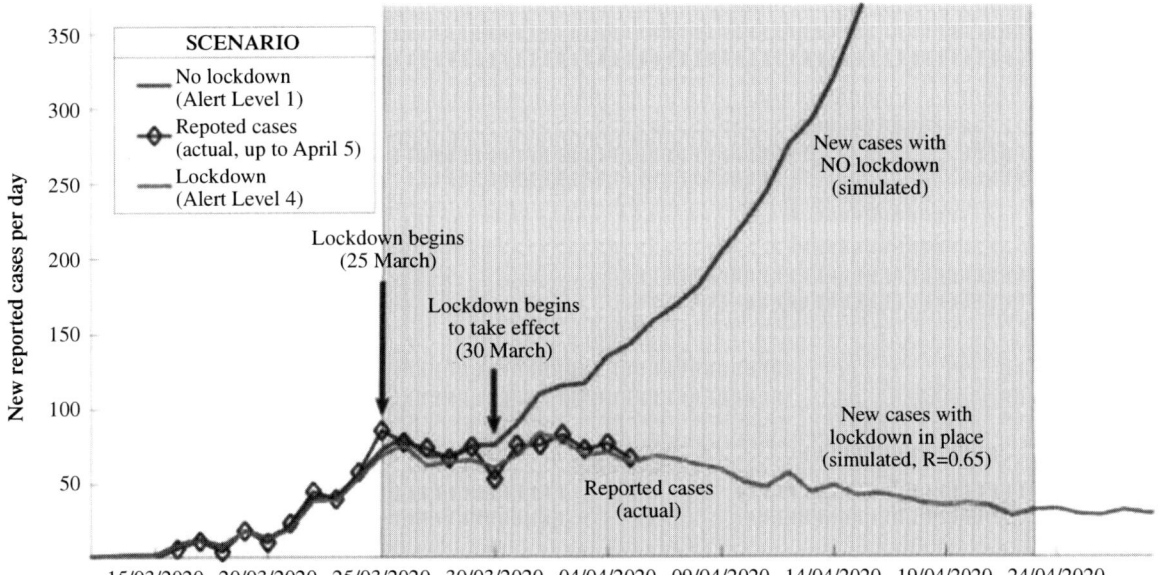

Figure 7.4 Age distribution of cases — Official Ministry of Health data

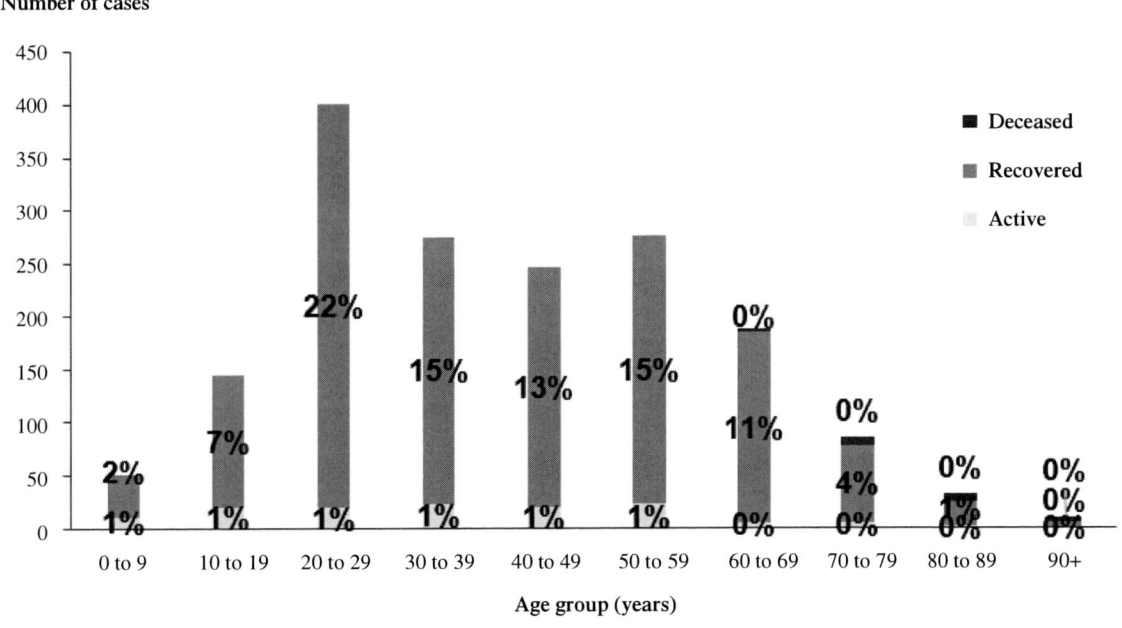

Figure 7.5 Gender distribution of cases — Official Ministry of Health data

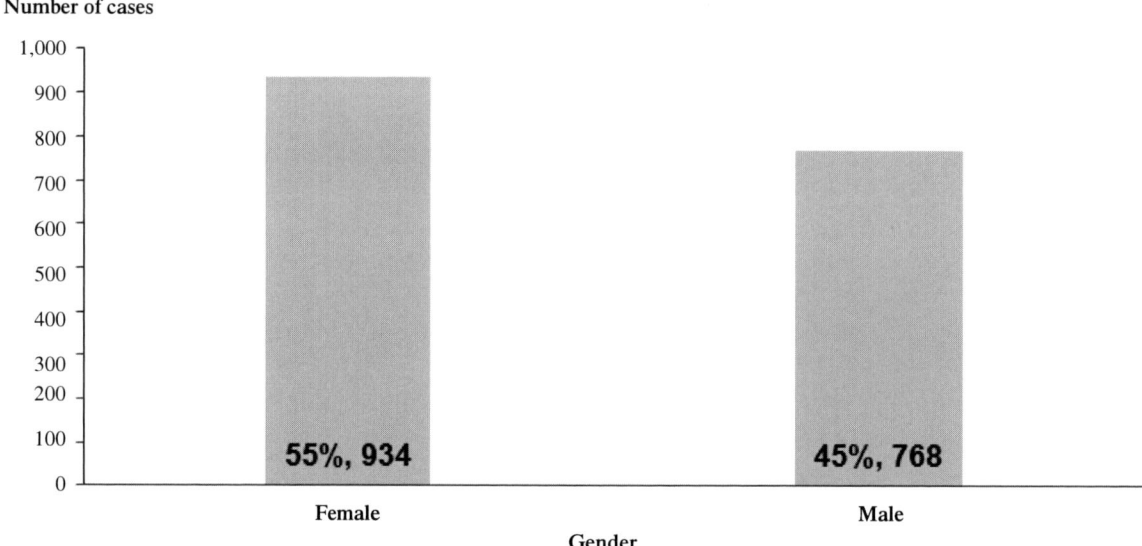

Number of cases

55%, 934 (Female)

45%, 768 (Male)

Gender

Rising numbers and political reassurance

The number of new Covid-19 cases in the country had been rising. On the day the level 4 lockdown began (25 March) there were 24 new cases, while since 23 January there had been a total of 156 new cases reported until the lockdown began. Over the seven days before lockdown there had been a total of 219. The peak period of new cases came during the nine consecutive days immediately after lockdown, when they totalled 435, the highest number, 65, having been recorded on 27 March (this being the highest daily number recorded in New Zealand so far). Numbers rapidly trailed off after this nine-day period. There were 180 new cases in the following 16 days, 155 of those recorded in the first eight days of this period. In the week before the end of level 4 there were 12 new cases, while 602 of a total of 1452 cases — 41.5% — had recovered. There had been five deaths.

Contact tracing was crucial in bringing several significant clusters, in various parts of the country, under control. In April, the MoH commissioned an academic to undertake a rapid review of the health sector's approach to Covid-19 contact tracing. The subsequent report made several firm recommendations for strengthening the system.[6] A government publicity programme, featuring posters and signs, including those on public footpaths, urged physical distancing, proper hand-washing with soap or santiser, exhorted people to stay at home if unwell, and urged them to seek a Covid-19 test if they were displaying relevant symptoms. However, the wearing of face masks was still not mandated by this time. Prime Minister Ardern emphasized what has come to be seen as her personal brand of politicking: "Be kind to one another", and stressed that, "People are not the problem, the virus is." This latter sentiment was born of compassion towards those who had contracted Covid-19, and while the overall response by New Zealanders was highly cooperative and supportive, there were many people who put others at greater risk. During the period of level 4 lockdown, there had been several highly publicised and — for the government, politically embarrassing — instances of people breaking the rules. The most publicised of these was the revelation that the Minister of Health, David Clark, had himself transgressed on at least two occasions while at his home in Dunedin. His offer to resign his portfolio was initially rejected by

---

6   www.health.govt.nz/publication/rapid-audit-contact-tracing-covid-19-new-zealand

the Prime Minister, but was accepted early in July. The health portfolio was then given to Chris Hipkins, who was already minister of education.

The incidence curve in the country had been flattened by the time the Prime Minister announced on 20 April that the level 4 lockdown would be extended for another week, to "lock in the gains" made. On 11 May the government declared that the country would move from level 4 to level 2 three days later. By this time the government's strategy had become one of elimination of the virus within New Zealand, rather than one of flattening the curve.

Although the impact of the lockdown on many thousands of New Zealanders continued to be severe, a poll conducted on 20-21 April showed that 87% of people were "satisfied" with the government's response to the Covid-19 crisis, with eight percent "not satisfied" and five percent "unsure". About a month later, 92% said they were satisfied, and only seven percent said they were unsatisfied, with two percent unsure. These were highly favourable political results for the government, particularly in a country with many sports-loving citizens, and in which all sporting activities had been stopped during the lockdown, bringing an abrupt — if temporary — end to the major rugby, rugby league, and football competitions.

In early May, Parliament passed, 63-57, an omnibus bill which became the Covid-19 Public Health Response Act (CPHRA), with a refreshment clause applying at least every 90 days. Among other things, the Act gave police the power to enter homes without a warrant in order to enforce the level 2 rules in the face of people who may have been congregating —e.g., partying — in defiance of the stipulations. The politics of the Covid-19 crisis were readily apparent during the passage of this bill. The centre-right and right-wing National and ACT parties, respectively, did not support it, claiming that it was an overreach of powers, showed distrust of New Zealanders, and did not allow for various mandatory orders to receive proper scrutiny. The country's statutory Human Rights Commission expressed "deep concern" over what it saw as an inadequate examination of the bill.[7]

Technocratic Governance

The Prime Minister, together with the Director-General of Health, Dr Ashley Bloomfield, gave daily televised updates and briefings to the nation during the lockdown, and responded to questions from attendant news media reporters. Bloomfield was exercising his emergency powers under the Health Act 1956, thus being able to command medical officers of health in each of the country's 20 District Health Boards (DHBs). The cabinet was heavily reliant on Bloomfield's expert advice. While this was perfectly appropriate under New Zealand's Westminster-styled parliamentary democracy, it represented a virtually unprecedented case of technocratic governance — that is, government by technical or scientific experts — as the cabinet was in no position to gainsay the epidemiological advice it was given.

---

7   www.hrc.co.nz/news/human-rights-commission-deeply-concerned-about-covid-19-public-health-response-bill/

Figure 7.6 Popular depictions of New Zealand prime minister, Jacinda Ardern, and director-general of health, Ashley Bloomfield

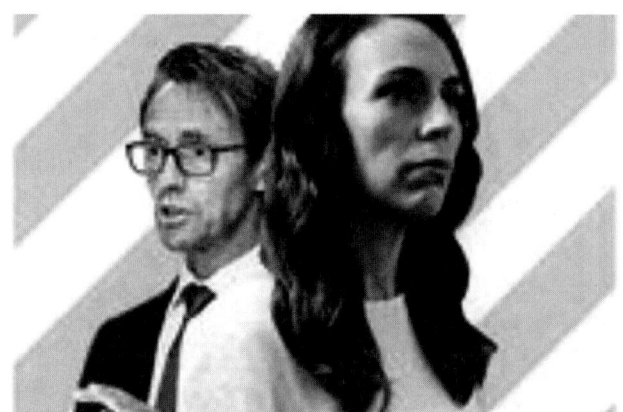 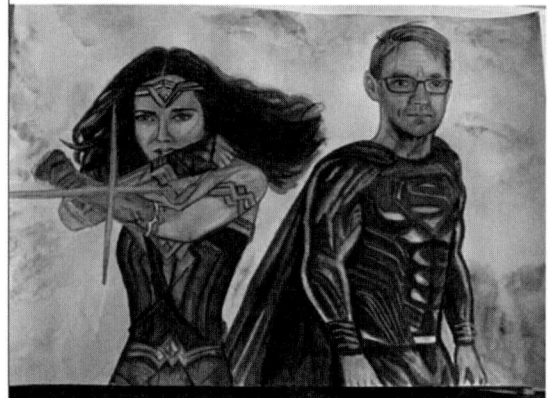

For its part, the government was acutely conscious of the need to strike an acceptable balance between public health imperatives, on the one hand, and the adverse economic impact, on the other. There was no indication at this stage that there were any working difficulties between the cabinet and its public health advisers, and no instance was reported of Bloomfield having vetoed a cabinet decision or intention by exercising his emergency powers. (Later, a private legal challenge was mounted, questioning Bloomfield's exercise of his powers under the Act, and claiming that the first nine days of the lockdown had been illegal. A judicial review panel of three High Court judges partly agreed with the challenge on narrow legal grounds, while being unsympathetic to the spirit of the challenge under the prevailing circumstances.[8])

Overt tension between government ministers and the Director-General of Health emerged later in the year. A few prosecutions had been brought under the CPHRA against individuals who had breached the rules after being placed in MIQs. These incidents sparked public concern and political debate about whether or not the security arrangements at these facilities were adequate. They also raised questions as to whether the testing regime in place for workers at these MIQ facilities was adequate. On 23 June, the government had announced its "enhanced strategy" for testing at the borders, including "regular health check and asymptomatic testing of all border facing workers." By August, however it had become clear that this policy intention had not been adequately implemented.

While the new Minister of Health, Chris Hipkins, and Bloomfield publicly played down any serious tension between themselves, the latter conceded that there had been some "dissonance". Both Ardern and Hipkins expressed their dissatisfaction with the scale and speed of the implementation of the testing strategy that the cabinet had approved in June. They had believed that the testing regime was operating more rigorously than it actually was. Despite New Zealand being a country of only five million people, its unwieldy public health system comprises 20 DHBs, with the MoH — headed by Bloomfield — being largely a policy-advice organisation, with only one operational function (the regulation of therapeutic products). So the management of border security and of MIQs rapidly became the diffuse responsibility of a multi-faceted bureaucratic arrangement which developed piecemeal in response to changing circumstances.

---

8   www.rnz.co.nz/news/national/423917/high-court-rules-some-of-covid-19-level-4-lockdown-was-unlawful

Bureaucratic Complexity

Despite the fact that implementation of the border testing regime was in the hands of DHBs, legislation ensured that they in turn could be directed by the Director-General of Health. However, Bloomfield's ability to exercise real, as distinct from formal, control was questionable. Although he had the power to direct DHBs it was difficult for him to directly monitor the implementation of the plan the government had announced on 23 June.[9] It may not have been helped by his apparent willingness to accept the "celebrity" status conferred on him by an increasingly admiring public (he was now nicknamed "The Terminator").[10] To complicate matters, the centre itself was fragmented among a number of offices and agencies, all of which bore some responsibility for the country's defences against Covid-19.[11] These included several other cabinet ministers apart from the Minister of Health: notably, the Ministers of Housing (made directly responsible for the MIQ system), Defence, and Police. An All of Government Controller (AGC) reported to the Prime Minister and cabinet; a Strategic Operations Command reported to the AGC, as did the National Controller and Director of Civil Defence and the Ministry of Business, Innovation and Employment's All of Government Strategy and Policy office, as well as Bloomfield himself (apart from his direct responsibility to his own minister). In turn, testing laboratories reported to the DHBs, which in turn were answerable to Bloomfield, while MIQs worked through the laboratories to the DHBs and thence to Bloomfield.

The situation became more fraught in July and August, when evidence emerged publicly of some security breaches at MIQs. Consequently, the government brought in the military, under the command of an air commodore, to assist in securing the border facilities, and ensured that at least one police officer (thus with power to arrest) was stationed at each facility. The government added to the complexity by creating a high-powered "testing oversight" group, reporting to Bloomfield.

COVID-19 and Cultural Identities

The leadership of this new oversight group was criticised by a group of Māori health experts as being inadequately informed or concerned about the health needs and status of Māori and Pasifika people.[12] The socio-political dimensions of the crisis came into sharper focus when a 50 year-old cool store worker was found to have been the source of the Auckland cluster that led the government to move the Auckland region to level 3 and the rest of New Zealand to level 2 beginning on 14 August. (At the time of writing, it was still not known how this man had contracted the disease. Tests indicated that it was highly improbable that it may have been carried on the surface of some imported goods in the cool store. False and racist social media stories — quickly and strongly denied by the government — circulated about how the virus spread from this one cool store worker.) The man lived in South Auckland, the most densely populated Polynesian area in the world, where people were considered to be more vulnerable to contracting Covid-19 because of their living conditions.[13] A research article published in the New

9   Allen, B. and Donadelli, F. (2020) "When Good Intentions Aren't Enough: Where New Zealand's Border Quarantine System Really Went Wrong", *The Conversation*, 27 August. https://theconversation.com/when-good-intentions-arent-enough-where-new-zealands-border-quarantine-system-really-went-wrong-145007

10 www.newshub.co.nz/home/new-zealand/2020/07/hundreds-turn-out-for-dr-ashley-bloomfield-s-rugby-match.html

11 www.stuff.co.nz/national/politics/300088617/coronavirus-who-runs-our-covid19-border-response

12 www.stuff.co.nz/national/politics/300086077/coronavirus-heather-simpson-to-spearhead-border-response-some-mori-health-leaders-gutted

13 www.stuff.co.nz/national/health/coronavirus/300080644/coronavirus-why-south-auckland-is-the-worst-place-for-the-return-of-covid19-community-transmission

Zealand Medical Journal estimated that Māori were 50% more likely to die from Covid-19 than Pakeha (European) New Zealanders.

During the main outbreak, Māori people had tested positive (0.12%) at a significantly lower rate lower rate than the overall population, as had Pasifika people (0.19%). However, in the Auckland outbreak, 60% of the cases were Pasifika people and 20% were Māori (Māori comprise 15% of the New Zealand population, and Pasifika people 7.5%.) The report attributed this disparity in part to "institutional racism", though it must also have reflected the fact that the outbreak had occurred in South Auckland.[14]

The government had set the maximum number of people allowed to attend gatherings at 10, until pressure from Māori and Pasifika people — unable to conduct their funerals according to custom — persuaded it to lift the limit to 50. Two Māori health commentators, both medical practitioners and researchers, argued that the government's decision to place all the positive cases from the Auckland cluster into MIQs, rather than requiring them to self-isolate at home, as had been the policy during the first community spread — when most of the victims were white — was racist.[15]

When the region moved down to level 2.5 children in South Auckland were slow to return after their schools re-opened, attendance at some schools dropping to 50%. This may have reflected nervousness about the possible spread of the virus, and might also have indicated that some older children had decided to seek work in difficult financial times for their families.

Local iwi (Māori tribes) in the north and east of the North Island set up roadblocks to stop foreign tourists in the country from entering their rohe (areas), with one Māori leader and former Māori Party MP criticising the government for not stopping tourists entering New Zealand earlier. These and similar moves elsewhere were not fully supported by the police.

To help ease the financial strain, the government invested $NZ 56.4 in Māori communities and businesses affected by the pandemic, $NZ 30 million of which was provided to Māori health workers. In doing so, the government was recognising its obligations under the Treaty of Waitangi, a bicultural agreement signed between the colonial government of New Zealand and many Māori chiefs in 1840, and officially recognised since the 1970s as an integral part of the country's constitutional framework.

Keeping Ahead of the Latest Curve

On 12 August the Prime Minister announced that after 102 days without any community spread being reported, a fresh outbreak had been discovered in New Zealand's largest city, Auckland (with 30% of the country's population). Level 3 was imposed on the region, its borders were sealed, and the rest of the country was moved from level 1 to 2. Gatherings of no more than 10 people were mandated for level 3 (with the exception of 50 being allowed for funerals), and a limit of 100 people for level 2. Schools in the Auckland region were closed. All rest homes throughout the country were put into lockdown mode, allowing no visitors.

By 25 August, 1,690 cases had been reported throughout New Zealand since February, of which 1,539 (91%) had recovered. There had been 22 deaths. From 12–25 August there had been a total of 116 positive cases of community spread, with no deaths, and 10 people had been admitted to hospital. A total

---

14   www.nzherald.co.nz/nz/news/article.cfm?c_id=1&objectid=12361484

15   www.stuff.co.nz/pou-tiaki/300082800/coronavirus-quarantine-policy-shift-is-racist-critics-say

of 160 persons linked to the Auckland cluster were in MIQs, 89 of them having returned positive tests. Genome sequencing had shown that these people were afflicted with a different form of the virus from the one that had circulated earlier in the year.

On 24 August the Prime Minister declared that the Auckland region would remain at level 3 until 11.59pm on Sunday 30 August, before moving to level 2.5, while all other parts of the country would stay at level 2 until at least 6 September. The newly coined level 2.5 meant that while those in the Auckland region were free to travel beyond it, gatherings could not exceed 10 people, as opposed to a maximum of 100 persons in the rest of the country. Funerals in the region could, however, be attended by up to 50 people.

The government's elimination strategy now focused on "keeping ahead of the curve" (as distinct from flattening it), or cornering the virus. More people across New Zealand were downloading and using the government's Covid-19 QR contact tracing app — which all businesses throughout the country were required to display at their doors or in their reception areas. Pressure was being exerted on government to speed up and improve digital capability in responding to the pandemic. Testing units were working overtime in monitoring MIQ workers and high risk border employees at ports and airports, and more than 100,000 people in the Auckland region had been tested since the outbreak was identified. The government planned to conduct 70,000 tests across the country over the week 26 August to 2 September, a total it considered to be a "gold standard". The wearing of face masks or coverings was mandated for everyone aged 12 and older on all public transport, except taxis and school buses, from 31 August.[16] There has been no mandating of face masks or coverings for all public exposure, in contrast to some other jurisdictions, and this reluctance by the government has been criticised by some New Zealand experts. Epidemiological critics have also challenged what they see as the inadequate testing and self-isolation requirements placed on international air crew coming into New Zealand.[17]

Figure 7.7 Covid-19 testing numbers — Official Ministry of Health data

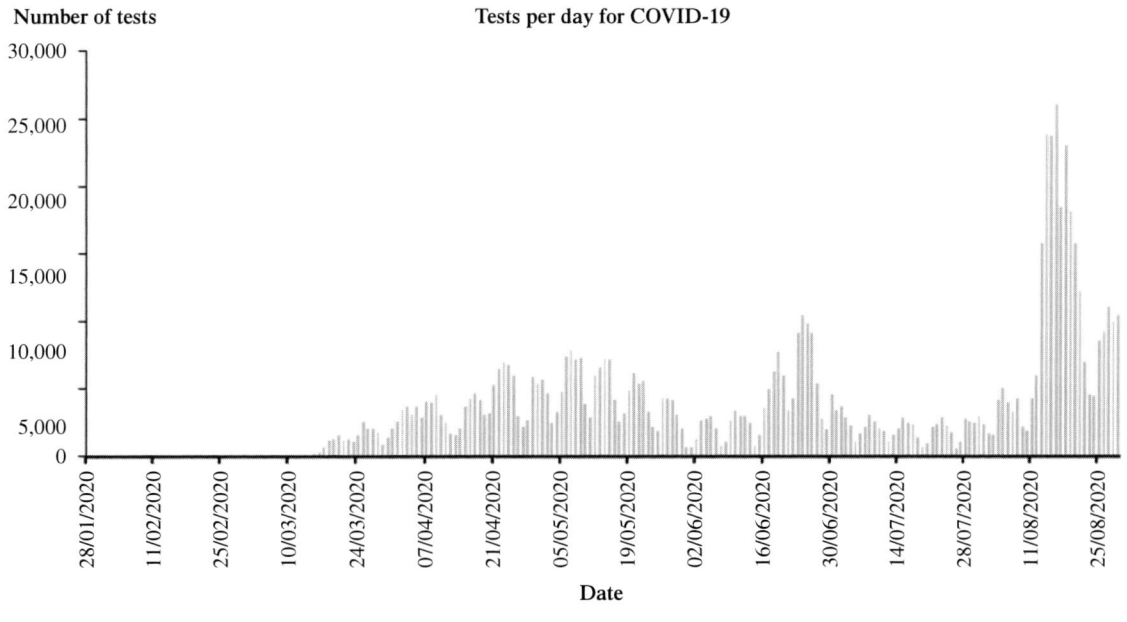

---

16 However, significant exceptions were permitted, which may prove to be problematic: www.stuff.co.nz/national/health/coronavirus/300092928/coronavirus-mandatory-facecoverings-wont-be-required-for-under12s-on-school-buses-or-for-uber-passengers

17 www.newshub.co.nz/home/new-zealand/2020/08/epidemiologist-michael-baker-calls-for-better-covid-19-testing-of-aircrew.html

Several criteria underpinned the government's decisions on changes to the alert levels. These included: the Director-General of Health's confidence in the data; the capability of the testing and contact tracing system; the effectiveness of self-isolation, MIQ and border measures; the capacity of the health system to shift between levels and cope with demand; the effects on the economy; and the extent to which people were following the rules.

In sum, between 22 January and 3 September a total of 797,990 Covid-19 tests were conducted throughout the country, while the daily testing rate peaked at more than 25,000 late in August during the Auckland outbreak. By the end of August a total of 268,000 people had been tested during this regional occurrence, tests being restricted to those who were symptomatic.

By early September a national total of 1,413 confirmed cases had been reported to the WHO, and 351 probable cases. Ninety-two percent of these confirmed and probable cases had recovered. There were 112 active cases in the country at this point, with six people in hospital.

On 4 and 5 September the latest deaths from the virus were reported — the Auckland cool store worker, in his 50s, who had been the initial case in the Auckland outbreak (the source of his infection remained unknown); and 82 year-old Dr Joe Williams, a former Prime Minister of the Cook Islands and an Auckland medical practitioner. Both died in Auckland. Their deaths, the first fatalities to occur in 98 days, brought the national mortality count to 24. All the other deaths were of people in their 70s, 80s or 90s, quite a number of whom had been in rest home Covid-19 clusters.

Economic Impacts and Responses

In March, the Minister of Finance, Grant Robertson, announced a $NZ12.1 billion business and income support package, declaring that the "rainy day" for which successive governments had committed to maintaining budget surpluses had now arrived. In 2018-19 the government had achieved an OBEGAL surplus of $NZ 7.3 billion, equivalent to 2.5% of GDP. New Zealand's public debt/GDP ratio had been for several years decidedly lower than the OECD average, and well below that of Western countries with whom it most closely identified. Borrowing money was not going to be a problem for the government at this critical time. The central bank, the Reserve Bank of New Zealand, effectively printed most of the money that the government was "borrowing".[18]

The day before the level 4 lockdown came into force, Parliament passed three bills, with strong cross-party support. These provided for $NZ52 billion of emergency spending, and the remission of interest on tax owing after 14 February. They enabled local authorities to meet remotely, the government to take control of schools, prevented no-cause evictions of tenants, and instituted a six-month freeze on rentals. Throughout the next month, a range of further financial measures were taken, including a grant of $NZ27 million to voluntary social service providers. By mid-July the demand on voluntary foodbanks had dramatically increased, especially in South Auckland.[19] There was also a $NZ87.7 million distance learning package for schools, including two educational television channels, one in English and the other in Māori. In mid-April, the prime minister announced a $NZ130 million support package for tertiary students. A media relief investment of $NZ50 million was also made.

---

18   www.stuff.co.nz/business/122410298/reserve-bank-expands-cap-on-quantitative-easing-to-100-billion

19   www.stuff.co.nz/national/122093506/coronavirus-demand-for-food-banks-double-precovid-levels-and-still-growing.

The country's national carrier, Air New Zealand Ltd, was severely hit, with most of its wide-bodied aircraft grounded. Its workforce was cut by 30% (about 4,000 staff). The government, the majority owner of the airline, made available a substantial financial support package for the company, to be used at its discretion. In August the airline disclosed an annual after-tax net loss of $NZ454 million, its first loss for 18 years.[20]

The government negotiated with banks to prevent people losing their homes through having to default on mortgage payments. All retail banks agreed to defer residential mortgage payments for up to six months for customers adversely affected financially by the pandemic, and offered customers special advice on financial management. However, it has been argued that the banks did not do enough.[21] Eleven thousand employees lost their jobs in the June quarter, disproportionately women in sales and hospitality work.[22] The Minister of Finance estimated that the Auckland level 3 lockdown had cost the region about $NZ500 million.

By the end of August, six months after the level 4 lockdown, the government had outlayed a total of $NZ48 billion on various income support, business maintenance, apprenticeship training, and other programmes. The wage subsidy, which had helped to keep about 240,000 people in employment since March, was extended to cover the August outbreak. Median incomes had fallen by 7.6%, the first such fall since records began in 1998, and the country experienced negative GDP growth for the first time in many years. In the June quarter the country's trade deficit narrowed, as imports fell sharply while exports "generally held up".[23] The unemployment rate also held up better than many had expected, but the "underutilisation rate" increased sharply. (This gauge is generally deemed to be just as important as the unemployment rate. It reflects the number of people who do not have a job but are seeking work — the official unemployed — are part-time employees who are available to work longer hours, potential jobseekers, and who are looking for a job which they will be able to start within the next month.[24])

Figure 7.8 GDP rates 2014–2020 — Statistics New Zealand

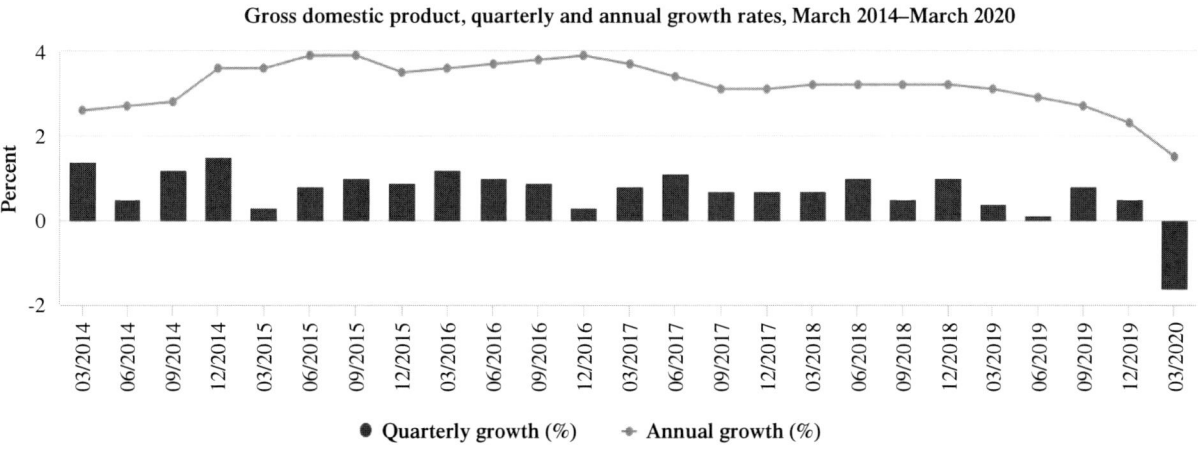

Gross domestic product, quarterly and annual growth rates, March 2014–March 2020

20 www.reuters.com/article/air-new-zealand-results/air-new-zealand-posts-first-annual-loss-in-18-years-forecasts-loss-in-2021-idUSL4N2FP0RN

21 www.rnz.co.nz/news/business/415838/banks-defend-covid-19-response-after-criticism-they-aren-t-doing-enough

22 https://thespinoff.co.nz/business/05-08-2020/11000-new-zealanders-have-lost-their-jobs-and-10000-of-them-were-women/

23 https://treasury.govt.nz/publications/weu/weekly-economic-update-28-august-2020-html

24 www.stats.govt.nz/indicators/underutilisation-rate

Political Realities

Prime Minister Ardern repeatedly appealed to and praised the cooperative efforts of what she called "our team of five million" (the New Zealand population) in responding to the lockdown despite the extensive hardships and inconvenience that it caused. It was a mostly successful political ploy, though in early September hundreds of people in various parts of the country demonstrated publicly against lockdowns and their associated rules. Clearly, the protestors did not consider themselves to be part of Ardern's "team", and may have been worried that this metaphorical device smacked of latent totalitarianism.[25] New Zealanders, a largely compliant people in any case, seemed enthusiastic about reporting to the Police any breaches of the lockdown rules. During the whole level 4 lockdown period there were nearly 55,500 more breaches reported than there were actions taken by the Police, which preferred to take an "educational" rather than a punitive approach.

As many thousands of New Zealanders found themselves in serious financial straits — about 75,000 people had gone on to welfare benefits since March — the Prime Minister announced that all government ministers and public sector chief executives would take a 20% pay cut. The leader of the opposition followed suit, reducing his salary by 20%. From 27 March Parliament adjourned for five weeks, but with agreement that the Leader of the Opposition would chair a cross-party Epidemic Response Committee — meeting remotely — to watch over the government's response to the pandemic.

The broad fault lines became clearer at this juncture. Debates focused in essence on the extent to which the economic costs to the country of the policies and actions designed to control the spread of the disease were justified. The arguments largely following partisan political lines: centre-right politicians tended to concentrate their attention on the economic costs, particularly on the decimation of the tourist industry (which by this time had ground to a virtual halt). Those on the centre-left, in support of the government, argued that without full and effective control of Covid-19 within New Zealand there would be no worthwhile economy at all.[26]

From about July strains had begun to appear in the coalition government itself, especially between the Labour and New Zealand First parties. The latter was led by veteran politician, Winston Peters, who was also the Deputy Prime Minister and Minister of Foreign Affairs. He had earlier advocated "travel bubbles" between New Zealand and other places where the virus had been kept under control or had been largely eliminated, like Taiwan, and Melbourne (before that city was hit with a major resurgence).

Although some commentators suggested that the government should have acted even earlier than it did, the lockdown met with widespread public approval. A mid-July poll had shown that the number of respondents who were satisfied with the government's ability to manage the pandemic had dropped to 82% from 92% in May. A poll taken in the latter part of August showed that 64% of respondents backed the Prime Minister to handle the pandemic, as against 18% who would have preferred the Leader of the Opposition, Judith Collins.[27] National — the main opposition party — had experienced two leadership changes within a month, damaging its standing in the political polls. Under Collins, it committed to establishing a single overarching authority to handle the management of Covid-19 at

---

25 www.nzherald.co.nz/nz/news/article.cfm?c_id=1&objectid=12362504

26 Tourism normally contributes about six percent of New Zealand's GDP, providing employment for 7.5% of the workforce.

27 www.stuff.co.nz/national/politics/300092282/election-2020-public-still-backing-government-and-jacinda-ardern-despite-second-outbreak-new-poll-shows?cid=app-iPhone

the border, were the party to lead the next government. She was critical of the "ad hoc" arrangements that had been progressively put in place by the government over the preceding months, saying the government had "dropped the ball", following on from the previous National Party leader's claim that the government's handling of the borders had been "shambolic".[28] These claims were derided by one academic commentator, who observed that, "From the tone and tenor of criticism in New Zealand, an otherwise uninformed observer would think that the performance of our leadership has been as bad as that of Donald Trump or Boris Johnson. Really?"[29]

Together with the opposition parties, Peters had argued that because of the pandemic the Prime Minister should postpone the election scheduled for 19 September. After consulting the Electoral Commission (which manages the general election) the Prime Minister announced that voting would be postponed from 19 September until 17 October.[30] This decision balanced a number of factors, not the least of which was the desire to remove any suggestion that to hold the election as scheduled could have significantly disadvantaged all but the Labour Party, given the Prime Minister's high public profile during the pandemic. The other parties acknowledged or accepted the Prime Minister's postponement.

Electioneering began soon after, with Peters claiming that New Zealand could have done "far better" had the Labour-led government accepted his urging that people coming into the country should have been quarantined at military bases. "If we could compare ourselves with Taiwan, we haven't done as well as we could have done." "Mistakes" had been made, according to Peters, and people needed to own up to that.[31]

Conclusion: Policymaking Theory and the New Zealand COVID-19 experience

The New Zealand government's response to the Covid-19 pandemic was driven by a steep learning curve, beginning early in 2020. The strategy of "Go hard, go early" to "flatten the curve" soon became a plan to eliminate the virus, in so far as this were possible. The level 4 national lockdown was successful in stopping what some statistical modelling showed could have been a calamitous spread of the disease. In deciding upon this approach the government, through its Director-General of Health, drew upon a great deal of scientific epidemiological advice and insight. In the process, Bloomfield, particularly through his daily lockdown television briefings, became the most high profile public servant in living memory. A technocrat had not been such a dominant figure in New Zealand government since the then Labour government's Minister of Finance, Roger Douglas, had led the implementation of the radical economic policies known eponymously as "Rogernomics", in the 1980s.[32]

The other person to receive widespread public acclaim was the Prime Minister, Jacinda Ardern, an able political communicator, who inspired high levels of public trust and reassurance. She and her

28   www.stuff.co.nz/national/politics/opinion/122522331/judith-collins-tough-times-calls-for-tough-border-measures

29   www.newsroom.co.nz/ideasroom/a-gap-between-criticism-and-reality

30   www.newsroom.co.nz/ardern-makes-call-on-election-date

31   www.stuff.co.nz/national/politics/300097515/election-2020-winston-peters-attacks-governments-coronavirus-response-as-he-relaunches-election-campaign

32   On technocracy, see F. Fischer (1990) *Technocracy and the Politics of Expertise*, Newbury Park, CA: Sage.

leading ministers fashioned an uncommonly impressive and effective relationship between scientific knowledge, on the one hand, and political judgment, on the other, with both policymaking strands evolving as the pandemic unfolded.[33]

The New Zealand case, especially in regard to the management of and testing at the borders, focused fresh academic attention on the perennial issue in public administration of centralization versus decentralization and the pros and cons of both. It also had theoretical relevance to public policymaking theory. It cannot be seen as an example of the so-called "rational" approach, so often promoted in much academic literature on public policymaking.[34] For a start, there is no known end point, since the goal of "eliminating" the virus — at least until a vaccine is produced and distributed — is likely to be unattainable, and so will not constitute any end game. Economic imperatives demand that the borders cannot remain closed indefinitely. So it will be some time before the proverbial fat lady sings in the New Zealand Covid-19 "opera".

Thus, anti-Covid-19 public policymaking currently differs from the "rational" public policies adopted internationally to control or eliminate diseases like smallpox, poliomyelitis or tuberculosis, simply because the means are not yet available, even though the political will generally is. Instead, the New Zealand experience, and probably that of other countries, exhibits many features which resonate with public policymaking understood as an on-going process of "muddling through". It involves coping with difficult and unpredictable circumstances and contingencies, with uncertain and limited knowledge, rather than solving clearly-defined problems characterised by scientific certainties. In so many respects it is a "wicked" rather than a "tame" public policy challenge, one in which the political values and perspectives of scientific experts themselves should not be ignored.

Above all, the scientifically-based responses to the pandemic in New Zealand were mediated within the political context of an election year. It will fall to New Zealand voters to demonstrate in October the extent to which they support the measures implemented and the leadership provided by the government in responding to the challenge of Covid-19.

---

33 On the relationships between science and politics, see B. S. Steel (ed) (2014) *Science and Politics: An A-to-Z Guide to Issues and Controversies*, Washington DC: CQ Press (a division of Sage Publishing).

34 Cf the seminal article, C. E. Lindblom (1959) "The Science of Muddling Through", *Public Administration Review*, 19, 2, pp. 79-88.

NEW ZEALAND

Robert Gregory
28.01–05.09 Total 1,413 cases / 351 probable cases / 24 deaths

01
Public Health Policies

28.01 the Ministry of Health (MoH) sets up the National Health Coordination Centre in response to the overseas outbreak of Covid-19.

02
Public Health Policies

03.02 the government announced that foreign travellers leaving China to be denied entry into New Zealand

05.02 a government-chartered flight operated by Air New Zealand arrived in Auckland from Wuhan, China, carrying 193 passengers, including 54 New Zealand citizens and 44 permanent residents. Thirty-five Australian passengers were transferred to an Australian flight, while the remaining 157 were quarantined in a military facility near Auckland, for 14 days.

07.02 MoH sets up a dedicated Healthline Freephone number for Covid-19-related calls.

28.02 New Zealand confirms its first case, a New Zealand citizen in her 60s who had flown into the country on 26 February. New Zealand now the 48th country to have a confirmed case.

03
Public Health Policies

04.03 second case confirmed, a New Zealand woman in her 30s returning from Italy.

05.03 third case confirmed, the first of local transmission, in Auckland.

14.03 sixth case confirmed, an Auckland man recently returned from America.

17.03 four more cases confirmed, bringing the total to 12.

20.03 11 new cases, all associated with overseas travel, making a total of 39.

21.03 the Prime Minister announced the introduction of a nation-wide alert system, levels 1 – 4.

24.03 40 new cases, making a total of 155 (including probable cases).

25.03 a national state of emergence declared by the civil defence minister. New Zealand enters alert level 4, full lockdown, at 11.59pm.

30.03 76 more cases bringing the total number of confirmed and probably cases to 589, 10 of which were cases of community-spread.

Twelve people were in hospital, two being in intensive care.

04
Public Health Policies

03.04 71 additional cases bringing the total to 868. Reported that there were 10 clusters of the virus, the biggest being at Marist College, Auckland.

07.04 54 new cases, with a total of 1,160 confirmed (943) and probable (217).

09.04 compulsory quarantining announced for all New Zealanders returning home from overseas.

10.04 first Covid-19 death reported, a woman in her 90s, at a rest home cluster in Christchurch.

11.04 two more deaths reported, a Wellington man in his 80s, and a man in his 70s, who was in the Christchurch rest home cluster.

13.04 another death, a man in his 80s from the Christchurch rest home cluster, bringing the national mortality count to five.

14.04 four more deaths, three of whom from the Christchurch rest home cluster,and a man in his 70s in Wellington. Total death toll now nine. Seventeen new cases, bringing a total of confirmed and probable to 1,366 (1,072 confirmed). 628 had recovered.

17.04 two further deaths, an elderly man and woman, both linked to clusters. The Wairarapa District Health Board became the first of the 20 DHBs to record zero active cases.

20.04 Prime Minister, Jacinda Ardern, announced that the country would drop down to level 3 at 11.59pm on 27 April, to be in force for at least two weeks, with a further decision to be taken by the government on 11 May.

21.04 five new cases, making a total of confirmed and probable of 1,445. One more death reported, an elderly woman in the Christchurch rest home cluster.

22.04 a further death, being an elderly woman in the Christchurch rest home cluster.

23.04 two more deaths, a woman in her 60s and a man who was in the Christchurch rest home cluster. This brought the total number of deaths to 17, of whom 10 were from this cluster.

25.04 another death, a woman in her 70s from

a rest home cluster in Auckland.

27.04 another death, an elderly woman from the Auckland rest home cluster.

05

Public Health Policies

01.05 three new cases, bringing the total of confirmed and probable to 1,479 (347 probable). Six people remained in hospital, and 11 new recoveries reported.

02.05 one further death, an elderly man in the Christchurch rest home cluster.

04–05.05 no new cases reported.

06.05 two new cases, and one further death – a woman in her 60s in the Christchurch rest home cluster. A record 7,323 tests completed nationally on this day.

11.05 the first day since 22 March in which the active count of cases was below 100.

14–16.05 14th and 16th – no new cases reported.

25–31.05 in the week of the 25th, no new cases, with the total at 1,504 confirmed and probable (350). The last hospitalised person discharged on 27th. Only one active case remaining in New Zealand on the 29th. One death from 24 May reclassified on 28 May as being related to Covid-19, and linked to the Christchurch rest home cluster. Death

toll stands at 22 (no more deaths occurred through to the end of August, the time of writing.)

06

Public Health Policies

16.06 two new cases reported, being arrivals from Britain, so no further community spread.

18.06 one new case, an incoming international traveller (quarantined at Auckland).

20–29.06 21 new cases, international travellers, none of community spread. Active cases now totalling 22.

30.06 no new cases; only one case remaining in hospital.

07

Public Health Policies

02–13.07 16 new cases, all of people in Managed Isolation Quarantine (MIQ) facilities, or in self-isolation.

14–21.07 11 new cases, all international travellers, no community spread. A total of 1,555 confirmed or probable cases (350), 27 active cases.

23.07 five new recoveries reported, no new cases.

24–31.07 five new cases, international travellers, no community spread. Total number of confirmed and probable cases stands at 1,560 (350 probable), with 1,518 (97%) having been classified as recovered.

08

Public Health Policies

01–05.08 nine new cases, all related to international travel, and in MIQ. No community spread.

06–10.08 no new cases of any kind.

11.08 one new case in managed isolation. This day marked 102 days since the last instance of community spread was recorded in New Zealand. Four cases of community transmission reported in Auckland, all being members of one family.

12.08 the government announced that from the 14th of August the Auckland region would move into level 3, and the rest of the country to level 2.

13.08 14 new cases confirmed, all but one related to the new Auckland community cluster. The other was detected at a border MIQ.

14.08 13 new confirmed or probable community cases reported, 11 in Auckland and two in the North Island's south Waikato town of Tokoroa. Levels 3 and 2 implemented as announced on the 12th.

15.08 seven new community cases reported, with active cases totalling 56. A record 23,846 daily tests conducted nationally, mainly in the Auckland region.

16–20.08 43 new cases reported, only two of

which were from the isolation of overseas travellers.

21–23.08 20 new cases reported, all community-spread except four that were imported and in MIQs.

24.08 Prime Minister Ardern announced that the Auckland region would remain at level 3 until 11.59pm on Sunday 30 August, when it would move to level 2.5, while the rest of the country would remain at level 2 until at least 6 September. Seven new community cases were listed on the 24th.

25–31.08 55 new cases reported, 16 of which were from border MIQs. The total number of cases since February stands at 1,738 (including 351 probable), with 131 active cases. Eleven people were in hospital with the disease.

09

Public Health Policies

03.09 a total of 797,990 tested throughout New Zealand since 22 January.

04.09 a man in his 50s dies from Covid-19. He's the youngest person to have died in New Zealand from the disease, bringing the total number of deaths to 23.

A total of 1,413 confirmed cases and 351 probable, with 112 active cases. Three new cases on this day, all related to existing clusters. Ninety-two percent of all cases since February had recovered.

The government decides that the alert levels 2.5 for Auckland and 2 for the rest of the country will remain until at least 14 September.

05.09 It's reported that 82 year-old Dr Joe Williams, a former Prime Minister of the Cook Islands and an Auckland doctor, died the day before from Covid-19 in Auckland. The number of deaths now stands at 24.

COVID-19 in Taiwan:
Some Crucial Experiences for Fighting the Pandemic

Bennis Wai Yip So

Facing a direct and immediate first wave of threat of COVID-19 from adjacent Mainland China and subsequent waves of impacts from other areas, Taiwan successfully avoid any community-wide diffusion of the virus. This should be attributed to its well-established healthcare infrastructure, a pro-active approach to the crisis, technocracy in decision making, effective containment measures, social collaboration and cooperation, and information transparency.

Up till 20 August 2020, accumulated confirmed COVID-19 cases in Taiwan reached 486 with deaths of 7 and total recoveries of 457. The mortality rate was 0.014% (See Figures 8.1 and 8.2)

Figure 8.1 Daily confirmed cases, deaths and recovered cases from 21 Jan. to 20 Aug. 2020

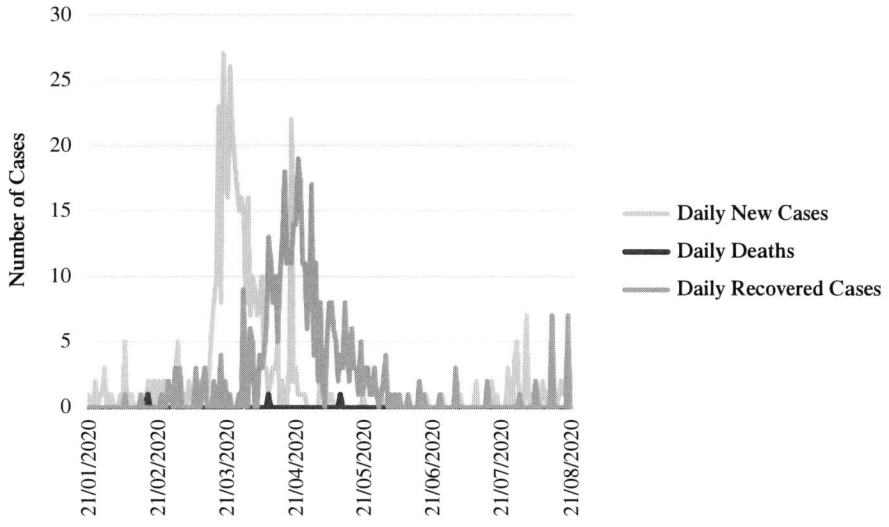

Figure 8.2 Accumulated and recovered cases from 21 Jan. to 20 Aug. 2020

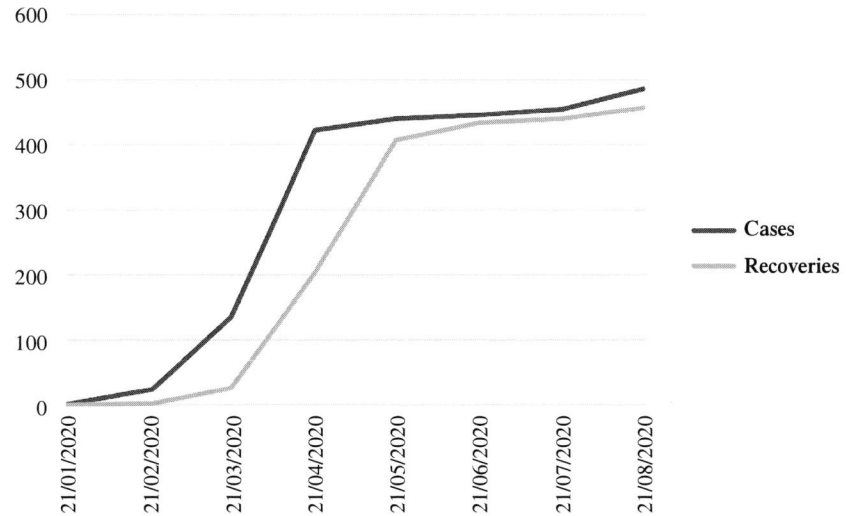

Success Story of Combating COVID-19: A Snapshot

Due to the proximity to and the frequent interpersonal connection with Mainland China, Taiwan was supposed to be a high-risk area of outbreak of COVID-19. Surprisingly, the performance of Taiwan's response has been very impressive, even though it is not perfect. Its response to the crisis not only avoids lockdown from which many western countries have suffered, but also minimizes the impact upon people's daily life. The most "disturbing" is requiring people to wear a mask in many public areas and it is imperative on public transport (from April 1 onward). Many body temperature check points are set up before various entrances to screen out all individuals with a fever symptom. Under the above premises, however, people can maintain their normal daily life. People keep working at office rather than work from home. Students in general can physically attend school rather than online classes, though sporadic cases of class suspension upon suspicion of COVID-19 occurred. People are allowed to dine out, though they have to keep a social distance from each other in restaurants. The regular-season play of the baseball league was already resumed on April 20.

Sporadic incidents might possibly cause community transmission,[1] including infected passengers from the Diamond Princess cruise liner who roamed around northern Taiwan in January; and the cluster infections on the naval supply ship Panshih that joined an overseas visit to Palau in March and returned to Kaohsiung in early April, its infected crew members had been in local communities for three days before being recalled for COVID-19 tests. The crowds clustering around tourist attractions during the Tomb Sweeping Festival, the Labor Day holiday and the Dragon Boat Festival were worrisome. Luckily, these incidents have not developed into a situation of community-acquired infection in Taiwan so far.

Luck, of course, cannot fully account for Taiwan's outstanding performance against the deadly virus. An early alert to the potential crisis was critical for taking precautions far ahead of most other countries which usually underestimated the situation or took a "wait and see" attitude before the outbreak. In response to the news about an outbreak of atypical pneumonia with unknown etiology in Wuhan, Taiwan Centers for Disease Control (CDC) under the Ministry of Health and Welfare (MOHW) launched inspection measures for inbound flights from Wuhan as early as on 31 December 2019.[2] By 5 January 2020, the CDC began monitoring all individuals who had travelled to Wuhan within 14 days and exhibited a fever or symptoms of upper respiratory tract infections. An early step to take a border control is the smartest measure to close the gap for virus intrusion. As a result, there is no need for Taiwan to adopt a mass testing exercise in communities, like the case in South Korea. Instead, Taiwan adopted a "precise identification strategy" to detect a limited number of infected individuals and trace their sources of infection and contact history case by case, subjecting all high-risk people to quarantine. In Taiwan, such detailed epidemiological investigation is considered a more appropriate measure to contain the virus contagion than mass screening.

The precise identification strategy cannot be shared by those countries that did not take an adequate border control in advance. Still, many useful lessons can be drawn from Taiwan. These include five dimensions: good medical infrastructure, professional decision making, effective containment, information transparency, and public collaboration.

---

1 Community transmission is when there is no clear source of origin of the infection in a new community. It happens when you can no longer identify who became infected after being exposed to someone who interacted with people from the originally infected communities.

2 The CDC was set up on 1 July 1999.

Infrastructures: Unified Epidemic Prevention and Control Mechanism, and National Health Insurance System

The severe acute respiratory syndrome (SARS) epidemic in 2003, which also spread from Mainland China to Taiwan and caused 73 deaths, was a painful experience for Taiwan, but Taiwan also drew a significant lesson from SARS, establishing a comprehensive epidemic prevention system to avoid such a catastrophe in future. First, the National Health Command Center was established under the CDC in 2005 to unify the leadership for epidemic prevention and control, and to facilitate a swift response and resource mobilization and coordination. Right before that, the Communicable Disease Control Act was amended in 2004 to authorize the setting-up of a cross-agency mechanism to handle any future epidemic. According to the act, an ad hoc taskforce Central Epidemic Command Center (CECC) can be set up with the approval of the Executive Yuan (i.e., the top executive state organ in Taiwan) in response to any epidemic crisis. The CECC can be authorized to command, supervise, and coordinate government agencies at all levels, state-owned enterprises, and private organizations in performing epidemic prevention work. More importantly, well-trained and experienced public health officers and experts occupy the key positions in the epidemic prevention system.

Another crucial infrastructure is its National Health Insurance (NHI) system that started from 2005. The system covers almost all citizens and non-citizen residents in Taiwan. People access any medical service with their own IC NHI cards. The NHI card becomes a convenient tool to track the suspected cases during the COVID-19 crisis. The government also uses the card to distribute state-supplied masks. People can purchase the masks with the NHI card through the NHI-contracted pharmacies and other (online) channels. The NHI also helped in developing a national health data base. The MediCloud System was set up in 2015 to collect and share the medical information scattered across Taiwan. In the early stage of the outbreak of COVID-19, in order to effectively avoid the flow of high-risk people and the risk of infection in medical institutions, the MediCloud System was adopted as a platform to share the travel and contact history of patients with front-line medical staff, under the premise of personal data security,[3] to judge infection risks and take relevant infection control measures.

Decision Making: Technocrats-in-command and Proactive Measures

Another distinctive feature of Taiwan experience is the decision-making mechanism and the central role of medical experts. Whilst in many countries politicians or top state leaders have played a key role in the anti-epidemic decision making, albeit being advised by epidemiologists, the voices of medical experts have had a pivotal role in COVID-19 decision-making in Taiwan, and their influence even outstripped those of the top leaders. President Tsai Ing-wen and the premier Su Tseng-chang play a minor role in the decisions directly related to the epidemic. The vice-president Chen Chien-jen promoted Taiwan COVID-19 experience in interviews with international media, but this is attributable to himself being an epidemiologist and a former minister of health during the SARS.[4] On the whole, Minister of Health and Welfare Chen Shih-chung and his professional team members in the CECC are the faces of the Taiwan anti-COVID-19 efforts. His swift and professional responses to the changing situations and 24/7 commitment to the anti-epidemic work were widely praised. When the CECC was upgraded to a level-1

---

3   The collection, processing and use of personal data were regulated by the Personal Data Protection Act enacted in 1995.
4   For example, see www.youtube.com/watch?v=XqFQW-SIV7Q; www.youtube.com/watch?v=G1potR0eXA4

setting on 27 February, the premier was supposed to be the chief commander (see Table 8.1). However, in the case of COVID-19, Chen, instead of Su, took command. The top executive leaders delegated most authority to the technocrats.

Technocrats-in-command can well account for the success of Taiwan experience. The technocrats refer to not only the public health officers but also an advisory specialist panel. The panel convener is Chang Shan-chwen, a professor of internal medicine and the executive vice president of National Taiwan University. The panel plays the role of think tank of the CECC, conducting data analysis and give policy advice. This does not argue that all decisions took no political factors into account, especially those concerning Mainland China, but professional judgment appeared more predominant.

In addition, a proactive approach to decision making is the hallmark of the technocracy. An action motto *chaoqian bushu* (literally "advanced deployment") has become very popular in Taiwan recently. It refers to the strategy the CECC took to address the outbreak. The typical example is the setting-up of the CECC. There are 4 setting-up levels for the CECC. The more serious the situation assessed is, the higher level the setting-up adopted. The higher the level is, the more authority is delegated to the CECC and a higher-ranking official would assume the chief commander (see Table 1). At the highest level-1 setting, all ministries and nationwide government agencies could be activated to assist this emergency function. Delegated senior staff of these ministries/agencies needs to be stationed at the CECC for coordinating tasks under the order of the chief commander of the CECC. As early as 20 January, a level-3 CECC was activated and quickly upgraded to level-2 on 23 January. On 27 February, it was further upgraded to level 1. In principle, the level-1 setting would be triggered by the emergence of community spreading. By February 27 (and even after that), Taiwan had not reached such a serious situation. However, in light of the mounting global urgency to contain the coronavirus, under Chen Shih-chung's recommendation, the CECC was upgraded to level 1.

Another case was the restriction on exporting masks as early as on 24 January. It was quite controversial when the measure was promulgated.[5] It seemed correct in retrospect when we saw the outbreak in neighboring countries, like Japan, but masks were in short supply partly caused by bulk purchasing by Mainland Chinese. Simply put, *chaoqian bushu* encourages "advanced preparations for worsening and even the worst conditions."

Table 8.1 Four levels of command unit activation protocols corresponding to different extent of outbreak and risk assessment

Level	Extent of Outbreak and Risk Assessment	Command Unit Action Protocol
4	COVID-19 epidemic confirmed in Wuhan, China	Organize contingency team
3	Evident ongoing community spread of COVID-19 in communities in Wuhan, China	Establish the CECC, appoint Taiwan CDC director as chief commander
2	Confirmed imported cases of COVID-19 in communities in Taiwan	Establish the CECC, appoint minister of health and welfare as chief commander
1	Community spreading of COVID-19 in Taiwan	Establish the CECC, appoint premier as chief commander

Source: www.cdc.gov.tw/File/Get/sR8H-GsvYkVS0nOVFXJ-4w

---

5   See www.scmp.com/comment/letters/article/3048434/coronavirus-outbreak-dont-blame-taiwan-export-ban-face-masks

Effective Containment

Border Control

Implementing border control in a timely manner, as noted above, is key to keeping the virus out. The imported source accounts for more than 80% of all confirmed cases. Only 12% are locally acquired (The rest are from a cluster infection on Panshih).[6] That means most infected cases had been identified and caught before they entered the local communities. The border control measures included tightening bans on traveler entry, and orderly evacuation of citizens from epidemic regions.

On 26 January, Mainlanders from Hubei were prohibited from entry, expanding to all Mainlanders and people from Hong Kong and Macao on 11 February. The prohibition further expanded to all foreign travelers on 19 March (except those holding a resident certificate or special entry permit). Transiting via Taiwan was also banned on 24 March. Beside the air travel, cruise ships were banned from docking from 6 February.

The above restrictions were first relaxed from June. Business travelers from low-risk and low-to-moderate risk countries or areas are now allowed to enter Taiwan. Transiting passengers are allowed for Taoyuan International Airport. Foreign nationals can now apply for entry except for reasons of tourism and social visits.

For the citizens stranded in foreign countries, the government took a careful step to evacuate slowly to avoid overloading of the medical system. So far, 19 charter flights have been arranged to carry citizens back to Taiwan.[7] All these inbound travelers avoided interpersonal contact on the flight and after arrival. They had to take a designated vehicle rather than ordinary public transport to the locations for home quarantine.

Community Transmission Prevention

The border controls alone were not sufficient to contain the virus contagion especially during the early period of the outbreak where the control had not yet been well established, and when the symptoms of the coronavirus were not well understood. Hence, not all potential cases could be detected upon their arrival and well isolated. For the first domestic case diagnosed on 28 January, a man was believed to have acquired the disease from his wife, who had traveled to Wuhan and was confirmed before him.[8] The first death on 16 February was a 61-year-old man who had not traveled overseas recently and no contact with COVID-19 patients.[9] A woman tested positive for the COVID-19 on 19 February 2020, but she had not travelled outside of Taiwan for two years.[10] Hence, measures to prevent community transmission are the key to further fill all loopholes.

The CECC kept abreast of any new findings concerning COVID-19 and frequently updated the criteria for reporting and testing. Apart from those who had travel history to China and other foreign countries, any person with a symptom that could be associated with the COVID-19 should be reported

---

6   See www.mofa.gov.tw/en/cp.aspx?n=AF816F475BFEFB99

7   See https://en.wikipedia.org/wiki/COVID-19_pandemic_in_Taiwan

8   See https://focustaiwan.tw/politics/202001285001

9   See https://focustaiwan.tw/society/202002160012

10   See https://focustaiwan.tw/society/202002200003

and took the COVID-19 test. The symptoms on the list were gradually expanded from pneumonia to abnormal olfactory and gustatory sense, and to diarrhea (see Fig. 3).

Sophisticated precautionary measures are applied to those who have travel history, had contacts with confirmed cases and those who are tested negative for COVID-19. They should be respectively subject to home isolation, home quarantine or self-health management for 14 days (for the criteria and procedures, see Fig. 4).

To ensure that people in home isolation/quarantine comply and at home, the Digital Fencing Tracking System was already built up by the end of February to accurately track whereabouts of people in quarantine. The location of people in home isolation/quarantine can be monitored by detecting electromagnetic signals of their mobile phone to determine whether they leave the range of their home.

Besides targeting the imported sources of transmission, minimizing close social contact in daily life is considered a commonsense method to reduce the risk of infection. While not resorting to a lockdown policy, wearing a mask was considered as an effective way to protect people from the virus. Different from many western countries, there is no social controversy over its effectiveness in Taiwan. The more critical issue is the guarantee of enough supply of masks. Apart from the restriction on export of masks, the government requisitioned all surgical face masks produced in Taiwan and implemented a rationing system for the public from early February. People can purchase a limited number of masks with the NHI card at a price of NT$5 per each (approximately US$ 0.17).[11] The production lines were expanded to ensure a stockpile to meet domestic needs. The rising production capacity allows Taiwan to export masks now (the ban on mask exports was lifted on June 1).[12]

Figure 8.3 Frequent adjustment of criteria for COVID-19 case reporting in response to international and domestic situations

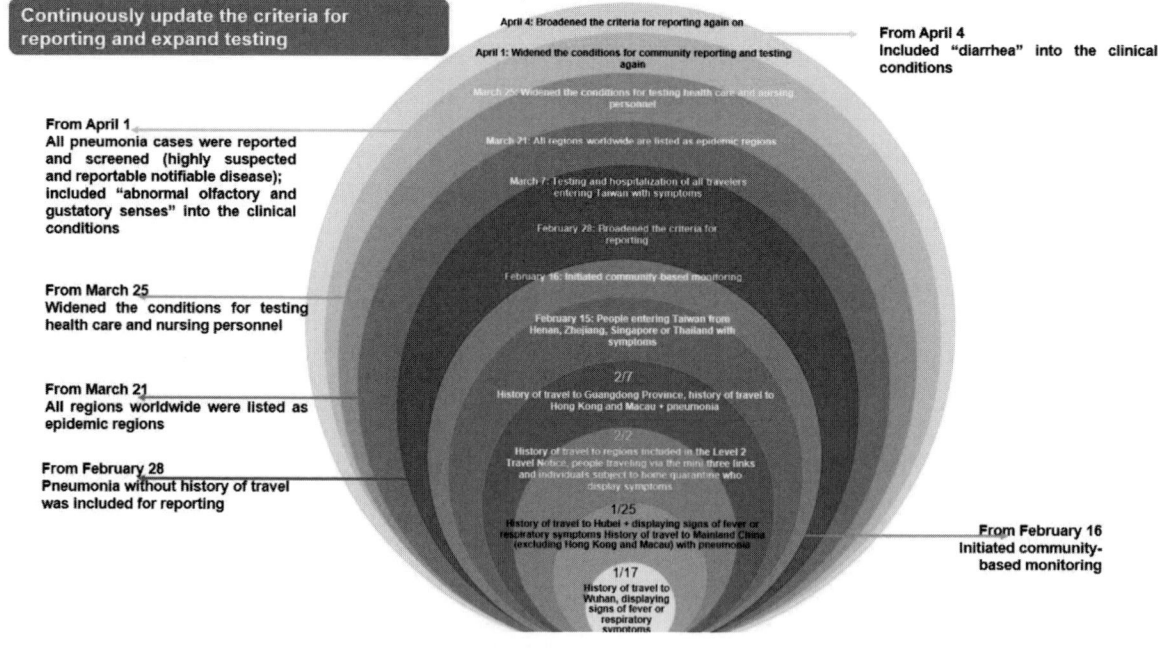

Source: https://covid19.mohw.gov.tw/en/cp-4775-53739-206.html

---

11 Each person could buy two masks each time and could not do it again within 7 days from February 6. From April 9 onward, the quota expanded to 9 adult-sized masks or 10 child-sized masks every 14 days.

12 See www.taiwannews.com.tw/en/news/3940506

Figure 8.4 Measures for monitoring potential infected targets

CECC Measures for Following Up on Persons at Risk of Infection   04/07/2020

Intervention	Home Isolation	Home Quarantine	Self-health management
Groups of persons	Persons who had contact with confirmed cases	People with travel history	1. Reported cases who have tested negative and met criteria for being released from isolation 2. People reported and tested for COVID-19 under "COVID-19 Community-based Surveillance"
Responsible authorities	Local health authorities	Local civil affairs bureau or borough chief	Central/Local health authorities
Enforcement	Home isolation for 14 days Active monitoring twice a day	Home quarantine for 14 days Active monitoring once or twice a day	Self-health management for 14 days
Notes concerning respective measures	• Health authority will issue a "Home (Self) Isolation Notice" • Health authority shall check health status of the individual twice a day • During the home isolation perios, the individual is to stay at home (or designated location) and not go out, and may not leave the country or use public transportation • Symptomatic individuals will be sent to the hospital for medical attention • Individuals not adhering to the CECC's prevention measures will be penalized under the Communicable Disease Control Act and be forcibly placed • After the home isolation period ends, the individual should conduct an additional 7-day period of self-health management	• Where the relevant authority has issued a Novel Coronavirus Health Declaration and Home Quarantine Notice, the individual is to wear a surgical mask and return home for home quarantine • The local borough chief or borough clerk shall call the individual every day during the 14-day period to ask about the individual's health status, and shall record the information obtained • During the quarantine period, the individual is to stay at home (or designated location) and not go out, and may not leave the country or use public transportation • Symptomatic individuals will be sent to designated medical facilities for tests, the relevant health authority will also begin active monitoring • Individuals not adhering to the CECC's prevention measures will be penalized under the Communicable Disease Control Act and be forcibly placed • After the home quarantine period ends, the individual should conduct an additional 7-day period of self-health management	• Asymptomatic individuals are to avoid public places, postpone any non-urgent medical care or examination, always wear a medical mask when going out, wash hands frequently, follow respiratory hygiene and cough etiquette, and take temperature twice a day, once in the morning and once in the evening • Individuals with fever or respiratory symptoms such as coughing or running nose are to wear a medical mask, seek medical attention immediately and not to use public transport; inform the physician of your contact histoy, travel history, and whether anyone else has similar symptoms; wear a surgical mask while returning home and avoid going out; and keep 1 meter away from others when talking to them • After being tested for COVID-19 and returning home, individuals are to stay at home and not to go out befor receiving results • Medical personnel are to halt work and not to come to work temporarily
legal basis	• Article 48, Communicable Disease Control Act • Paragraph 1, Article15, Special Act for Prevention, Relief and Revitalization Measures for Severe Pneumonia with Novel Pathogens	• Article 58, Communicable Disease Control Act • Paragraph 2, Article15, Special Act for Prevention, Relief and Revitalization Measures for Severe Pneumonia with Novel Pathogens	• Article 48, Communicable Disease Control Act; Article 58, Communicable Disease Control Act • Article 67, Communicable Disease Control Act; Article 69, Communicable Disease Control Act

Source: https://covid19.mohw.gov.tw/en/cp-4786-53904-206.html

Many large-scale public gathering functions were canceled after the outbreak. Crowd management measures were further enforced. On March 25, the CECC recommended that indoor events that are attended by more than 100 people and outdoor gatherings attended by more than 500 people be suspended, in order to prevent cluster infections. The center further announced social distancing measures on 1 April to encourage the general public to maintain social distancing. Furthermore, from 10 April, night markets, traditional markets and shopping areas were required to enforce social distancing and to have only one point of entry.

The CECC also sent warning messages to people at crowded locations (especially during weekends and holidays) via cell phones to remind them of maintaining a safe social distance and wearing masks. The public was also advised to implement 14 days of self-health management after returning from a crowded place.

The above containment measures were effective in preventing a further outbreak of the epidemic. Since 12 April, Taiwan has not recorded any locally transmitted cases: all recent cases were of imported infections. This was during a time when many epidemic prevention measures at the community level started to be relaxed, beginning in early June (including passengers allowed to remove masks on train/ Mass Rapid Transit (MRT) System if proper social distancing can be observed; and no limit on number of people in some indoor gathering points such as movies theaters and art exhibitions). It implies the border control and associated quarantine measures are doing enough to block the virus intrusion at the current stage.

Information Transparency

People in Taiwan are well informed of the updated situation of the epidemic. Starting from 22 January, the CECC hosted a daily press briefing and published at least one press release every day to establish a transparent, immediate, and professional platform for communication with the media and the public. This daily press became a weekly press from June 7 onward given the success of containment effort, but a provisional briefing is immediately organized if any new case is confirmed.

Data on the outbreak situation and disease survey results are provided on the official Line and Facebook accounts. Any new policies or clarifications of disinformation related to the epidemic are immediately announced through these channels.[13] As a result, no social panic due to lack of information or spread of misinformation has been evident during the outbreak to date.

The CDC has also produced numerous videos to promote some new social manners in response to the prevention of COVID-19, such as appropriate hand washing procedures and encouraging social distancing. These videos were broadcast frequently on TV to remind people to observe new social norms under the epidemic.[14]

---

13   For the fake news problem related to the COVID-19, see https://focustaiwan.tw/cross-strait/202004080010
14   See www.cdc.gov.tw/Category/ListMovie/DWSgB84e8MEvXgBqiQmR6A

Public Collaboration

Last but not least, the above measures could not be well implemented without the engagement of the private sector and voluntary assistance from the communities.

First of all, manufacturers and technicians were mobilized to help expand the capacity of mask production. In one month from 5 February, daily mask production jumped from 4 million to 10 million.[15] Some factories adjusted their production lines to work with the government to produce 75% rubbing alcohol.

The pharmacies that sell state-supplied masks to the public spent much time and manpower to package the masks and handle the long queue of buyers before June.

Tens of thousands of volunteers in communities helped provide food to people under quarantine and check their conditions on site. In many popular gathering places such as night markets, patrollers were organized to control the flow of crowds. Sanitizers are usually available in shopping malls, restaurants and lift lobbies. The public may clean their hands at their convenience.

Concluding Remarks and Challenges

Taiwan took advantage of its unique institutional context (SARS experience and the NHI) to pre-empt the first wave of the coronavirus intrusion. The government was prudent in coping with subsequent waves of crises and kept the island relatively safe in the first half of 2020. The achievement received a high recognition across the world. The secretary of health and human services of the United States, Alex Azar, further paid a landmark visit to Taiwan in early August, signing a memorandum of understanding with the MOHW to expand cooperation on global health security, infectious disease control and vaccine development on 10 August.[16]

However, the pandemic is not vanishing but keeps sweeping across the world without the availability of COVID-19 vaccine in near future. Challenges are expected in the second half of the year when close social contacts are resumed and people are relaxing alertness due to no locally transmitted case reported for a long time. It is possible for the undetected infected to spread the virus, especially in the case of asymptomatic transmission. Four unusual cases from June to August remain unexplainable up to now. These confirmed cases were all foreigners (a Japanese student, a Thai migrant worker, a Belgian engineer and a Malaysian with a Taiwanese wife) who stayed in Taiwan for a while and tested positive upon their return to home countries, but those having contacted with them in Taiwan have tested negative so far.[17] Do these cases imply there are many undetected cases in local communities? Is it necessary to carry out a mass testing?

A mass testing program for COVID-19 antibodies is being conducted in Changhua County by its government in collaboration with College of Public Health, National Taiwan University. Some positive cases have been detected. That reflects the existence of hidden domestic cases but it seems they cause

---

15 See https://focustaiwan.tw/society/202003240015

16 See https://focustaiwan.tw/politics/202008100020

17 See https://focustaiwan.tw/society/202006260007; www.cdc.gov.tw/En/Bulletin/Detail/hxfI2-iPAw0D5a2BDDW8lw?typeid=158; www.taiwannews.com.tw/en/news/3978550 ; https://focustaiwan.tw/society/202008170010

no community outbreak. The local healthcare authority is optimistic about this situation, because the detected antibodies suggests there should be a certain level of immunity in the community.[18]

The CECC still resists the application of a mass testing (including for all inbound travelers) and argues that it may cause overload of the healthcare system.[19] Nevertheless, epidemic prevention measures are being tightened again after moderate relaxation in June. People must wear a mask on the MRT now and may be required to do so in some crowded and indoor areas, such as certain chain supermarkets and department stores.

References

1. Cheng, Hao-Yuen. et al. "Initial rapid and proactive response for the COVID-19 outbreak: Taiwan's experience." *Journal of the Formosan Medical Association*, 119.4 (2020), pp. 771–773.

2. Huang, Irving Yi-Feng. "Fight COVID-19 through government initiatives and collaborative governance: The Taiwan experience." *Public Administration Review*, 80.4 (2020), pp. 665–670.

3. For the crucial policies and measures to combat COVID-19, see a specific official website for the COVID-19 under the Ministry of Health and Welfare: https://covid19.mohw.gov.tw/en/mp-206.html

4. For detailed government information for the COVID-19, see www.cdc.gov.tw/En/Category/List/fl7pveR6ZcoetNProjyY-g

---

18 See https://focustaiwan.tw/society/202008090003
19 See https://focustaiwan.tw/society/202008250017

TAIWAN

Bennis Wai Yip So

19.01–15.08 Total 482 cases / 7 deaths

19.01 – 25.01 (3)*
Public Health Policies

20.01 In response to the outbreak of coronavirus disease (COVID-19), Taiwan Centers for Disease Control (Taiwan CDC) announced the establishment of the "Severe Special Infectious Pneumonia Central Epidemic Outbreak Command Center", with its Director, Chou Jih-Haw, as the commander.

21.01 The Central Epidemic Command Center (CECC) announced the first confirmed imported case of 2019 novel coronavirus infection(2019-nCoV) in Taiwan, thus raising the travel alert level for Wuhan, China.

22.01 The CECC organized manpower across government agencies to strengthen quarantine measures at international (including cross-strait) airports and ports, to enhance the public alertness towards the disease and at the same time to reduce public panic. Such efforts also included planning and conducting drills for future infection control at healthcare institutes.

23.01 In light of the expanding outbreak revealed by shutting down public transport in Wuhan, the command level of the Central Epidemic Command Center (CECC) was escalated to a level-2 setting and that Minister of Ministry of Health and Welfare (MOHW) Chen Shih-Chung (陳時中) acted as the Commander.

26.01 – 01.02 (10)*
Public Health Policies

30.01 People who entered any hospital were required to wear a mask.

02.02 – 08.02 (17; 1 recovery)*
Public Health Policies

02.02 In response to the demands of epidemic prevention, the CECC requisitioned face masks, allocating them to the health bureau of local governments.

People who had visited China in the last 14 days were advised to temporarily avoid visiting hospitals and other healthcare institutes and to postpone nonessential medical care or checkups; and for the medical staff who had visited China in the last 14 days were advised to temporarily halt work and to stay at home and conducted self-health management for 14 days.

06.02 A real-name rationing of face masks was executed from 6 February. Citizens could purchase the masks from pharmacies with their health ID cards. Each person could buy two masks each time and could not do it again within 7 days.

07.02 National Health Research Institutes under the MOHW launched the development on a vaccination for the new coronavirus.

As of February 10, a 14-day home quarantine was required for travelers transiting through China, Hong Kong and Macau. The number of direct flights between Taiwan, and China, Hong Kong and Macau was reduced. Flights from certain airports were suspended.

Socio-Economic Policy Packages

02.02 The CECC resolved that the start of second term of all elementary and high schools was delayed for 2 weeks, starting from 25 February.

03.02 To prevent the spread of the deadly novel coronavirus (2019-nCoV), the CECC decided that Taiwan university students would begin their second semester after February 25; all Mainland students were not allowed to enter Taiwan after February 9.

Due to the delay of start of the second term for elementary and high schools, parents with children under 12 were allowed to apply for a "special childcare leave" from the 11th to 24th February.

09.02 – 15.02 (18; 2 recoveries)*
Public Health Policies

11.02 Travelers entering Taiwan were required to complete health declaration form.

12.02 The MOHW set up the Call Center on Febru-

---

* Source: Taiwan Centers for Disease Control: www.cdc.gov.tw/

   Source: Ministry of Health and Welfare: www.mohw.gov.tw/mp-1.html

   Source: Executive Yuan: www.ey.gov.tw/

ary 11 for to give regular phone calls to those subject to home isolation and home quarantine to ensure them remain in quarantine.[1]

16.02 – 22.02 (26/1; 3 recoveries)*

Public Health Policies

16.02 To strengthen community-based surveillance, people with foreign travel or foreigner contact or other potential risks would be included in COVID-19 testing procedures.[2]

Socio-Economic Policy Packages

21.02 In order to assist students whose family income was affected by COVID-19, the Ministry of Education (MOE) required schools at all levels to initiate student assistance measures based on the student's case situation and needs after the start of school, such as providing emergency bailout bursary in accordance to the "School Assistance Program for Vulnerable Students in Colleges and Universities" bailout bursaries, or providing counseling and scholarships through the "Higher Education Program for Higher Education Program Assistance Mechanism."

23.02 – 29.02 (39/1; 9 recoveries)*

Public Health Policies

24.02 In response to health concerns arising from COVID-19, overseas travel of medical personnel was restricted. Traveling to China, Hong Kong and Macau was banned. For other regions in the list of travel alert issued by the CECC, official approval must be obtained beforehand.

Travelers from the regions in the list of travel alert level-1 or level-2 must be subject to 14-day self-health management.

26.02 The MOHW issued the "Guidelines for the Management of Outsourcing Personnel of Medical Institutions in response to Severe Special Infectious Pneumonia." In order to strengthen crowd control of hospitals for avoiding in-hospital transmission of COVID-19, all hospitals were required to implement the following crowd control measures: (1) Patient segregation (2) Visitor control management (3) Outsourcing worker management.

27.02 In order to strengthen the resource integration of the central ministries and departments and localities, the Premier decided to raise the CECC to command level 1 and the Minister of MOHW, Chen Shih-Chung remained as the commander.

28.02 Travelers from China, Hong Kong, Macau, South Korea and Italy were required to undergo home quarantine for 14 days.

Socio-Economic Policy Packages

27.02 Executive Yuan (EY) approved a special budget to fund COVID-19 response and relief measures.

01.03 – 07.03 (45; 12 recoveries)*

Public Health Policies

05.03 In light of the rise of production capacity of masks, citizens could buy 3 adult-sized masks and 5 child-sized masks each time (real-name rationing). Still, each person could buy the masks once a week.

The normal operation of some domestic manufacturing and service industries were affected by the COVID-19. In order to reduce the impact of the epidemic on business operations, the CECC and various ministries would jointly formulate the

---

1   If an individual was already identified as a contact of a confirmed case, such an individual was subject to a 14-day period of home isolation. The individual should record their temperature and health status twice per day, and has mobile phone turned. The health authority would contact the individual twice a day to follow up the individual's health status. During the home isolation period, people should stay at home or within the area specified by the health authority; moreover, they were forbidden from leaving the house or the specified area and going abroad, and they were not allowed to take public transportation as well. If people in home isolation have symptoms of COVID-19, they would be arranged to seek medical care. Those who violate the home isolation regulations and leave the house or take public transportation will be fined.

2   In order to strengthen the detection of suspected cases of COVID-19 and to prevent the spread of the virus, the CECC formulated screening criteria for COVID-19 test: (1) People with foreign travel or foreigner contact within 14 days as well as fever and respiratory infections suspectedly caused by COVID-19. (2) People with fever and respiratory syndrome. Anyone who filled one of the two criteria, s/he should take a screening test. If the result was negative, s/he should take a self-health management at home. There was no need to take a second test unless the symptoms worsened; if the result was positive, s/he had to be reported as a confirmed case for further treatment.

3   Those in self-health management should avoid leaving the house or going abroad, and they should wear the masks when going outside. If people in self-health management had symptoms of COVID-19, they would be arranged to seek medical care.

"Guidelines for Enterprises to Maintain Operation in Response to Serious Special Infectious Pneumonia (COVID-19)".

The CECC issued the Guidelines for Large-Scale Public Gatherings in the Wake of the COVID-19 Outbreak. Those activities with crowd clustering (more than 1000 people) should be postponed or suspended. Those activities with close inter-personal contacts were advised to be postponed or suspended.

08.03 – 14.03 (53; 20 recoveries)*

Public Health Policies

10.03 The CECC launched the "Real-name mask system 2.0". In addition to existing physical channels such as health insurance chartered pharmacies and health centers, people could pre-order masks online with health ID cards, natural person certificates, or through health insurance Mobile APP.

11.03 Those who were quarantined for COVID-19 and their caregivers would be compensated with NT$1,000 per person per day.

Socio-Economic Policy Packages

12.03 In response to the outbreak of COVID-19, from February 13 to 27, Ministry of Transportation and Communications (MOTC) approved three

relief measures formulated by the Tourism Bureau, subsidizing travel agencies for their losses caused early departure of Mainlander tour group, and the suspension of outbound and inbound tour groups.

13.03 The EY approved a relief measure formulated by the MOTC. That subsidized the major operating costs of catering outlets, duty-free shops, shops, commercial advertisements, etc., including building use fees, land use fees, and royalties.

15.03 – 21.03 (153/2; 28 recoveries)*

Public Health Policies

15.03 Setting up a "Traveler Entry Health Declaration and Home Quarantine Electronic System." If one entered Taiwan from abroad, one could use the mobile phone to enter the system in advance; in this situation, you could fill in the health situation and travel history, and speed up the entry process.

Travelers from Europe through March 5-14 were required to notify local district offices of their travel history; banning entry of all foreign citizens; those entered had to be subject to 14-day home quarantine upon entry.

An intelligent electronic fence system was set up to monitor and trace the people in quarantine

through a cellphone to ensure the enforcement of anti-epidemic measures.

17.03 People with a travel history to the countries in the list of alert level 3 must be subject to home quarantine.

20.03 Inbound travelers could purchase face masks at duty free shops in airports upon their arrival by presenting their boarding passes.

The travel alert level of all regions across the world was escalated to level 3. People should avoid any non-essential overseas travel.

Socio-Economic Policy Packages

16.03 The MOTC formulated relief measures for the transport and freight industry, subsidizing 50% of automobile fuel usage fee for 2020 for business vehicles in the small car rental industry, small truck rental industry, automobile freight industry, automobile route freight industry and automobile container freight industry.

From March 17 to the end of the school term, students and teachers from elementary to high schools were not allowed to go abroad. Those who had an urgent demand for it could apply for an exceptional approval.

17.03 In order to assist the domestic airlines affected by the COVID-19, the Civil Aviation Administration of the MOTC sub-

sidized the airlines loan interest and other costs caused by anti-epidemic measures.

The Ministry of Labor (MOL) expanded the "Work-Life Balance Subsidy Program": (1) Increase the amount of subsidies (2) Increase the hourly pay for child temporary care (3) Extend the application period.

22.03 – 28.03 (283; 30 recoveries)*

Public Health Policies

25.03 The CECC recommended suspending indoor gatherings of over 100 people and outdoor gatherings of over 500 people to prevent cluster infections.

Socio-Economic Policy Packages

23.03 Those who had been quarantined and got no salary or other equivalents during the quarantine, if no violation of quarantine regulations, they might apply for a compensation for NT$ 1,000 per day.

24.03 The MOHW offered allowance for staff working in special wards, negative pressure isolated wards or intensive care units. Allowance standards: (1) Physician NT$10,000 per day. (2) Nursing staff NT$10,000 per shift. (3) Radiation operators NT$10,000 per month. (4) infection control staff NT$10,000 per month.

25.03 In order to mitigate the impact of the COVID-19, the MOE allocated NT$100 million from the extra budget for relief and offered another NT$300 million, i.e., NT$400 million in total to subsidize the teaching, training and epidemic prevention and other anti-epidemic measures colleges and universities.

The Ministry of Finance allowed the extension of tax payments or payments by instalments if taxpayers was impacted by the COVID-19.

In response to the impact of the COVID-19 that caused unemployment problems, the MOL involved the unemployed at the age over 20 in the "micro business loan scheme." For those already in the scheme, they could apply for suspension of interest payment for one year and extended the repayment for one year. The interest incurred by the suspension/extension would be subsidized by the Ministry.

27.03 The EY assigned the Ministry of Economic Affairs (MOEA) to set up a relief and revitalization hotline for giving consultative services to people and businesses.

*29.03 – 04.04 (355/5; 50 recoveries)**

Public Health Policies

01.04 The CECC redefined the symptoms of the COVID-19 and expanded the targets for screening test.[4]

Those in home quarantine/isolation home had to abide by the law, and offenders would be severely punished.

To meet the demand of epidemic prevention, the CECC publicly released information on confirmed cases.

The CECC announced social distancing measures on April 1 to encourage the general public to maintain a social distance in the public area.

Those inbound travelers who were subject to home quarantine were forbidden to take public transportation.

02.04 Inbound passengers who had symptoms of fever or respiratory tract in the past 14 days, in addition to taking a screening test at the airport or hospital, the passengers should take designated vehicles to the designated place for home quarantine.

03.04 The CECC promulgated access control

measures for hospitals. Except for the following circumstances, all kinds of visits were prohibited: (1) The patient's need for medical operations such as surgery, invasive examination or treatment; (2) Special units such as emergency department, intensive care unit or hospice, taking account of the needs of a patient's condition; (3) Upon the requirement and agreement of other medical institutes.

Socio-Economic Policy Packages

31.03 Universities and colleges were allowed to adjust the arrangement of teaching. For the classes that have more than 100 students, students should wear masks during the lesson, or adopting a small group teaching by splitting the class, or adopting distance teaching. These arrangements could be executed on a trial basis and in a small scale. Classes or departments took turn to practice.

01.04 In order to assist local governments in providing transportation to medical service for home isolation and home quarantine, subsidies were offered: taxies for epidemic

prevention - NT$ 3,500 per vehicle per day, and isolation epidemic prevention compensation - NT$ 2,100 per vehicle per day, and 50% of the cost for local governments.

02.04 As the pandemic was exacerbated across the world, Taiwan amended the COVID-19 relief act to add another NT$150 billion to the special budget, which was combined with NT$140 billion from other government budgets and funds and NT$700 billion in loans, bringing the total relief package to NT$1.05 trillion.

*05.04 – 11.04 (385/6; 99 recoveries)**

Public Health Policies

07.04 Patients in medical institutions were mostly vulnerable groups with low immunity, and medical staff had close direct contact with patients, the risk of disease transmission was higher. In order to ensure the response and preparation of medical institutes to the epidemic situation, the CECC took the following six strategies: (1) expanded screening tests (2) community monitoring (3) expanded admission (4) monitoring the avail-

---

4   Under one of the following conditions, if a doctor thought it was necessary to carry out a screening test, they could report and took a tests: (1) fever (>=38 degrees Celsius) or acute respiratory infection or abnormal sense of smell and taste. (2) showing symptoms of pneumonia clinically, radiographically or pathologically. (3) without history of travel, suspectedly a phenomenon of local transmission.

ability of hospital beds (5) continuous requisition (6) patient segregation.

08.04 In order to grasp the health status of those in home quarantine/isolation, the CECC established a two-way communication mechanism, using chat robot "Epidemic Stop Magic" LINE Bot to keep in touch with those in "home quarantine/isolation. They could actively report their health status through the robot.

09.04 The arrangement of real-name rationing of face masks was further adjusted. Each citizen could buy 9 adult-sized masks or 10 child-sized masks every 14 days.

Socio-Economic Policy Packages

07.04 The MOEA offered subsidies to the catering industry to encourage the development of food delivery service.

10.04 The Civil Aviation Administration of the MOTC launched the "Relief 2.0 scheme" to the civil aviation industry. The government provided credit guarantees, and the loans and interest subsidies amounting to NT$ 50 billion.

In order to reduce the burden of schooling for

the children of involuntarily unemployed workers, the MOL announced the expansion of the "School Subsidy for Unemployed Workers' Children" for the second school term.

12.04 – 18.04 (398; 178 recoveries)*

Public Health Policies

14.04 The CECC revised the "Severe Special Infectious Pneumonia Notification Case Handling Process"

and "Community Monitoring, Notification, Acquisition and Case Handling Process".[5]

Socio-Economic Policy Packages

16.04 The Tourism Bureau, MOTC had launched the Tourism Industry "Relief 2.0 scheme", offering salary subsidies to tour guides, tour escorts and other employees in the tour industry, and business subsidies to travel agencies, hotels and homestay businesses for the period from April to June.

19.04 – 25.04 (429; 275 recoveries)*

Public Health Policies

22.04 The real-name mask 3.0 system was

launched. Citizens could pre-order face masks through the multi-media kiosks in the four major supermarket chain shops.

24.04 The CECC established a "new coronavirus screening and analysis technology support platform" involving the Biosafety level-3 laboratory (BSL-3 laboratory) to provide Virus testing, imitation specimen testing, specimen testing, virus melting spot inhibition experiment and other services.

Socio-Economic Policy Packages

20.04 The MOL gave a 3-month allowance to those self-employed labors or labors without a specific employer. It amounted to NT$10,000 per month.

22.04 In order to assist difficult enterprises to overcome difficulties and maintain employee livelihoods, the MOEA issued a new relief measure for the workers in manufacturing and technical service industries. Those enterprises in the industries whose turnover had declined by 50%, the government subsidized 40% of the regular salary of the employees for 3 months (Maximum NT$20,000),

and offered a one-time capital subsidy amounting to the number of full-time employees multiplied by NT$10,000. 23 April

The Sports Department launched the sports industry relief and revitalization scheme, firstly subsidizing sports lottery dealers and sports groups. Sports group subsidies amounted to about NT$30 million. In addition to subsidies for specific sports groups, the Sports Department also received a second wave of a special budget of NT$1.95 billion from the EY to support the sports industry affected by the COVID-19.

In order to reduce the impact of the COVID-19 on fishermen's livelihoods, the fishermen could apply for subsidies, NT$10,000 per person per month, for 3 months each time.

24.04 In order to alleviate the burden of lessees who leased lands or buildings owned by Taiwan Power and Chinese Petroleum Corporation or Taiwan Power Company (affiliated with the MOEA), the lessees could apply for delaying rent payment. If the rent could

5   In order to well inform doctors of the negative test cases or the community sampling targets, the screening procedures were revised as follows: For the first sampling test: (1) if it was positive (a confirmed case), the Center of Disease Control (CDC) would arrange admission to hospital for isolation. (2) if it was negative but with mild symptoms, one could continue a home quarantine; if the symptoms were mild but there was a continuous unimproved or worsening condition, one should actively inform the healthcare unit to arrange a second sampling test. If the second test result was positive, the CDC should arrange admission to hospital for isolation; if the result remained negative, then one could continue the home isolation, home quarantine or self-health management.

not be paid off by the end of 2020, it was allowed to be done in 3 years. They could also apply for the rent reduction, in principle 20% off for year 2020.

26.04 – 02.05 (432; 332 recoveries)*

Public Health Policies

30.04 In order to let the people gradually return to normal life, a "new attitude towards epidemic prevention and LOHAS" campaign was launched. It promoted that the public could safely participate in various outdoor activities while maintaining personal epidemic prevention measures (washing hands frequently, wearing a mask while taking public transportation and being unable to maintain social distance) Activities, such as watching outdoor concerts, artistic performances and sports events, or sports, tourism and other activities that were beneficial to physical and mental health. In addition, when people went out for a meal, they could choose shops with appropriate dining distances, partitions, and set menus to enjoy the food.

People should maintain a social distance of 1.5 meters indoors and more than 1-meter outdoors when they went out. If they could not maintain it, they should wear masks.

01.05 In light of the mitigation of COVID-19 transmission, people were allowed to visit long-term care accommodations. Visits were recommended to use an appointment system to manage the number of visitors, thus logging in with real names to manage visitor's personal information, health statement and travel history information. Each resident could be visited once a day, and at the same time, a group of visitors was limited to a maximum of 3 people (including children). Visitors and residents must wear masks throughout the visit.

03.05 – 09.05 (440; 366 recoveries)*

Public Health Policies

08.05 Businesses that were currently suspended might be opened for business after being evaluated by the county and city governments to meet the epidemic prevention and safety requirements.[6]

09.05 In order to boost the market supply of medical equipment and epidemic prevention materials, Taiwan Food and Drug Administration actively assisted manufacturers to submit applications for the manufacture of medical equipment, such as surgical masks, isolation clothing, protective clothing and forehead (ear) temperature guns and other important epidemic prevention materials.

Socio-Economic Policy Packages

06.05 The MOL encouraged workers to take advantage of temporarily reduced working hours to participate in training courses, and continued to develop job skills, and offered them training allowances.

10.05 – 16.05 (440/7; 395 recoveries)*

Socio-Economic Policy Packages

11.05 The MOEA offered a subsidy for 40% of a monthly salary (maximum NT$20,000) to employees. An allowance of NT$10,000 was given to each peasant or fisherman.

16.05 For the hotels that provided legal quarantine accommodation for home quarantine or home isolation, Tourism Bureau under the MOTC subsidized the hotels for NT$ 1,000 per room per day to increase the willingness of hotels join the epidemic prevention accommodation.

17.05 – 23.05 (441; 414 recoveries)*

Public Health Policies

22.05 In light of the stable domestic epidemic situation, the CECC allowed paid testing for COVID-19 in some designated medical institutes for emergency demands, work and study abroad. Each person was allowed to apply for it once in three months.

23.05 The CECC promoted various scientific and technological epidemic prevention measures. Among them, Taiwan Centers for Disease Control used the Google Assistant service to build an "epidemic prevention expert" Chinese and English smart chat robot, so that Taiwanese and foreigners in Taiwan could use multiple channels to obtain the latest information for epidemic prevention.

24.05 – 30.05 (442; 423 recoveries)*

Public Health Policies

25.05 The CECC eased the restriction of some

---

6   (1) Maintain social distance, such as 1.5 meters indoors and 1 meter outdoor, with "socially distant" seating arrangements or additional partitions. (2) Implement personal hygiene protection, such as wearing masks, measuring body temperature, providing hand-washing supplies or equipment in entrances and places. (3) Establish a real-name system, and indeed implement flow control and environmental clearance. (4) Fire safety inspection and building public safety inspection were qualified.

epidemic prevention measures. Visits to hospitals were allowed with keeping a record of visitors and all visitors should observe personal protection measures. Disease prevention restrictions on all walks of life were eased, but people were required to follow the principles:

1. To maintain social distancing of 1.5 meters indoors and 1 meter outdoors.
2. To wear masks
3. To install partitions.

31.05 – 06.06 (443; 430 recoveries)*

Public Health Policies

01.06 The inventory of masks was sufficient to meet the demand. From June 1, a fixed amount of 8 million masks per day would be requisitioned, and the remaining would be opened for domestic or foreign sales.

Socio-Economic Policy Packages

02.06 The EY released the implementation content of "Triple stimulus voucher", paying NT$1,000 for NT$3,000 in return, increasing the value by 3 times to stimulate consumption. For the underprivileged groups, the government remitted NT$1,000 to redeem the triple stimulus voucher.

07.06 – 13.06 (443; 431 recoveries)*

Socio-Economic Policy Packages

11.06 In order to revitalize the development of the arts and culture industry, the Ministry of Culture announced that on July 22, a total of 2 million copies of NT$600 of "art fun coupons" would be issued, which was earmarked for any arts and cultural consumption across Taiwan. It could be used in more than 10,000 outlets and was expected to create an output value for more than NT$ 5 billion.

The MOTC launched a travel subsidy scheme for the period from July 1 to October 31. During the period, you could enjoy accommodation subsidies of NT$1,000 for travel accommodation in Taiwan, and up to NT$2,000 dollars for travel accommodation in outlying islands.

14.06 – 20.06 (446; 434 recoveries)*

Public Health Policies

17.06 To ensure the safety of inbound flights with infected cases and minimize the risk of community transmission, the CECC stipulated that only those met one of the following two criteria could board the plane: 1) It had to be more than 2

months between the onset date and the boarding date, and the symptoms had been alleviated; 2) It had already reached 10 days since the onset date, and two negative tests for respiratory tract specimens were obtained.

Socio-Economic Policy Packages

15.06 The MOL provided an employment reward for up to NT$30,000 for 15-to-29- year-old-graduates in 2019, encouraging the freshmen to actively seek jobs and to stabilize their employment.

21.06 – 27.06 (444; 435 recoveries)*

Public Health Policies

22.06 Taiwan and the United States, Japan and Australia held an online workshop on "New Coronavirus: Preventing the Second Wave of Epidemic Situation" to jointly improve the capacity of epidemic prevention and suppress the threat of the infectious disease to the world.

23.06 International air passengers were allowed to transit through the Taoyuan International Airport from June 25.

28.06 – 04.07 (449; 438 recoveries)*

Public Health Policies

29.06 Entry measures to be gradually relaxed for

foreign nationals, Hong Kong and Macao residents; eligible travelers must present negative COVID-19 test result at check-in and undergo 14-day home quarantine upon entry.

30.06 The CECC said mask expropriation policy would be extended to the end of December this year, the real-name mask policy would continue to apply.

Socio-Economic Policy Packages

02.07 The Chinese Taipei Basketball Association announced on 2 July that the 2020 William Jones Cup would not be held due to the pandemic.

05.07 – 11.07 (451; 438 recoveries)*

Public Health Policies

07.07 Inspection and examination of imported medical masks was officially launched.

08.07 The CECC further relaxed restrictions concerning attending funerals and visiting people in home isolation or quarantine

Socio-Economic Policy Packages

09.07 The Sports Administration, MOE allocated NT$2 billion to issue 4 million copies of vouchers - an electronic purse worth 500 dollars per person, for sports consumption.

12.07 – 18.07 (454; 440 recoveries)*

Public Health Policies

16.07 Mainland Chinese children who were under the age of 2 and holding a residence permit apply for entry, they must be accompanied by their parents. After entry, they must complete a 14-day home quarantine in accordance with the regulations.

19.07 – 25.07 (458; 440 recoveries)*

26.07 – 01.08 (474; 441 recoveries)*

Public Health Policies

26.07 All passengers who arrived in Taiwan from the Philippines had to complete a screening test at the airport. Symptomatics were sent to the centralized quarantine station to wait for the test results, and asymptomatics returned home or went to the epidemic prevention hotel to complete a 14-day home quarantine.

29.07 The CECC said that mass screening might find asymptomatic people, but at present, all visitors from abroad needed to stay home for 14 days. Quarantine measures, after the expiration of the quarantine period for asymptomatic people, they still had to manage their own health for another 7 days, which could effectively prevent congestion. As for the spread of the community epidemic caused by asymptomatic cases abroad, the reason was that the 14-day quarantine measures had not been implemented, or the 14-day home quarantine measures had not been adopted for contacts of confirmed cases, which was different from the current situation in Taiwan.

Socio-Economic Policy Packages

31.07 The Tourism Bureau announced that the "Measures for the suspension of outbound tour groups and inbound tour groups" remained valid until August 31, and the announcement would be adjusted in due course according to the subsequent development of the epidemic.

02.08 – 08.08 (479; 443 recoveries)*

09.08 – 15.08 (482; 450 recoveries)*

Public Health Policies

10.08 Alex Azar, the United States secretary of Health and Human Services, met with President Tsai Ing-Wen and expressed his recognition of Taiwan's success in combating COVID-19 and attributed it to an open and democratic society.

Taiwan and the United States signed their first memorandum of understanding (MOU) on health cooperation with the MOHW. The cooperation includes medical and health supplies and technical cooperation.

Travelers arriving in Taiwan from the Philippines had to undergo a 14-day quarantine at a group quarantine facility after the entry.

13.08 The CECC announced that starting from 00:00 Taipei Standard Time on August 13, Mainland Chinese children aged 2 to 6 years might apply for entry into Taiwan and their parents might accompany them. Mainland Chinese children under 6 years old and their parents accompanying them were allowed to return to Taiwan. These children and parents had to undergo a 14-day home quarantine as required after entry.

Socio-Economic Policy Packages

14.08 The Tourism Bureau, MOTC launched "Relief 3.0 Scheme" to offer salary subsidies to travel agencies, hotels, and tour guides and tour escorts for the period from July to September.

COVID-19 in the United Kingdom:
Capability Development, Deficits and Discontents

Yifei Yan

Notwithstanding piecemeal measures since the end of January 2020, the UK government only launched its high-level, strategic *Coronavirus action plan* in early March, and waited two more weeks to announce a national lock-down. Prioritising the development of capabilities of NHS during this period was effective to some extent. However, inadequate understanding of how various socio-economically disadvantaged populations are being affected and lackluster measures to address public discontent can pose perturbing ramifications on both the equity and the efficiency of the government's management of the ongoing pandemic, especially as the new and more deadly variant of the virus is spreading rapidly since December 2020.

Overview

As of September 1, 2020, 16,273,209 tests have been conducted in the U.K. (Figure 9.1), of which 337,168 people have tested positive (Figure 9.2), and 41,504 have sadly died (Figure 9.3).

Figure 9.1 Cumulative testing performed by date reported, U.K. (as of September 1, 2020)*

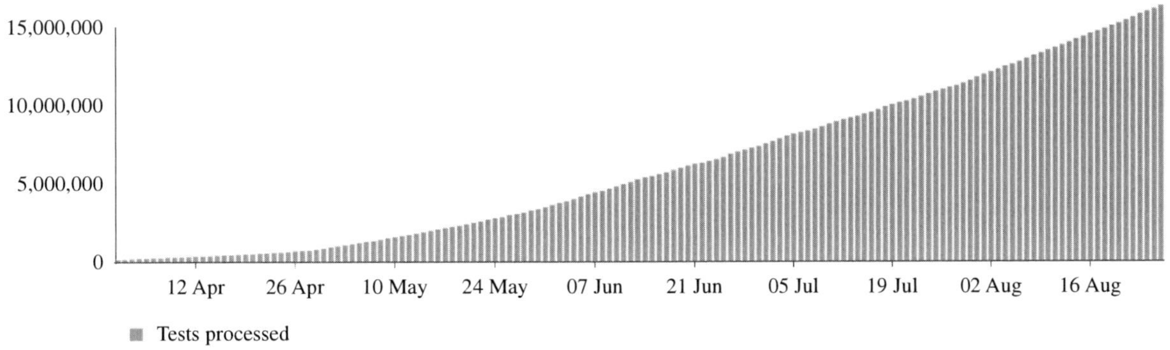

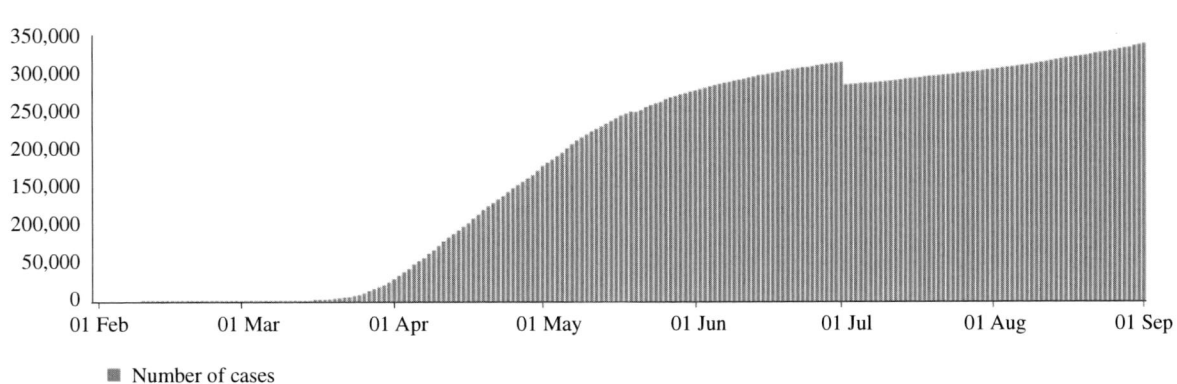

■ Tests processed

Source: https://coronavirus.data.gov.uk/testing, accessed 2020-09-01

Figure 9.2 Cumulative positive cases by date reported, U.K. (as of September 1, 2020)*

■ Number of cases

Source: https://coronavirus.data.gov.uk/cases, accessed 2020-09-01

*Number of individuals who have had at least one lab-confirmed positive COVID-19 test result, by date reported. On 2 July, case data from pillars 1 and 2 of the testing programme were combined and de-duplicated, resulting in a step decrease in the cumulative number of cases reported.

**Figure 9.3 Cumulative deaths within 28 days of positive test by date reported, U.K.
(as of September 1, 2020)**

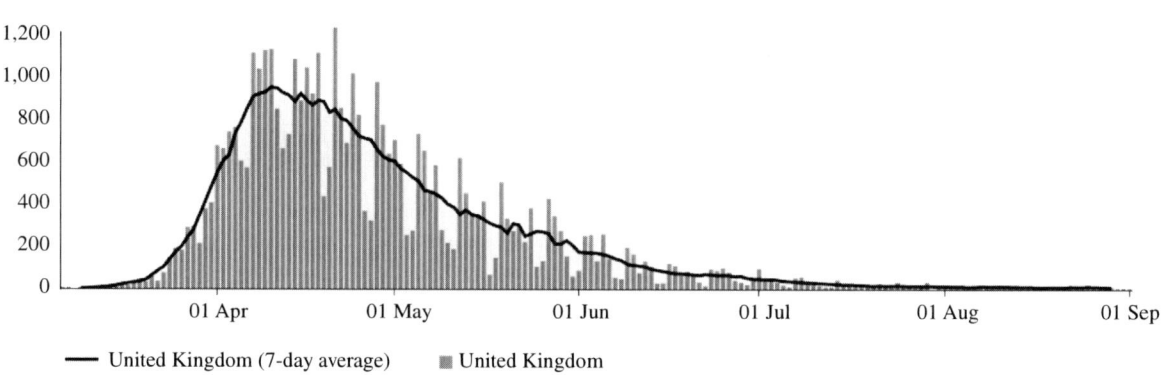

Source: https://coronavirus.data.gov.uk/deaths, accessed 2020-09-01

According to the data from the end of January, when the first cases were reported, it can be said that the first wave of the ongoing pandemic peaked in the month of April.[1] Since then, there has been a steady decline of the number of both positive cases and deaths, leading the government to ease the lockdown on June 1. Other restrictive measures were gradually eased over the next two months, though not without exceptions: since the end of June, local lockdowns of various durations were imposed due to more recent spike of cases in places like Aberdeen,[2] Greater Manchester,[3] Leicester[4] etc.

U.K.'s policy response to COVID-19 pandemic is largely led by the national government, although the four nations of England, Scotland, Wales and Northern Ireland enjoy substantial autonomy regarding their reactions. In particular, as will be shown later, *Coronavirus action plan* issued on March 3 specified the responsibilities of government entities across different levels (such as the Department of Health and Social Care, Chief Medical Officer or CMO, National Health Services or NHS, Public Health England, etc.), both in separation and when coordinated to work together. It is also mentioned in this official document about soliciting expert advice and guidance in policymaking, exemplified by the reliance on the Scientific Advisory Group for Emergencies (SAGE). "Chaired by the Government Chief Scientific Adviser and co-chaired by the CMO for England", this expert group "provides scientific and technical advice to support government decision makers during emergencies."

A comparison with international experiences may suggest that UK government's response so far to the current COVID-19 episode is far from remarkable. While the number of total cases are behind countries such as the United States, Brazil, Russia and Spain, U.K. recorded the second highest number of total deaths as of the end of May, second to only the United States. Further calculation shows that U.K. suffered highest death rate from coronavirus among all countries.[5] In an editorial published by the

---

1   For the sake of space, the focus of this chapter is mostly on the first wave of the pandemic in the U.K. After the first wave, the number of cases started to rise substantially again since September, leading the government to first come up with a new three-tier system of restrictions in mid-October, and then to announce a second national lockdown from October 31 to December 2, 2020. Yet as the new variant of Coronavirus continued to spread rapidly since then, a third lockdown was announced on January 4, 2021 which is expected to last till mid-February.

2   https://news.sky.com/story/coronavirus-lockdown-to-be-reimposed-in-aberdeen-after-spike-in-cases-12042945

3   www.bbc.co.uk/news/uk-53602362

4   https://assets.publishing.service.gov.uk/government/uploads/system/uploads/attachment_data/file/897128/COVID-19_activity_Leicester_Final-report_010720_v3.pdf

5   www.ft.com/content/6b4c784e-c259-4ca4-9a82-648ffde71bf0 The number is calculated as the people killed directly or indirectly by the virus per million. Accessed 2020-05-28.

BMJ in May, 2020, effectiveness of U.K.'s policy response was sharply and explicitly criticised as being "too little, too late, [and] too flawed".[6]

Apart from effectiveness, U.K.'s response to COVID-19 also appears to have alarming deficits in terms of equity. Although the economy and employment is hit hard in general,[7] and despite the official rhetoric of "being in this together", evidence reveals that not all populations in the U.K. are affected equally, as acknowledged in one official report published in June 2020.[8] In particular, people of black backgrounds are most likely to be diagnosed with the disease, whereas the death rates in black and Asian communities are also higher than white Britons.[9] The increase of domestic violence during lockdown suggests that victims (mostly women) are another group for which emergency support is in shortage,[10] whereas scholars further point out how inadequate disability access provisions may affect the life of the disabled people during the pandemic.[11] Behind these less-than-encouraging pictures, citizen distrust, disappointment and discontent over the government's response to COVID-19 is increasingly reported.[12]

The rest of the report narrates the policy response to COVID-19 in the U.K. in a chronological order. Key features of the policy response are highlighted for each stage, together with a preliminary discussion on its effectiveness, limitations, issues and controversies.

Early Response: January to February

The UK government was alerted to the COVID-19 outbreak, especially in China and East Asia, at the end of January. For example, the FCO advised against "all but essential" travel to mainland China on January 28.[13] Two days later, the four UK CMOs raised risk to the public from low to moderate, following WHO's announcement of the disease as a Public Health Emergency of International Concern.[14] On January 31, 83 British nationals and 41 foreign nationals flying back from Wuhan to the U.K. were all put to a 14-day quarantine in different places.[15]

The first positive case within U.K. was also reported on January 31. Hence, fresh measures were taken in February which included a public information campaign advising the public on how to slow the spread of coronavirus and reduce the impact on NHS services (February 2), the pass of the *Health*

6   Scally, Gabriel, Bobbie Jacobson, and Kamran Abbasi. "The UK's public health response to covid-19." *BMJ 2020*; 369 (2020). https://doi.org/10.1136/bmj.m1932.

7   www.theguardian.com/business/2020/aug/12/uk-economy-covid-19-plunges-into-deepest-slump-in-history. Accessed 2020-09-01.

8   Public Health England. "Beyond the data: Understanding the impact of COVID-19 on BAME groups." (2020). London: PHE Publications. https://assets.publishing.service.gov.uk/government/uploads/system/uploads/attachment_data/file/892376/COVID_stakeholder_engagement_synthesis_beyond_the_data.pdf Accessed 2020-09-11.

9   www.theguardian.com/world/2020/jun/02/covid-19-death-rate-in-england-higher-among-bame-people. Accessed 2020-07-07.

10 www.nytimes.com/interactive/2020/07/02/world/europe/uk-coronavirus-domestic-abuse.html. Accessed 2020-07-09.

11 https://blogs.lse.ac.uk/socialpolicy/2020/09/21/how-services-responses-to-the-pandemic-are-exposing-the-uks-inadequate-disability-access-provisions/. Accessed 2020-09-20.

12 A recent manifestation of such discontent is over the decision to reopen schools on September 1, see www.theguardian.com/education/2020/aug/01/now-teachers-sound-alarm-over-plans-to-reopen-schools

13 www.gov.uk/government/news/fco-advises-against-all-but-essential-travel-to-mainland-china. Accessed 2020-05-28.

14 www.gov.uk/government/news/statement-from-the-four-uk-chief-medical-officers-on-novel-coronavirus. Accessed 2020-05-28.

15 www.bbc.co.uk/news/uk-51318691 Accessed 2020-05-28. The practice of arranging flights for UK citizens to fly back from COVID-19 infected areas also continued later in the cases of Japan's Diamond Princess (February 20), Peru (March 27), India (April 4 and April 30), the Philippines (April 21), and so forth.

Protection (Coronavirus) Regulations 2020 which grants authority to forcibly subject any at-risk individual considered by health professionals under quarantine (February 10), and the pilots of home testing by the NHS (February 22). Besides that, the government pledged financial commitments to tackling the pandemic globally. £20m of new funding was announced on February 3 that will go to the Coalition for Epidemic Preparedness Innovations (CEPI). Five days later, a further £5 million of UK aid was announced which will support the WHO in helping developing countries most at risk of coronavirus quickly identify cases and care for patients.

From "Herd Immunity" to Lockdown: March

Those early-stage measures and commitments were not adequate to prevent the pandemic from spreading. The number of cases rose sharply from the last week of February (February 23–29) to the first week of March (March 1–7) from 51 to 387. On March 5, the CMO for England announced the first death of patient with COVID-19 in the U.K..[16] It was till then that a more systematic response was formulated. The main manifestation was the *Coronavirus action plan: A guide to what you can expect across the U.K.* published on March 3.[17]

This official document shows that the government was initially quite affirmative about its capacity to handle the situation, optimistic that "[t]he UK government and the devolved administrations... have planned extensively over the years for an event like this, and the U.K. is therefore well prepared to respond in a way that offers substantial protection to the public". In addition to specifying the division of responsibilities and coordination amongst government entities and illustrating expert involvement, this document envisioned U.K.'s response into four distinctive phases. (Table 9.1).

Just one day after its publication, NHS declared the spread of coronavirus as a Level-4 incident, the highest category of emergency, in light of the 12 new cases on that day which drove the total number of cases up to 51. With this exacerbated situation, it was announced on March 12 that U.K. has moved from the phase of containment to that of delay. However, rather than following suit of France, Spain and Italy which had imposed lockdown measures in light of similar spike of cases by that time, U.K. remained restriction-free as the SAGE believed that lockdown won't be acceptable to the population.[18] Instead, the expectation was, in the words of the government's Chief Science Officer Patrick Vallance, that if the population can "build up some kind of herd immunity" by being infected and then recovering from mild to moderate symptoms, then the transmission of the disease can be reduced as "more people are immune".[19] As such, the government only needs to "protect those who are most vulnerable to it".[20] Reflecting such thinking, Prime Minister Boris Johnson announced on March 12 that the government would no longer try to track and trace the contacts of every suspected case, and it would test only people who are admitted to hospitals.[21]

---

16   www.gov.uk/government/news/cmo-for-england-announces-first-death-of-patient-with-covid-19. Accessed 2020-07-07.

17   www.gov.uk/government/publications/coronavirus-action-plan/coronavirus-action-plan-a-guide-to-what-you-can-expect-across-the-uk. Accessed 2020-09-11.

18   Scally, Jacobson and Abbasi 2020.

19   On how "herd immunity" may be an inappropriate concept and measure for pandemic such as coronavirus, see Adam Oliver "Separating behavioural science from the herd", https://blogs.lse.ac.uk/covid19/2020/05/26/separating-behavioural-science-from-the-herd/. Accessed 2020-07-08.

20   www.washingtonpost.com/world/europe/uk-coronavirus-herd-immunity/2020/03/16/1c9d640e-66c7-11ea-b199-3a9799c54512_story.html. Accessed 2020-07-08.

21   www.theatlantic.com/health/archive/2020/03/coronavirus-pandemic-herd-immunity-uk-boris-johnson/608065/. Accessed 2020-07-08.

Table 9.1 Four phases of COVID-19 response outlined in the *Coronavirus action plan*

Phase	Description
Contain	Detect early cases, follow up close contacts, and prevent the disease taking hold in this country for as long as is reasonably possible.
Delay	Slow the spread in this country, if it does take hold, lowering the peak impact and pushing it away from the winter season.
Research	Better understand the virus and the actions that will lessen its effect on the UK population; innovate responses including diagnostics, drugs and vaccines; use the evidence to inform the development of the most effective models of care
Mitigate	Provide the best care possible for people who become ill, support hospitals to maintain essential services and ensure ongoing support for people ill in the community to minimise the overall impact of the disease on society, public services and on the economy

Source: Coronavirus action plan

Subsequent measures were launched to fulfill this commitment of protecting the most vulnerable, notably the elderlies, who were also the priority of receiving testing over this period. On March 12, the government advised elderlies over 70, and those with underlying health condition to avoid going onto cruises, schools to cancel overseas trips, and people who were showing symptoms to self-isolate for 7 days. The next day, it further advised that anyone suspected of having COVID-19 should not visit care homes or people receiving home care.

Judging from the continuous sharp spike of confirmed cases and deaths (from 2,274 cases in the week of March 8-14 to 7,848 cases in the following week of March 15–21; and from 21 deaths to 233 deaths), response at this stage seemed to have been miscalculated. It remained unclear on what basis was "herd immunity" expected to be acquired or on what basis was the idea of four phases delineated. In contrast, a report by researchers at the Imperial College London, released on March 16, made a powerful case from both modeling and drawing lessons from China and South Korea that "population-wide social distancing combined with home isolation of cases and school and university closure" would have the largest impact on rapidly reducing case incidences.[22]

The decision of lockdown was finally conveyed in a speech by Boris Johnson on the evening of March 23, although measures already started to get tightened before this broadcasted statement.[23] Within the lockdown period, the population was expected to "stay home",[24] the violation of which would incur penalties ranging from fines to arrest, as the police was now granted power of enforcement by the *Coronavirus Act 2020* passed on March 25.[25] More broadly, this Act grants the government discretionary emergency powers in multiple areas including police, social care, schools, local councils that are unprecedented since World War II. Earlier, business closure was similarly consolidated through the *Health Protection (Coronavirus, Business Closure) (England) Regulations 2020* that came into force

---

22 Ferguson, Neil, Daniel Laydon, Gemma Nedjati Gilani, Natsuko Imai, Kylie Ainslie, Marc Baguelin, Sangeeta Bhatia et al. "Report 9: Impact of non-pharmaceutical interventions (NPIs) to reduce COVID19 mortality and healthcare demand." (2020). https://doi.org/10.25561/77482

23 For instance, Johnson announced earlier on March 18 that households where an occupant has symptoms of COVID-19 are recommended to undertake self-isolation for 14 days; all citizens should begin practising "social distancing"; mass gatherings such as sporting events should also be suspended; schools closure would start next Monday, except for children of key workers and vulnerable children until further notice. On March 20, the closure of all social venues was further announced. Non-essential domestic and international travel was advised on March 22 and March 17 respectively.

24 Going out is only allowed for specific purposes, such as one form of exercise a day, buying food and medicine.

25 www.legislation.gov.uk/ukpga/2020/7/contents Accessed 2020-07-08.

on March 21. Under this Regulation, the closure shall last until a direction is given by the Secretary of State, subjected to a review every 28 days. Businesses that do not follow COVID-19 restrictions will be issued with prohibition notices.

Restoring and Enhancing the Capabilities of NHS: April

As the slogan "Stay Home, Protect NHS, Save Lives" suggests, ensuring that NHS, one of the most important frontline agencies that deals with the treatment of COVID-19, has enough capacity to do so, is the immediate purpose of asking people to stay home. This, in turn, is expected to serve the ultimate goal of saving lives during the pandemic.

Efforts of strengthening NHS in tackling COVID-19 were ongoing throughout this episode. For instance, in announcing the setting out of the *Action plan*, Boris Johnson mentioned on March 2 that a new NHS 111 online service has been put in place to help people get quick advice about coronavirus. The NHS in England is also ploughing an initial extra £1.7 million in to 111 to offer more clinical advice over the phone. Further funding will provide 50 additional initial call responders with the capacity to answer around 20,000 more calls every day. Expansion of coronavirus testing capacity was mentioned on March 11, with enhanced labs helping the health service carry out 10,000 tests daily. On March 17, NHS England announced that NHS Hospitals across the country are freeing up 30,000 of the overall 100,000 beds available by postponing non-urgent operations and providing care in the community for those who are fit to be discharged. The NHS also sourced up to 10,000 from independent and community hospitals as part of the preparation.

However, it was primarily during the lockdown that this frontline agency got the much-needed and most precious breathing space to furnish capabilities.

On April 2, a five-pillar plan was announced by the Health Secretary to build up, among others, NHS's mass-testing capacity, so that the country "can carry out 100,000 tests for coronavirus every day by the end of this month." A concrete step towards that was the infrastructural development through the establishment of new special-purpose hospitals, with the help of private airlines such as easyJet and Virgin Atlantic. The first of its kind, the NHS Nightingale hospital at the ExCeL conference centre in East London, was announced on March 24 and officially opened on April 3, with up to 500 beds equipped with ventilators and oxygen. Several other NHS Nightingale hospitals at various place such as Birmingham, Bristol, Exeter, Harrogate, Manchester and Sunderland were at different levels of progress over the next one month or two. Testing capacity was further enhanced with the opening of the Lighthouse Labs, the largest network of diagnostic testing facilities in British history, located in Milton Keynes (opened on April 9), Alderley Park (opened on April 20) and Glasgow (opened on April 23) respectively. On April 16, a drive-through coronavirus testing facility was opened at Edinburgh Airport, as part of the government's UK-wide drive to increase testing for thousands more NHS and other key workers.

Thanks to the progress on increasing testing capacity, the government announced on April 15 that all symptomatic care home residents will be tested for COVID-19. All social care staff who need a test will now have access to one with the Care Quality Commission (CQC) to contact all 30,000 care providers to offer tests. Over the next two weeks, the coverage plan further extended to include all essential workers in England and members of their households showing symptoms, and subsequently all symptomatic members of the public aged 65 and over.

In bolstering the capacity of NHS for handling the demand of the situation, the role of technology cannot be underestimated. To illustrate, people staying at home suffering from suspected coronavirus symptoms started to get regular check-ins from a new NHS messaging service launched on March 28, for which daily texts are sent by the NHS to new patients who register their COVID-19 symptoms and contact details with the 111 online service. On April 14, an initial £2.6 million was announced to fund a number of hi-tech projects in a joint initiative with the European Space Agency (ESA) in support of NHS England, such as using satellite data and drone technology to help deliver test kits, masks, gowns and goggles during outbreaks.

The usefulness and relevance of technology is not confined to testing and treatment only. Since early March, NHS started working closely with tech giants such as Google and social media platforms such as Twitter and Facebook in fighting coronavirus-related fake news and helping the public get easy access to accurate information. On March 25, the government launched a free and automated "chatbot" service on Whatsapp to provide access to official and trustworthy information and advice about COVID-19 in a timely manner. On April 30, novel technology which could dramatically cut the time of cleaning ambulances was tried out at the Defence Science and Technology Laboratory. A further example of innovation involves the use of technology in the criminal justice system. Also on April 30, the government introduced a new video platform which enables all parties in a criminal hearing to take part remotely, allowing all magistrate and crown courts in England and Wales to hold secure hearings.

In making all these capacity-building efforts work, workforce development of the NHS staff is crucial. On March 21, nearly 20,000 fully qualified staff from the independent sector were reported to be joining the NHS to help manage the expected surge in cases. On April 15, the government announced the re-launch of a national recruitment campaign aiming to attract 20,000 people into social care to relieve pressures in the care workforce. As a gesture of support, the government promised to cover the costs of providing free car parking to NHS staff working in hospitals. Doctors, nurses and paramedics as well as their family members with visas due to expire before October 1, 2020 will also have them automatically extended for one year. Last but not least, to provide much needed financial support during the pandemic as well as to enhance the financial sustainability of NHS, over £13 billion of its debt would be scrapped from April 1, as announced by the Health Secretary on April 9.

Beyond the First Lockdown: May and June onward

Notwithstanding these capacity-building efforts, COVID-19 cases continued to spike sharply since lockdown the lockdown that started in late March. Overall, April's record of over 140, 000 positive cases is more than five times the record for March (Figure 9.4), whereas the death record of over 24,000 cases are 6.5 times the figure for March (Figure 9.5). It was also during this period (April 21) that the highest number of deaths on a single day in the first wave of pandemic was reported, whereas nearly one-third of the months (9 days) had a daily record of more than 1,000 deaths.

Hence, not surprisingly, the lockdown which was originally envisioned to be "at least three weeks"[26] got extended. In his speech on a Sunday evening (May 10), Boris Johnson further clarified the five conditions of easing lockdown: only by fulfilling the following "five tests" shall "moving forward" be considered: (1) sufficient critical care capacity across the U.K., (2) sustained and consistent fall in daily deaths, (3) rate of infection (known as "R Rate") decreasing, (4) testing and PPE able to meet the demand, and (5) adjustments to measures will not risk a second peak that overwhelms the NHS.

---

26 www.itv.com/news/2020-03-23/boris-johnson-downing-street-coronavirus-update/. Accessed 2020-07-08.

Figure 9.4 Daily positive cases by date reported, U.K. (as of September 1, 2020)*

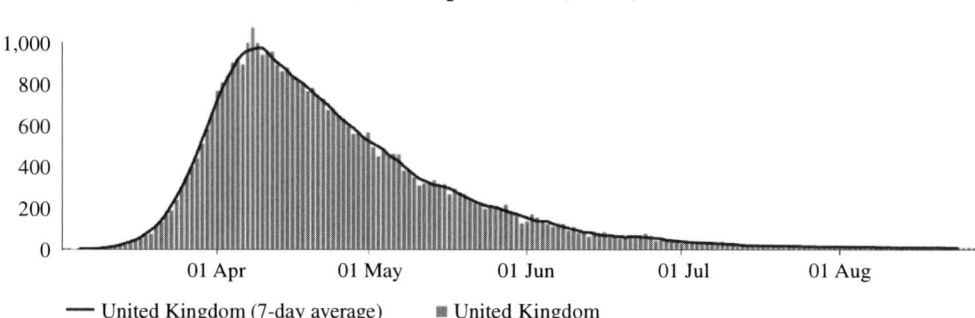

■ Number of cases   —— Cases (7-day average)

Source: https://coronavirus.data.gov.uk/cases, accessed 2020-09-01

Figure 9. 5 Daily deaths within 28 days of positive test by date reported, U.K. (as of September 1, 2020)*

—— United Kingdom (7-day average)   ■ United Kingdom

Source: https://coronavirus.data.gov.uk/deaths, accessed 2020-09-01

Together with the "five tests", Johnson introduced in the speech a new COVID Alert System run by a new Joint Biosecurity Centre. Alert level within the System depends jointly on the R rate and the number of cases, and this level in turn determines the social distancing measures taken accordingly.[27] According to his interpretation, the highest level (Five) was what could have happened without lockdown measures, whereas Level Four was the situation since the beginning of the lockdown. By the time of the speech, U.K. was "in a position to begin to move in steps to Level Three."

The actual move from Level Four to Three happened only a month later (one June 19),[28] after which Johnson announced further (and gradual) lift of lockdown restrictions on June 23.[29] While this move is believed to be also (if not primarily) driven by the dire need to revive the economy that was hit hard by the pandemic, the daily new cases were indeed in steady decline since May, till the surge of the second wave. Confirmed cases in May, slightly above 100,000, is nearly 45,000 lower than the record of April. Death incidences had a similarly decreasing trend and the figure was less than half of the death record of April.

---

27   www.gov.uk/government/speeches/pm-address-to-the-nation-on-coronavirus-10-may-2020. Accessed 2020-07-08.

28   www.gov.uk/government/news/update-from-the-uk-chief-medical-officers-on-the-uk-alert-level. Accessed 2020-07-08.

29   www.nytimes.com/2020/06/23/world/europe/uk-coronavirus-reopening.html. Accessed 2020-07-09.

Discussion: Capacity Deficits and the Erosion of Public Trust

Going through U.K.'s response in the first wave, it seems reasonable to suspect that measures taken by the government needed time to take effect. Yet acknowledging this does not mean that some more fundamental limitations of the response so far can be conveniently overlooked. To begin with, despite the hope and hypes of its efforts, the government does not always have enough operational capacity to carry them forward. The new test, track and trace programme introduced in May, and its flagship contact tracing App in particular, is a good example. After the piloting in the Isle of Wight in early May, the App was rolled out across U.K. on May 28. However, it was reported that the system crashed on that same day, as tracers cannot log on to the system and had no support accessible.[30] Furthermore, while the App is offered in multiple languages,[31] the requirement to download it on smartphones as the only way to access it still confines its accessibility, especially for those with less technological competence, such as some of the elderly. In contrast, a similar app offered in Singapore[32] has both smartphone version and a physical token availability to cater to the needs of different population.

This is far from the only manifestation of capacity deficits of the government. Those emergency capacity-building measures mentioned earlier, albeit laudable and much-needed, can hardly be expected to close all the capacity gaps faced by the system, especially when considering that since the passage of the *Health and Social Care Act 2012*, close to £1bn has been cut from public health budgets.[33] Capacity deficits were also reflected in the imbalanced composition of the expert groups, whose advice the government claimed to rely on. Dominated by modellers and epidemiologists, public health experts, communicable disease experts, women, and ethnic minorities were underrepresented in the group, whose advice may have otherwise been crucial in helping the government better analyse and accordingly address the socio-economic and equity implications of the pandemic.[34]

Lack of well-rounded analytical capacity in understanding ground reality and equity implications in turn brings into question the effectiveness of existing relief and stimulus packages. Indeed, as early as on March 11, the UK government announced in its annual budget that 12 billion pounds will be provided for temporary, timely and targeted measures to provide security and stability for people and businesses. Various subsequent measures were planned which aimed to help furloughed workers, the self-employed and small businesses from different sectors to cope with the disruptions of COVID-19. A notable example was the "Plan for Jobs" statement by Chancellor Rishi Sunak on July 8.[35] While up to 25 billion pounds of extra public spending or lower taxes may look ambitious, this amount was commented as small "both compared to the current government support that will be withdrawn through the autumn and to what other governments elsewhere have done".[36]

One of the more specific measures was the "Eat Out to Help Out" scheme. Ran in the month of August, it was designed to encourage people to visit restaurants, cafes and pubs after the ease of lockdown by

---

30 www.thesun.co.uk/news/11726771/coronavirus-test-and-trace-system-shambles/. Accessed 2020-07-08.

31 www.nhs.uk/apps-library/nhs-covid-19/. Accessed 2021-01-24.

32 www.tracetogether.gov.sg/. Accessed 2021-01-24 08.

33 Scally, Jacobson and Abbasi 2020.

34 Scally, Jacobson and Abbasi 2020.

35 For a summary of the measures, see www.instituteforgovernment.org.uk/explainers/governments-post-covid-19-stimulus-package. Accessed 2020-09-01.

36 To illustrate, the current furlough scheme, which stands at £10bn a month, is to be ended in October and replaced by a new Job Retention Bonus paid to employers who keep employees on until at least the end of January 2021, which is estimated to be £9.4bn at the maximum and very likely to be much less. See www.instituteforgovernment.org.uk/blog/sunak-speech-reaction. Accessed 2020-09-15.

giving 50% discount for food and non-alcoholic drinks (capped at 10 pounds per person) for dine-in.[37] Despite its popularity, critics found it hard to reconcile the programme's "underpinning rhetoric—the appeal to do the right thing by spending money" and "the reality for families in poverty who struggle to afford the essentials".[38] A similar line of criticism was that it ignored the interests of small businesses at the cost of mainly supporting large chains.[39] In practice, the programme even received withdrawal from the restaurants it intended to help, as their staff suffered from physical and mental stress due to handling the surge of customers during the programme period.[40]

Fundamentally, to what extent NHS can be protected and lives saved also depend on the compliance and cooperation of citizens. According to a survey conducted ten days after the announcement of lockdown, only 83% of respondents were practising sensible social distancing measures; in contrast, 30% reported to be continuing to go outside for non-essential purposes.[41] In another survey that reported largely similar findings, it was further concluded that citizen compliance is more out of "a sense of common fate, a shared identity, and acting for the common or the social good"—in short, social norms—than the "fear of the virus, police or law".[42]

In that light, compared with the impression of an incompetent government that abovementioned examples may create, even more detrimental would be the impression of a government whose associated members break such norms. This was what happened with the controversy surrounding Dominic Cummings towards the end of May.[43] To many of the public, what Cummings did, as well as the subsequent defence offered by himself and government leaders including Boris Johnson, precisely eroded public trust.[44] So much so that when the government reminded citizens of the "civic duty" to observe social distancing and take precautionary measures, it seemed that these reminders were no longer taken as seriously compared with early stages of the first lockdown. Although this lockdown already started to ease by June 25, one of the hottest days of the year, the crowds that flocked to the beach of Bournemouth still looked so appalling that the authorities there announced it to be a "major incident". The celebration of Liverpool FC fans of their team's winning championship of this year's Premier League on the same day had similarly ignored the pandemic guidelines.[45] A day earlier, "[a]t least 22 officers were injured" from attacks with bottles and other objects as they tried to maintain law and order in breaking up an unauthorized music event.[46]

By the end of April, Boris Johnson already stated in a press conference that the U.K. had passed the peak of its outbreak.[47] Yet even as shops and businesses started to reopen and with the official

---

37 www.gov.uk/guidance/get-a-discount-with-the-eat-out-to-help-out-scheme. Accessed 2020-09-01.

38 www.theguardian.com/society/2020/aug/04/eat-out-to-help-out-a-forlorn-dream-for-those-struggling-to-feed-a-family. Accessed 2020-09-01.

39 www.cambridge-news.co.uk/news/uk-world-news/insulting-eat-out-help-out-18726884. Accessed 2020-09-01.

40 www.telegraph.co.uk/news/2020/08/19/hundreds-restaurants-pull-eat-help-staff-suffer-physical-mental/. Accessed 2020-09-01.

41 https://theconversation.com/coronavirus-lockdown-fresh-data-on-compliance-and-public-opinion-135872. Accessed 2020-07-09.

42 https://blogs.lse.ac.uk/politicsandpolicy/lockdown-social-norms/. Accessed 2020-07-09.

43 For a summary of what happened, see www.theguardian.com/politics/2020/may/27/who-is-dominic-cummings-coronavirus-covid-19-lockdown-car-trip-uk-politics. Accessed 2020-07-09.

44 www.theguardian.com/commentisfree/2020/may/27/public-health-trust-dominic-cummings-second-wave. Accessed 2020-07-09.

45 www.nytimes.com/2020/06/26/world/europe/uk-coronavirus-lockdown.html. Accessed 2020-07-09.

46 www.nytimes.com/2020/06/26/world/europe/uk-coronavirus-lockdown.html. Accessed 2020-07-09.

47 www.bbc.co.uk/news/uk-52493500. Accessed 2020-07-03.

announcement of stimulus packages in the hope of an economic "reset" months after that statement, the high R number remains a serious reminder that it is not over yet: with number of cases started to rise substantially in early September, the R number was raised to between 1 and 1.2 for the first time since March, further arousing the fear for a second wave of outbreak.[48] More importantly, whatever is achieved in curbing the first wave also comes at a heavy price, not only in terms of the number of confirmed and death cases, but also in the huge economic losses faced by sectors from hotels and retailing to higher education, as well as the erosion of public trust on the government. Insofar as the "battle" against COVID-19 will still be a prolonged one, fixing the capacity deficits and restoring public trust remain essential to improving policy effectiveness and equity. Gaining more in-depth understanding of the international experience, among others, may offer especially useful insights in this regard.[49]

---

48 www.bbc.co.uk/news/health-54116939. Accessed 2020-09-15. On September 22, Johnson announced new and tighter restrictions including ban on indoor team sports, doubled fines on violation of rules of wearing masks, etc., considering that the UK is at a "perilous turning point". www.theguardian.com/world/2020/sep/22/coronavirus-boris-johnson-sets-out-new-covid-restrictions-at-perilous-turning-point. Accessed 2020-09-23.

49 See, for example: Capano, Giliberto, Michael Howlett, Darryl SL Jarvis, M. Ramesh, and Nihit Goyal. "Mobilizing policy (in) capacity to fight COVID-19: Understanding variations in state responses." *Policy and Society* 39, no. 3 (2020): 285–308.

UNITED KINGDOM

Yifei Yan and Cleo Wong

02.02.2020–20.01.2021 Total 3,505,754 cases / 93,290 deaths

02.02 – 28.02

Public Health Policies

02.02 A UK-wide public information campaign was launched to advise the public on how to protect themselves from infection, slow the spread of coronavirus and reduce the impact on NHS services.*

03.02 The Government pledged £20 million to develop new vaccines to combat covid-19. The new funding will support work developing new vaccines for epidemics with the aim to advance vaccine candidates into clinical testing as quickly as possible. The new funding will go to the Coalition for Epidemic Preparedness Innovations (CEPI) – an innovative global partnership between public, private, philanthropic, and civil society organisations launched in Davos in 2017 to develop vaccines to stop future epidemics.*

08.02 The International Development Secretary Alok Sharma pledged £5 million of UK aid to support the WHO to help respond to the global coronavirus outbreak. On top of that, additional experts funded by UK aid are expected to be deployed to the WHO.*

10.02 The novel coronavirus diagnostic test developed by PHE was rolled out to laboratories across the UK to accelerate the country's testing capabilities.* The Health Protection (Coronavirus) Regulations 2020 were put in place with immediate effect to impose restrictions on any individual considered by health professionals to be at risk of spreading the virus. People with coronavirus can now be forcibly quarantined and could be sent into isolation if they pose a threat to public health.*

22.02 The NHS started pilots of home testing for coronavirus where NHS staff, including nurses and paramedics, will visit people in their own homes rather than them having to travel.#

26.02 A new surveillance system to detect cases of COVID-19 in England was established by PHE and the NHS to strengthen existing systems and to prepare for and prevent wider transmission of the virus. Samples will be tested from patients with severe respiratory infections who do not meet the current case definition for COVID-19.*

28.02 The NHS rolled out services on NHS sites to test people for coronavirus, including a new service in action in west London, offering 'drive through' coronavirus testing. The new service, provided by Central London Community Healthcare NHS Trust in Parsons Green, was only accessed through a referral from NHS 111.#

Major Development

PM Boris Johnson has been revealed missing 5 Cabinet Office Briefing Rooms briefings; as well as shipping China PPEs.[1]

03.03 – 31.03

Public Health Policies

03.03 Government's action plan to tackle the spread of coronavirus was published:

- Every government department having a designated Ministerial virus lead to oversee the response to the global threat of the virus, for instance on schools or businesses.

- A war room set up in the Cabinet Office, bringing together communications experts and scientists from across government and the NHS to roll out the public information campaign.

- Coronavirus being a standing item on the weekly Cabinet agenda, with the PM continuing to oversee the Government approach.

- The option, should the virus spread, to encourage more home working and discourage unnecessary travel as part of a 'social distancing' strategy that could delay the peak of the outbreak until later in the year, potentially helping combat the virus in warmer weather conditions.

- A new NHS 111 online service was put in

---

* denotes gov.uk

\# denotes england.nhs.uk

** where shown, the number in brackets is the accumulated number of confirmed cases and death cases respectively.

1 www.thetimes.co.uk/article/coronavirus-38-days-when-britain-sleepwalked-into-disaster-hq3b9tlgh

place to help people get quick advice about coronavirus, as enquiries to the health service about the outbreak have surged.

- The NHS in England is also ploughing an initial extra £1.7 million in to 111 to offer more clinical advice over the phone.#

05.03 A statutory was made into law that adds COVID-19 to the list of notifiable diseases and SARS-COV-2 to the list of notifiable causative agents. This change was made by adding them to the Health Protection (Notification) Regulations 2010. This change requires GPs to report all cases of COVID-19 to Public Health England.*

06.03 PM announced a new funding of £46 million, made up of:

- Up to £20 million for the Coalition for Epidemic Preparedness Innovations (CEPI) to support vaccine development. This is in addition to the £30 million commitment that the UK has already made to CEPI, bringing the UK's total commitment to £50 million.
- Up to £5 million through the Joint Initiative on Research for Epidemic Preparedness in collaboration with Wellcome to develop quicker diagnosis methods and perform other essential research

for disease control. This is in addition to the £20 million rapid response research call for novel coronavirus research launched on 4 February 2020.

- Up to £16 million for humanitarian partners to help the most vulnerable countries prepare for coronavirus. This includes £5 million to the International Federation of the Red Cross and Red Crescent Societies; £5 million to UNICEF to support infection prevention and access to safe water; and £6 million for extra support for other partners, including for medics and supplies.
- £5m for the WHO's flash appeal. This is in addition to the £5 million commitment that the UK has already made to the appeal.*

09.03

- The government extended delivery hours for supermarkets and other food retailers to support the industry response to the coronavirus. Food retailers can increase the frequency of deliveries to their stores and move stocks more quickly from warehouses across the country to replenish their shelves.*
- Local Government Secretary launched a new taskforce to strengthen local plans to help tackle the

outbreak of coronavirus. The taskforce will bring together senior experts from across key sectors – including resilience, local government, public health and adult social care fields – who will assess Local Resilience Forum (LRF) plans and provide support and advice to ensure they are robust.*

10.03 The NHS has unveiled a package of measures to counter coronavirus fake news – working with Google, Twitter, Instagram and Facebook – to help the public get easy access to accurate NHS information and avoid myths and misinformation.#

11.03

- Up to £150 million of new UK aid will go to the International Monetary Fund's Catastrophe Containment and Relief Trust (CCRT) to help developing countries deal with the short term economic disruption caused by coronavirus, allowing them to focus their spending on tackling the outbreak.*
- The NHS with Public Health England (PHE) was undertaking an expansion of coronavirus testing, with enhanced labs helping the health service carry out 10,000 tests daily. Approximately 1,500 tests were being processed every day at PHE labs with the great majority of

tests being turned around within 24 hours. As more people come forward to be tested, the NHS is now scaling up tests by 500%.#

12.03 The government announced that UK is moving out of the contain phase and into delay. The UK Chief Medical Officers raised the risk to the UK from moderate to high. The government advised elderlies over 70, and with underlying health condition avoid going onto cruises, schools to cancel overseas trips, and people who are showing symptoms to self-isolate for 7 days. *

13.03

- The Foreign & Commonwealth Office advised against all but essential travel to parts of Spain.*
- Government advised anyone who is suspected of having COVID-19, with a new continuous cough or high temperature, should not visit care homes or people receiving home care, and should self-isolate at home. People receiving care will be isolated in their rooms if they have symptoms of coronavirus.*

14.03 PHE together with NHS England and the Department of Health and Social Care (DHSC) agreed on the need to prioritise testing for those most at risk of severe illness from the virus. The goal is to save lives, protect the most vulnerable, and relieve pressure on our NHS. Tests will primarily be given to: all patients in critical care for pneumonia, acute respiratory distress syndrome (ARDS) or flu like illness; all other patients requiring admission to hospital for pneumonia, ARDS or flu like illness; where an outbreak has occurred in a residential or care setting, for example long-term care facility or prisons.*

15.03

- Next stage of the public information campaign was launched. Members of the public will see advice in TV adverts featuring Chief Medical Officer Professor Chris Whitty and voiced by actor Mark Strong to ensure everyone knows the best way to limit and delay the spread of the COVID-19.*

- From tomorrow, daily press conferences will be hosted by the Prime Minister and senior Ministers on the coronavirus pandemic, supported by scientific and medical experts including the Chief Medical Office and Chief Scientific Adviser.*

16.03

- The government published new and updated guidance to provide affected sectors with the latest advice on managing the threat from COVID-19.*

- UK Government announced at least £1.5 billion to the devolved administrations for their COVID-19 response: this means £780 million for the Scottish Government, £475 million for the Welsh Government and £260 million for the Northern Ireland Executive.*

17.03

- Government advised people to stay at home for 14 days if someone in the household has symptoms of COVID-19.*

- The Foreign & Commonwealth Office (FCO) advised against all non-essential international travel, initially for a period of 30 days. This advice takes effect immediately.*

- Routine inspections of schools, colleges, early years settings, children's social care providers and local authorities were temporarily suspended to reduce the burden on staff who are providing vital services to the nation in response to coronavirus.*

- Four new implementation committees focusing on health, public sector preparedness, economy and international response, will feed into a new daily meeting, which will be chaired by the Prime Minister. The four implementation committees are: Healthcare

(chaired by the Health Secretary to focus on the preparedness of the NHS, notably ensuring capacity in the critical care system for those worst affected, the medical and social package of support for those to whom we will be providing the new shielding regime); General Public Sector (chaired by the Chancellor of the Duchy of Lancaster to look at preparedness across the rest of the public and critical national infrastructure); Economic and Business (chaired by the Chancellor, with the Business Secretary as deputy chair, to consider economic and business impact and response, including supply chain resilience); International (chaired by the Foreign Secretary, to consider our international response to the crisis through the G7, G20 and other mechanisms).

- Rough sleepers, or those at risk will be supported by £3.2 million of initial emergency funding if they need to self-isolate to prevent the spread of coronavirus (COVID-19). The funding will be available to all local authorities in England and will reimburse them for the cost of providing accommodation and services to those sleeping on the streets to

help them successfully self-isolate.

- An emergency bill to give ministers powers to take the right action at the right time to respond effectively to the progress of the coronavirus outbreak will be introduced to Parliament.

- To ensure the NHS and adult social care have the additional staff capacity they need to respond to increasing demands on services during the outbreak, the powers enabled by the bill will allow recently retired NHS staff and social workers to return to work without any negative repercussions to their pensions. NHS staff will also be covered by a state-backed insurance scheme to ensure they can care for patients if, for example, they are moving outside their day-to-day duties while making use of their skills and training.

- NHS England announced that NHS Hospitals across the country are freeing up 30,000 of the overall 100,000 beds available by postponing non-urgent operations and providing care in the community for those who are fit to be discharged. The NHS is also sourcing up to 10,000 in independent and community hospitals.#

278

18.03

- The Prime Minister recommended that all citizens should begin practising "social distancing", including where possible working at home and stopping unnecessary travel; More vulnerable groups should avoid social contact for around 12 weeks; The suspension of mass gatherings, such as sporting events.*

- Manufacturers of hand sanitisers and gels will have their applications for denatured alcohol fast-tracked during the coronavirus (COVID-19) outbreak*

- The government will increase the number of people tested for COVID-19 to 25,000 hospital patients a day. The increased capacity was expected to be ready within 4 weeks, with highest-priority cases being tested first.*

- Emergency legislation will be taken forward as an urgent priority so that landlords will not be able to start proceedings to evict tenants for at least a 3 month period.*

- Homeowners who are struggling to pay interest fees on their Help to Buy equity loans will be offered payment holidays.*

- Schools will close from Monday, except for children of key workers and vulnerable children until further notice.*

19.03

- The Ministry of Defence (MOD) announced that it will put an additional 10,000 military personnel at a higher readiness and place Reserves on standby to support public services as part of a new "COVID Support Force". This is on top of the 10,000 already held at higher readiness. *

- The Government published guidance for schools giving them the flexibility to provide meals or shop vouchers to the 1.3 million disadvantaged children entitled to free school meals if they are no longer attending school, either due to closures or as a result of self-isolating at home.*

- Funding was announced to help patients who no longer need urgent hospital treatment to return home, making at least 15,000 beds available during the coronavirus outbreak.

- £1.6 billion will go to local authorities to help them respond to other coronavirus (COVID-19) pressures across all the services they deliver. This includes increasing support for the adult social care workforce and for services helping the most vulnerable, including homeless people.

- £1.3 billion will be used to enhance the NHS discharge process so patients who no longer need urgent treatment can return home safely and quickly.*

- The government temporarily relaxed elements of competition law as part of a package of measures to allow supermarkets to work together to feed the nation. The move allows retailers to share data with each other on stock levels, cooperate to keep shops open, or share distribution depots and delivery vans. It would also allow retailers to pool staff with one another to help meet demand.*

- Health bodies were reaching out to recent leavers and final year medical students and student nurses to join the front line after surveying on how much time they can dedicate to dealing with the impact of the pandemic. Staff will be able to 'opt in' to a register to fill a range of clinical and non-clinical roles across the NHS, based on their skills and time away from practice. Those who join the 'NHS army' will be given a full induction and online training to help them to hit the ground running.#

20.03

- Government and rail operators across the UK agree reductions in service levels following reduced passenger demand as people change their travel patterns to help tackle spread of COVID-19 starting 23 Mar.*

- All pubs, restaurants, gyms and other social venues across the country are ordered to close their doors for the foreseeable future.*

21.03

- Nearly 20,000 fully qualified staff will be joining the NHS to help manage the expected surge in cases. The deal with the independent sector includes the provision of 8,000 hospital beds across England, nearly 1200 more ventilators, more than 10,000 nurses, over 700 doctors and over 8,000 other clinical staff.#

- The Health Protection (Coronavirus, Business Closure) (England) Regulations 2020 came into force. Most restaurants, cafes and bars were now required not to sell food or drink for consuming on the premises. The following businesses must remain closed: Public houses. Cinemas. Theatres. Nightclubs. Concert halls. Museums and galleries, etc. The closure lasts until a direction is given by the Secretary of State. The Secretary of State is required to keep the need for these restrictions under review every 28 days.* Local government will be responsible for enforcing regulations requiring those businesses asked to close.*

22.03 Government advised to avoid non-essential travel in the UK. Essential travel does not include visits to second homes, camp sites, caravan parks or similar, whether for isolation purposes or holidays. People must remain in their primary residence.*

23.03

- The government and the UK's Chief Scientific Adviser backed the UK's leading clinicians and scientists to map how COVID-19 spreads and behaves by using whole genome sequencing. Through a £20 million investment, the consortium will look for breakthroughs that help the UK respond to this and future pandemics, and save lives. COVID-19 Genomics UK Consortium will deliver large scale, rapid sequencing of the cause of the disease and share intelligence with hospitals, regional NHS centres and the government.*

- £500,000 of funding is available for technology companies who come up with digital support solutions for people who need to stay at home because of coronavirus. The 'Techforce19' challenge aims to support those who need to stay at home for several weeks and need help through digital solutions that can be launched in the next few weeks.*

24.03

- Leave extended to 31 May for individuals who are currently unable to return home at the end of their visa.*

- A new hospital will open to provide support for thousands more patients with coronavirus, NHS England announced. The NHS Nightingale Hospital, London, will be ready for use from next week. The hospital will initially provide up to 500 beds equipped with ventilators and oxygen. The capacity will then continue to increase, potentially up to several thousand beds, should it be required.#

25.03

- The UK Government has launched a GOV.UK Coronavirus Information service on WhatsApp. The new free to use "chatbot" service aims to provide official, trustworthy and timely information and advice about coronavirus (COVID-19) and further reduce the burden on NHS services.*

- The Health Secretary pledged that the government will cover the costs of providing free car parking to NHS staff working in hospitals. Councils will set up local arrangements so NHS and care workers and volunteers can provide suitable evidence that they can display in their windscreen to ensure they avoid parking tickets.*

26.03

- From today, if members of the public do not comply with lockdown restrictions of staying at home and avoiding non-essential travel, the police may: instruct them to go home, leave an area or disperse; ensure parents are taking necessary steps to stop their children breaking these rules; issue fixed penalty notice for offence; Individuals who do not comply could be taken to court and potentially face fines and police arrest.

- New UK aid funding consists of £210 million was announced to help develop a vaccine. This new funding for the Coalition for Epidemic Preparedness Innovations is in addition to the £40 million already given to the organisation.*

27.03 NHS staff will be first in line for a new coronavirus (COVID-19) testing programme being developed in collaboration with government and industry that aim to boost testing capacity for frontline NHS staff. Dozens of universities, research institutes and companies across Britain are lending their testing equipment to 3 new hub laboratories which will be set up for the duration of the crisis.

28.03

- Business Secretary eased requirements to ensure hand sanitiser and PPE reaches NHS staff more quickly. Efforts to boost availability of essential supplies involve temporary measures including: asking the Health and Safety Executive (HSE) and Local Authorities to fast-track PPE through the product safety assessment process and prioritise this activity over other market surveillance activity; allowing PPE equipment providing protection against COVID-19 which lack the CE mark onto the market provided products meet essential safety requirements; providing new guidance for local authorities and ports and borders enforcement officers on the import and safety testing of hand sanitizer.*

- People staying at home suffering with suspected coronavirus symptoms will get regular check-ins from a new NHS messaging service launched today. Daily texts will be sent by the NHS to new patients who register their Covid-19 symptoms and contact details with the 111 online service. The messages will check how people are, and ensure that those who need help to get them through the isolation period receive it. #

30.03

- The Foreign & Commonwealth Office announced a new government partnership with airlines to fly back more tourists stranded abroad due to the coronavirus pandemic.*

- The Home Secretary announced that effective immediately, during the coronavirus outbreak, prospective renters and workers are now able to submit scanned documents, rather than originals, to show they have a right to rent or right to work.*

31.03

- Children eligible for free school meals will benefit from a national voucher scheme allowing them to continue to access meals whilst they stay at home. Schools can now provide every eligible child with a weekly shopping voucher worth £15 to spend at supermarkets while schools are closed due to coronavirus.

- Doctors, nurses and paramedics with visas due to expire before 1 October 2020 will have them automatically extended for one year. The extension will also apply to their family members, demonstrating how valued overseas NHS staff are to the UK.*

- Chancellor waives import taxes on vital medical equipment: NHS suppliers will no longer have to pay customs duty and import VAT on specific medical goods coming from outside the EU, including ventilators, coronavirus testing kits and protective clothing.*

- The NHS has enlisted easyJet and Virgin Atlantic to work alongside NHS clinicians at new Nightingale hospitals as part of the fight against coronavirus. The airlines are asking staff who have not been working since the COVID-19 grounded some planes to consider helping the thousands of doctors, nurses and other medics at the new hospitals being built across the country.#

Major Development

27.03

- PM Boris Johnson tested positive for Covid-19.[2]

- Health Secretary Matt Hancock tested positive[3]

29.03 Chris Whitty, the Government's Chief Medical Officer, has been forced to self-isolate after suffering from coronavirus symptoms.[4]

02.04 – 30.04

Public Health Policies

02.04 The UK will carry out 100,000 tests for coronavirus every day by the end of this month, Health Secretary Matt Hancock pledged today. Increased testing for the NHS will form part of a new 5-pillar plan, bringing together government, industry, academia, the NHS and many others, to dramatically increase the number of tests being carried out each day.*

03.04 For this summer's awards, schools and colleges are being asked to provide centre assessment grades for their students. These should be fair, objective and carefully considered judgements of the grades schools and colleges believe their students would have been most likely to achieve if they had sat their exams, and should take into account the full range of available evidence.*

04.04 A new Coronavirus Status Checker that will help the NHS coordinate its response and build up additional data on the COVID-19 outbreak was launched today by Health and Social Care Secretary Matt Hancock. People with potential coronavirus symptoms are now being asked to complete the status checker and answer a short series of questions which will tell the NHS about their experience.*

06.04 Over five million items of PPE were being delivered by the UK Government to Northern Ireland so that front line workers can safely care for patients and the public in hospitals and communities.*

07.04 Government would close down all other businesses for two and a half days over the Easter Break. Over this Easter period, essential businesses that have

2   www.bbc.com/news/uk-52060791

3   www.independent.co.uk/news/uk/politics/coronavirus-matt-hancock-boris-johnson-test-positive-covid-19-symptoms-a9430031.html

4   www.express.co.uk/news/uk/1261367/chris-whitty-coronavirus-test-postive-chief-medical-officer-self-isolate-covid19

been operating during this period of lockdown may operate on Saturday 11 April and Easter Monday 13 April.*

08.04

- A £1million fund to fast-track innovation to aid the Armed Forces in the fight against Coronavirus was launched by the Defence and Security Accelerator (DASA). The call is open to any idea or novel approach that could boost the Ministry of Defence's capabilities and work as part of the national effort against Coronavirus or similar future threats.*

- The NHS launched a mental health hotline as part of a package of measures to support the NHS' 1.4 million staff as they help people deal with the coronavirus.#

09.04 Health Secretary Matt Hancock has today officially opened the biggest diagnostic lab network in British history at the launch of a new site in Milton Keynes. The site in Milton Keynes is the first of 3 mega-labs that will be integrated into the new national testing infrastructure, with new sites being set up each day across the country to take patient samples.*

10.04 A UK-wide plan was announced to ensure personal protective equipment (PPE) gets to where it is needed most.

The government already coordinated deliveries of PPE directly to health and care providers and to 38 local resilience forums across England to ensure appropriate distribution of critical PPE.*

13.04 HM Treasury confirmed that more than £14 billion from the Coronavirus emergency response fund will go towards public services, including the NHS and local authorities involved in the fight against Coronavirus. HM Treasury support will also enable home delivery of medicines to the most vulnerable people in the country, and it has helped support medical and nursing students and retired doctors and nurses to join the front line. Alongside £1.6 billion of new funding for Local Authorities, this health service funding means that HM Treasury has provided £2.9 billion to support local services and hospital discharge, reinforcing care for the vulnerable, and meaning that those who are strong enough can leave hospital more quickly, freeing up bed space for patients that need it.*

14.04

- An initial £2.6 million was made available to fund a number of projects to develop hi-tech solutions to these challenges, in a joint initiative with the European Space Agency (ESA) in support of NHS

England.*

- The UK Government has committed a further £350m to support the devolved administration in Wales tackle coronavirus. As a result of a boost to the Coronavirus emergency response fund, the devolved administration in Wales will receive an additional £350 million on top of the £250 million allocated from the £5 billion fund.*

15.04

- Government announced all symptomatic care home residents will be tested for COVID-19 as testing capacity continues to increase. All patients discharged from hospital to be tested before going into care homes as a matter of course. All social care staff who need a test will now have access to one with the Care Quality Commission (CQC) to contact all 30,000 care providers in the coming days to offer tests.*

- Care providers unable to get PPE from their usual suppliers will be supported by a 24/7 hotline and a dedicated, in-house team at the National Supply Disruption Response (NSDR), who can rapidly pack and deliver PPE to providers. The government is going to pilot a website which will allow care homes to order PPE online, us-

ing NHS Supply chains and shipped directly via Royal Mail.*

- To attract 20,000 people into social care over the next three months to relieve pressures in the care workforce, in the next few weeks the government will re-launch a national recruitment campaign to run across broadcast, digital, and social media. The campaign will highlight the vital role that the social care workforce is playing right now, during this pandemic, along with the longer-term opportunity of working in care. *

16.04 A drive-through coronavirus testing facility has opened at Edinburgh Airport as part of the Government's UK-wide drive to increase testing for thousands more NHS and other key workers. Those tested will receive their results within 48 hours.*

18.04

- Councils across England will receive another £1.6 billion in additional funding as they continue to respond to the coronavirus pandemic, the Local Government Secretary has announced today.*

- As a result of the UK Government's funding boost for councils across England announced by Local Government Secretary Robert Jenrick, the

Northern Ireland Executive will receive an additional £50 million. This takes the total funding the UK Government has made available to the Northern Ireland Executive to support its efforts to tackle coronavirus to almost £1.2 billion.*

- Scotland will receive an additional £155 million in funding from the UK Government to help tackle coronavirus.*

21.04 The UK Government committed a further £95m to support the devolved administration in Wales tackle coronavirus, the Local Government Secretary has announced. As a result of the UK Government's funding boost for councils across England announced by Local Government Secretary Robert Jenrick, the devolved administration in Wales will receive an additional £95 million. This takes the total given by the UK Government to support the effort in Wales to almost £2 billion.

23.04

- 20,000 households in England were contacted to take part in the first wave of a major new government study led by the Department for Health and Social Care (DHSC) and the Office for National Statistics (ONS) to track coronavirus (COVID-19) in the general population. The results will help scientists and the

government in the ongoing response to the coronavirus outbreak, with initial findings expected to be available in early May.*

- All essential workers in England, and members of their households who are showing symptoms of coronavirus will now be able to get tested, the government announced.*

25.04 A clinical trial was approved to determine if plasma donated by patients who have recovered from COVID-19 can help those battling the illness. If effective, a scaled-up national programme will deliver up to 10,000 units of convalescent plasma per week to the NHS. This would provide enough convalescent plasma to treat 5,000 patients each week.*

26.04 A new and innovative UK business developed a collection of digital flashcards to address the problems healthcare workers wearing PPE were having in transferring vital information to deaf, blind and critically ill coronavirus patients.*

28.04 The government announced that anyone in England with symptoms of coronavirus who has to leave home to go to work, and all symptomatic members of the public aged 65 and over, will now be able to get tested after booking a test using an online portal. This will mean people

who cannot work from home and those aged 65 and over can know for sure whether they have coronavirus and need to continue isolating. Members of their households with symptoms will also be eligible for testing.*

29.04

- The Health and Care Secretary announced that thousands of patients could benefit from potential treatments for COVID-19 that will be fast-tracked through a new national clinical trial. This platform will accelerate the development of new drugs for patients hospitalised with COVID-19, reducing the time taken to set up clinical studies for new therapies from months to just weeks and helping to ease pressure on the NHS and ultimately save lives.*

- The Home Secretary announced that free visa extensions will be automatically granted to more crucial overseas health and care frontline workers. Those with visas due to expire before 1 October 2020 will receive an automatic one-year extension.*

- A new method of reporting daily COVID-19 deaths was developed by Public Health England (PHE). The new daily count includes deaths in all settings with COVID-19 for the first time. Data will

complement the new Care Quality Commission (CQC) and Office for National Statistics (ONS) figures on care homes*

- The government announced that a major new programme of home testing for coronavirus commissioned by the Department of Health and Social Care will track the progress of the infection across England. It will help improve understanding of how many people are currently infected with the virus, and potentially how many have been infected and recovered since the outbreak began.*

30.04

- Government brought in a new video platform to enable all parties in a criminal hearing to take part remotely – allowing all magistrate and crown courts in England and Wales to hold secure hearings, making it easier to make sure justice continues to be served.*

- From tomorrow, PPE purchased by care homes, businesses, charities and individuals to protect against Covid-19 will be free from VAT for a three-month period.*

Socio-Economic Policy Packages

02.04 Community pharmacies are receiving a £300 million cash boost to ensure they can continue to carry out essential services during the coronavirus outbreak and protect community health during a period of unprecedented demand.

03.04

- Transport Secretary Grant Shapps announced that England's buses will continue to serve those who rely on them thanks to a funding boost totalling £397 million for vital bus operators. The package will keep key routes running to provide a lifeline for those who cannot work from home, including those travelling to jobs on the frontline of the UK's fight against COVID-19, such as NHS staff.*

- Food redistribution organisations across England will benefit from £3.25 million of government funding to help them cut food waste and redistribute up to 14,000 tonnes of surplus stock during the coronavirus outbreak.*

- Businesses could help boost the UK's resilience to the long-term impact of the coronavirus outbreak and similar situations in the future, as a result of £20 million government funding announced. Grants of up to £50,000 will be available to technology and research-focussed businesses to develop new ways of working and help build resil-

ience in industries such as delivery services, food manufacturing, retail and transport, as well as support people at home in circumstances like those during the coronavirus outbreak.

07.04

- The Government was to make extra funding available for schools to cover the unique challenges and financial costs of the coronavirus outbreak. The money will cover unforeseen additional costs including for cleaning and keeping schools open over Easter.*

- The basic element of Working Tax Credit was increased by £1,045 to £3,040 from 6 April 2020 until 5 April 2021. The amount a claimant or household will benefit from will depend on their circumstances, including their level of household income. But the increase could mean up to an extra £20 each week. The government is also uprating Child Benefit, other tax credits rates and thresholds, and Guardian's Allowance by 1.7% with effect from 6 April 2020.*

- The Department for Digital, Culture, Media and Sport (DCMS) launched a new £1.3 million scheme to give financial support to Destination Management Organisations at

risk of closure due to the coronavirus pandemic.*

08.04

- Airlines will be able to temporarily defer the payment of air navigation charges, saving them tens of millions of pounds, following action from UK government, to provide financial relief to airlines struggling during the pandemic.*

- Chancellor Rishi Sunak announced that charities across the UK will receive a £750 million package of support to ensure they can continue their vital work during the coronavirus outbreak.*

09.04 From 1 April, over £13 billion of NHS debt will be scrapped as part of a wider package of NHS reforms announced by the Health Secretary today. The changes will provide much needed financial support during this unprecedented viral pandemic, as well as laying secure foundations for the longer-term commitments set out last year to support the NHS to become more financially sustainable.*

10.04

- Adoptive families will be offered emergency support including online counselling and couples therapy as the Government expands the scope of the Adoption Support Fund to

meet needs arising from the outbreak of coronavirus (COVID-19).

- The Education Secretary announced that up to £8 million will be available to pay for different types of therapeutic support for families whose adopted children may have already suffered trauma and be made more anxious owing to the uncertainty of the effects of the virus.*

16.04

- The government announced that councils will be allowed to defer £2.6 billion in business rates payments to central government, and £850 million in social care grants will be paid up front this month in a move aimed at helping to ease immediate pressures on local authority cash flows.*

- Companies House will temporarily pause the strike off process to prevent companies being dissolved. This will give businesses affected by the coronavirus outbreak the time they need to update their records and help them avoid being struck off the register.*

- The Chancellor announced a government-backed loan scheme for large businesses affected by coronavirus has been expanded to cover all viable firms. Outlining further details of the Coronavirus Large Business Interruption Loans Scheme (CLBILS) ahead of its launch on Monday, Sunak said all firms with a turnover of more than £45 million will now be able to apply for up to £25 million of finance, and up to £50 million for firms with a turnover of more than £250 million.*

17.04

- Coronavirus Job Retention Scheme extended by one month to reflect continuing social distancing measures.*
- A £9m fund will target those adversely affected by the Covid-19 pandemic. It will contribute to fixed business costs for under-24m vessels. A further £1m grants fund will support local projects to promote locally caught fish, by application.*

19.04 Disadvantaged children across England were set to receive laptops and tablets as part of a push to make remote education accessible for pupils staying at home during the coronavirus outbreak. The government will also provide 4G routers to make sure disadvantaged secondary school pupils and care leavers can access the internet.*

20.04

- The Chancellor announced that UK businesses driving in-

novation and development will be helped through the coronavirus outbreak with a £1.25 billion government support package, including a new £500 million loan scheme for high-growth firms, called the Future Fund, and £750 million of targeted support for small and medium sized businesses focusing on research and development. To be eligible, a business must be an unlisted UK registered company that has previously raised at least £250,000 in equity investment from third party investors in the last five years.*

- The Environment Secretary George Eustice and Chief Secretary to the Treasury Steve Barclay announced that over 1,000 fishing and aquaculture businesses in England will receive direct cash grants through a fisheries support scheme, in which up to £9 million will be available for grants to eligible fishing and aquaculture businesses. A further £1 million will be made available to support projects to assist fishermen to sell their catch in their local communities.*

- A new 'support finder' tool will help businesses and self-employed people across the UK to quickly and easily determine what finan-

cial support is available to them during the coronavirus pandemic.*

22.04 Businesses were expected to receive almost £10 billion in business rate relief as part of the government's comprehensive package of support for the economy during the coronavirus pandemic.*

23.04

- Social distancing measures mean that some charities can no longer offer face-to-face support, and must transfer to mainly remote based services to provide victims with the practical and emotional help they need. £600,000 will be reallocated to services immediately, allowing helplines to stay open longer and employ more support workers to handle calls. It will also help fund the technology needed for other forms of contact. Six organisations that together cover the whole of the United Kingdom will benefit from the funding, meaning victims of crimes, in particular sexual and domestic abuse, can still access this essential support.*

- The Government confirmed that councils will temporarily be able to use the funding they receive for the free entitlements for two, three and four-year-olds differently, redistributing it where absolutely

necessary for the benefit of critical workers and the parents of the most vulnerable children, when their usual arrangements are no longer possible as a result of Coronavirus. This is to make sure sufficient childcare places are available for vulnerable children and those of critical workers, and will build on existing commitments to continue paying free entitlement funding – worth £3.6 billion a year – to local authorities throughout the Coronavirus outbreak. Childcare businesses will also benefit from other support schemes, including a business rates holiday, the Small Business grant for those that don't pay business rates, the Self-Employment Scheme and the Coronavirus Job Retention Scheme (CJRS).*

24.04

- A multimillion government support package for essential freight services was announced to keep the flow of goods and services running smoothly in and out of the UK, and around the country, throughout the pandemic.*

- Vulnerable children most at risk of neglect, violence or exploitation will benefit from extra support to keep them safe during the Coronavirus outbreak. More than £12 million will be spent to tackle the increased risk some children and young people are facing as they stay at home to reduce the spread of Coronavirus.*

- People who may be particularly vulnerable or isolated during the coronavirus outbreak, including new parents, the homeless, unpaid carers, young people and cancer patients, could soon benefit from a range of innovative digital solutions selected as part of the TechForce19 challenge.*

- Thousands of schools will benefit from a partnership with tech giants to gain access to education platforms. Expert technical support to access Google and Microsoft's education platforms, along with free training on how to use the resources most effectively, will be available for schools immediately. This will include online resources, support getting set up, webinars and peer to peer support between schools.*

25.04 The majority of landlords and tenants are working well together to reach agreements on debt obligations, but some landlords have been putting tenants under undue pressure by using aggressive debt recovery tactics. To stop these unfair practices, the government will temporarily ban the use of statutory demands (made between 1 March 2020 and 30 June 2020) and winding up petitions presented from Monday 27 April, through to 30 June, where a company cannot pay its bills due to coronavirus. This will help ensure these companies do not fall into deeper financial strain. The measures will be included in the Corporate Insolvency and Governance Bill, which the Business Secretary set out earlier this month.*

28.04

- A new online learning platform to help boost the nation's skills while people are staying at home, was launched by Education Secretary Gavin Williamson. Free courses are available through a new online platform hosted on the gov.uk website. The new platform gives people access to free, high-quality digital and numeracy courses to help build up their skills, progress in work and boost their job prospects.*

- Today the Home Office announced £3.1 million will go to specialist services for children who have both been directly and indirectly affected by domestic abuse. This can include one-to-one and group counselling sessions to improve the mental health of children affected and early intervention schemes.*

- The government was extending deadlines to ten consultations and calls for evidence currently underway by three months – including the Plastic Packaging Tax, a call for evidence on Vehicle Excise Duty and a consultation on the HMRC Charter – and also a short delay to the publication of other documents announced at Budget 2020. The extension will give all stakeholders, who are facing disruption due to COVID-19, more time to submit their views and allow them to fully engage with these documents and contribute to the tax policy making process.*

29.04 The government announced that the £400,000 Community Radio Fund administered by Ofcom will be used to provide a lifeline for radio stations hit hardest by the coronavirus. Relevant stations will be invited to bid for emergency grants through Ofcom to help meet their core costs*

Major Development

02.04 UK's Health Secretary Matt Hancock, who had been self-isolating after his COVID-19 diagnosis last week, returned to the frontline to address the daily Downing Street briefing.[5]

04.04 250 China ventilators arrived U.K.[6]

05.04 PM Boris Johnson admitted to hospital.[7]

06.04

- PM moved into intensive care.[8]

- Chris Whitty recovered from his symptoms of coronavirus and is out of isolation.[9]

- Chief medical officer Prof Chris Whitty admitted that the 2 million home test kits ordered

5   www.ndtv.com/world-news/uk-health-minister-matt-hancock-back-at-work-after-covid-19-recovery-pledges-more-tests-2205259

6   www.theguardian.com/uk-news/2020/apr/30/entire-order-of-250-chinese-ventilators-were-useless-despite

7   www.bbc.com/news/uk-52177125

8   www.bbc.com/news/uk-52192604

9   https://metro.co.uk/2020/04/06/chris-whitty-isolation-coronavirus-symptoms-12517276/

from China for £20 mil. were faulty in a press conference.[10]

12.04 PM Boris Johnson discharged from hospital[11]

24.04 Both Dominic Cummings and Ben Warner, government advisors, were revealed to have taken part in the SAGE meetings.[12]

29.04 The UK government has flown over 22 million pieces of PPE and more than 1000 ventilators to the NHS and Social Care Services from China over the last three weeks.*

30.04 A group of senior British doctors and medical managers voiced concern over 250 ventilators purchased in China in a letter to Health Secretary Matt Hancock.[13]

01.05 – 26.05

Public Health Policies

01.05 Local Government Secretary Rt Hon Robert Jenrick MP wrote to all councils in England thanking them for their efforts in the battle against coronavirus and reminding them of their eligibility for testing: council workers with symptoms of coronavirus are now able to be tested for the virus, and can re-

turn to work if the results are negative.*

04.05

- New measures to protect students and universities, including temporary student number controls, was announced by the Education Secretary, which intended to stabilise university admissions this autumn and to help the universities and students are safeguarded at a time of unprecedented uncertainty.*

- Isle of Wight residents will be the first to be offered access to a new contact tracing app, as part of government action to test, track and trace to minimise the spread of COVID-19 and move towards safely reducing lockdown measures. Everyone on the island will receive access to the official NHS COVID-19 contact tracing app from this Thursday. The app will work together with enhanced contact tracing services and swab testing for those with potential COVID-19 symptoms to help minimise the spread of COVID-19.*

06.05 A new dedicated app for the adult social

care workforce in England was launched to support staff on-the-go through the coronavirus pandemic. New mental wellbeing guidance will soon be published to further support the care sector with bespoke advice for care workers.*

Socio-Economic Policy Packages

01.05

- The Rugby Football League (RFL) will receive a £16 million cash injection to safeguard the immediate future of the sport for the communities it serves, the Government has announced.*

- Transport Secretary Grant Shapps announced that air passenger services between Great Britain and Northern Ireland will be safeguarded through a £5.7 million government investment.

- High Streets Minister Simon Clarke MP confirmed that hundreds of local business partnerships across England will share £6.1m of funding to spend on projects that will help their local economies through the uncertainty of the coronavirus pandemic.*

04.05

- New support for SMEs during coronavirus has today been launched in the form of nearly 100 expert-led webinars. The webinars will offer practical advice to SMEs and focus on issues businesses trading internationally are facing.*

- The government launched a £14 million support fund for zoos and aquariums in the latest step to protect businesses affected by the coronavirus pandemic. Establishments covered by the Zoo Licensing Act will be able to bid for a portion of the £14 million that has been made available.*

- A £5.4m boost will be distributed through not for profit organisations and Law Centres across England and Wales, to help organisations continue to provide vital legal advice throughout the pandemic to people seeking help with housing, debt, discrimination and employment problems.*

06.05

- England's dairy farmers will be able to access up to £10,000 each to help them overcome the impact of the

---

10   www.nytimes.com/2020/04/16/world/europe/coronavirus-antibody-test-uk.html

11   www.aljazeera.com/news/2020/04/british-pm-boris-johnson-discharged-hospital-200412125215780.html

12   www.theguardian.com/world/2020/apr/24/revealed-dominic-cummings-on-secret-scientific-advisory-group-for-covid-19

13   www.newsweek.com/british-doctors-say-ventilators-purchased-china-could-kill-coronavirus-patients-1501286

coronavirus outbreak. The new funding will help support dairy farmers who have seen decreased demand for their products as bars, restaurants and cafes have had to close. Eligible dairy farmers will be entitled to up to £10,000 each, to cover 70% of their lost income during April and May to ensure they can continue to operate and sustain production capacity without impacts on animal welfare.*

- A revaluation of business rates will no longer take place in 2021 to help reduce uncertainty for firms affected by the impacts of coronavirus, Communities Secretary Rt Hon Robert Jenrick MP has announced.*

Major Development

05.05 UK Home Office facing questions about the lack of interventions at the border before the coronavirus lockdown after the government's chief scientific adviser revealed the UK received a "big influx of cases" from Europe that "seeded right the way across the country". Figures revealed that just 273 out of the

18.1 million people who entered the UK in the three months prior to the coronavirus lockdown were formally quarantined.[14]

06.05 Heathrow will start using thermal cameras to carry out temperature checks on passengers within the next fortnight, as it called for common health screening standards around the world for air travellers. The UK's busiest airport said it would trial thermal cameras capable of monitoring the temperature of people in the immigration halls, initially in Terminal 2. If successful, it will install the equipment in the departures, connections and staff search areas. Similar technology is in place at many Asian airports, for example at Singapore Changi.[15]

26.05 Journalist and presenter Emily Maitlis opened Tuesday's Newsnight with a monologue about the ongoing lockdown row involving Boris Johnson's top aide Dominic Cummings. In a statement, the BBC said Maitlis' comments did not meet the broadcaster's standards of due impartiality.

01.06 – 29.06
Public Health Policies

01.06 Lockdown was eased, although the risk level was still at 4.

09.06 It was announced that face coverings will become compulsory on public transport in England from 15 June.[16]

19.06 UK Alert Level has moved down from 4 to 3: "The Joint Biosecurity Centre has recommended that the COVID-19 alert level should move from Level 4 (A COVID-19 epidemic is in general circulation; transmission is high or rising exponentially) to Level 3 (A COVID-19 epidemic is in general circulation). The CMOs for England, Scotland, Wales and Northern Ireland have reviewed the evidence and agree with this recommendation to move to Level 3 across the UK."[17]

29.06 Matt Hancock announced that due to the spike of COVID-19 cases, Leicester will be under UK's first local lockdown for four weeks: from Tuesday, June 30, non-essential shops in the city would have to close, and from Thursday, July 2, schools would shut to

all but the most vulnerable children. This local lockdown was gradually and partially released one month later.[18]

Major Development

04.06 UK hosted the Global Vaccine Summit.

20.06 Premier League football game series are back this weekend.

27.06 UK hosted Unite for Our Future event, demonstrating the commitment to international collaboration on vaccines, treatments and tests. Johnson made a speech on the event.

04.07 – 30.07
Public Health Policies

04.07 businesses began to reopen; hairdressers and barbers, museums and galleries; pubs, restaurants, bars, and cafes too.

24.07 New face covering rules are enforced in England. From this day on, Coverings are mandatory in enclosed public spaces such as supermarkets, indoor shopping centres, transport hubs, banks and takeaways. Police can hand out fines of up to £100 to those who do not comply.[19]

---

14   www.theguardian.com/world/2020/may/05/just-273-people-arriving-in-uk-in-run-up-to-lockdown-quarantined?CMP=Share_iOSApp_Other

15   www.theguardian.com/uk-news/2020/may/06/heathrow-to-carry-out-temperature-checks-on-passengers?CMP=Share_iOSApp_Other

16   https://twitter.com/DHSCgovuk/status/1270256817625378817

17   www.gov.uk/government/news/update-from-the-uk-chief-medical-officers-on-the-uk-alert-level

18   www.thesun.co.uk/news/12053926/leicester-lockdown-end-coronavirus-rules-restrictions/

19   www.bbc.co.uk/news/uk-53522129

30.07 Matt Hancock announced new local lockdown measures on parts of Northern England including Greater Manchester, east Lancashire and parts of West Yorkshire, due to spike of cases.[20]

Socio-Economic Policy Packages

08.07 Rishi Sunak announced a stimulus package for job search, for employers to bring back furloughed employees, train young people, boost investment, and so forth.[21]

Major Development

04.06 UK hosted the Global Vaccine Summit.

02.07 schools are announced to reopen from 1 September. Guidance is published by the Government to provide schools, colleges and nurseries with the details needed to plan for a full return, as well as reassuring parents about what to expect for their children.[22]

03.08 – 24.08
Public Health Policies

03.08 Scottish First Minister Nicola Sturgeon announced local lockdown in Aberdeen, Scotland, after 54 cases had been reported in recent days as part of a cluster of infections in Aberdeen.[23]

13.08 Boris Johnson has announced a series of tough new enforcement measures targeting the most serious breaches of social distancing restrictions.[24]

15.08 According to the plan set out in the government document 'roadmap to recovery', except for specific areas where local restrictions are still in place, the rest of England will resume national easements on indoor performance, weddings, sporting events etc.[25]

Socio-Economic Policy Packages

03.08 The program of "Eat Out to Help Out" officially begins, which will run through August till August 31. The scheme was announced in early July,[26] and is designed to encourage people to visit restaurants, cafes and pubs, which have been badly hit by the lockdown. It applies to eat-in food and drink on Monday to Wednesdays at more than 72,000 venues, in which customers enjoy 50% of discount capped at £10 per person (does not apply to alcohol).

Major Development

24.08 Seventeen members of staff and two pupils have tested positive for coronavirus at a school in Dundee, Scotland in less than two weeks after Scottish schools returned.

14.10 – 31.10
Public Health Policies

14.10 New three-tier restrictions came into force in England as a response to the surge of number of cases and deaths since September. Under this new system, most part of England is on medium alert (lowest tier in the scheme), whereas "millions of people in the North and the Midlands" are under high alert with extra curbs on households mixing. The Liverpool City Region, with "very high alert" (highest tier), will face even more strict restrictions.[27]

31.10 Boris Johnson announced a second national lockdown for England, which will last for four weeks, to prevent a "medical and moral disaster" for the NHS. Under the new restrictions, people are being told to stay at home unless they have a specific reason to leave, such as work which cannot be done from home, and education. The announcement is made on a day with 21,915 new cases, bringing the total since the pandemic began to 1,011,660. This also makes the U.K. the ninth country to reach the milestone of a million confirmed cases, after the US, India, Brazil, Russia, France, Spain, Argentina and Colombia.[28]

16.11 – 29.11
Public Health Policies

16.11 The Business Secretary announced that the UK government has secured 5 million doses of Moderna vaccine which, if approved by the medicines regulator, are expected to be delivered to the U.K. from Spring 2021. This new deal increases total number of doses secured by the U.K. to 355 million, as part of

20   www.bbc.co.uk/news/uk-53602362

21   www.gov.uk/government/speeches/a-plan-for-jobs-speech

22   www.gov.uk/government/news/schools-and-colleges-to-reopen-in-full-in-september

23   https://news.sky.com/story/coronavirus-lockdown-to-be-reimposed-in-aberdeen-after-spike-in-cases-12042945

24   www.gov.uk/government/news/prime-minister-announces-stronger-enforcement-measures-as-easements-resume

25   Ibid.

26   www.bbc.co.uk/news/business-53337170

27   https://www.bbc.co.uk/news/uk-54533924

28   https://www.bbc.co.uk/news/uk-54763956

government's strategy to build a diverse portfolio of promising vaccines.[29]

29.11 The UK government has signed a deal for a further 2 million doses of Moderna's promising vaccine candidate, bringing the total to 7 million doses for the U.K.. This new deal means that the U.K. now has access to a total of 357 million doses of vaccines from 7 different developers.[30]

02.12.2020 – 20.01.2021

Public Health Policies

02.12 Margaret Keenan in the UK became the first person in the world to be vaccinated.[31]

04.01 Boris Johnson announced a third national lockdown, expected to be lasting at least till mid-February, in light of the rapid spread of the new variant of the Coronavirus.[32]

09.01 The Queen and the Duke of Edinburgh were vaccinated by a household doctor at the Windsor Castle. They are among the 1.5 million people in the UK to have had at least one dose of a COVID-19 vaccine so far.[33]

20.01 1,820 deaths within 28 days of a positive COVID test was reported today. Not only is this the highest number reported since the start of UK's third and ongoing lockdown, but it is also the record high since the start of the pandemic.[34]

---

29   www.gov.uk/government/news/government-secures-5-million-doses-of-moderna-vaccine

30   www.gov.uk/government/news/uk-government-secures-additional-2-million-doses-of-moderna-covid-19-vaccine

31   www.bbc.co.uk/news/uk-55227325 Accessed 2021-01-24

32   www.standard.co.uk/news/politics/pm-national-lockdown-covid19-b683912.html Accessed 2021-01-24

33   www.bbc.co.uk/news/uk-55602007 Accessed 2021-01-24

34   https://news.sky.com/story/covid-19-1-820-more-coronavirus-deaths-in-uk-highest-number-reported-on-a-single-day-12193513 Accessed 2021-01-24

UNITED STATES

Yamin Xu

05.01–31.10 Total 9,077,689 cases / 222,316 deaths

05.01– 11.01 (0 / N/A)

Public Health Policies

07.01 Centers for Disease Control and Prevention established the Coronavirus Incident Management System. (*D)

11.01 Centers for Disease Control and Prevention updated Level 1 Travel Notice for China. (*D)

12.01– 18.01 (0 / N/A)

Public Health Policies

17.01 Airport sceenings: The CDC began implementing public health entry screening at San Francisco (SFO), New York (JFK) and Los Angeles (LAX) airports. The CDC would later add screening at two more airports Atlanta (ATL) and Chicago (ORD). (*U)

21.01– 24.01 (1 / N/A)

Public Health Policies

21.01 The United States announced its first confirmed coronavirus case — a man in his 30s in Washington state. (*N)

24.01 Sen. Rick Scott, R-Fla., urged the Trump administration to declare a public health emergency and sent a letter to the CDC requesting information about the agency's plan to combat the virus. "We have to get serious about the threat of coronavirus coming from China," Scott said in a press release.

Americans told 'risk is low' Anthony Fauci, head of the National Institute of Allergy and Infectious Diseases, commented on the risk to Americans. "We don't want the American public to be worried about this because their risk is low," Fauci said. "On the other hand, we are taking this very seriously and are dealing very closely with Chinese authorities."

Many health professionals argued that the flu posed a greater threat than the coronavirus. (*U)

26.01– 01.02 (1 / N/A)

Public Health Policies

28.01 'Monitoring' since December

Alex Azar, secretary of Health and Human Services and chairman of the coronavirus task force, told reporters during a press briefing that the U.S. had "been monitoring this virus and preparing a response since back in December." (*U)

29.01 195 Americans returned from China

The first group of passengers returned to the U.S. from China. They were expected to remain under observation for up to three days as they were screened, a CDC official said. The American passengers flew into California from Wuhan, with a stopover in Anchorage, Alaska, where they had also been screened. (*U)

Wuhan, China, repatriation flight #1 arrived in Alaska and transits to March Air Reserve Base, Calif.

DOD approved Health and Human Services request for assistance (RFA#1) for March Air Reserve Base providing

---

- Majority of the contents were drawn from NBC, USA TODAY, Department of Defense Coronavirus Timeline, ABC, New York Times and CNN. Other sources listed individually. Cumulative cases and deaths were drawn from the Covid Tracking Project, which are under daily automated updates. Numbers might be adjusted later on, thus possibly different from when they were first recorded here, and they should be used as estimate.

(*N)=NBC timeline:

    www.nbcnews.com/health/health-news/coronavirus-timeline-tracking-critical-moments-covid-19-n1154341

(*U) =USATODAY:

    www.usatoday.com/in-depth/news/nation/2020/04/21/coronavirus-updates-how-covid-19-unfolded-u-s-timeline/2990956001/

(*A)=ABC timeline:

    https://abcnews.go.com/Health/timeline-coronavirus-started/story?id=69435165

(*D)=DOD (Department of Defense) timeline:

    www.defense.gov/Explore/Spotlight/Coronavirus/DOD-Response-Timeline/

(*NYT)=New York Times: Coronavirus Timeline

    www.nytimes.com/article/coronavirus-timeline.html

(*C)=CNN Coronavirus Timeline Fast Fact

    www.cnn.com/2020/02/06/health/wuhan-coronavirus-timeline-fast-facts/index.html

approximately 200 beds for State Department officials evacuated from Wuhan, China. (*D)

30.01 US reported first case of person-to-person transmission

The CDC reported that the first case of person-to-person transmission in the U.S. was the husband of a Chicago woman who developed symptoms after visiting China. "We understand this may be concerning, but based on what we know now, our assessment remains that the immediate risk to the American public is low," said Robert Redfield, director of the CDC. (*U)

POTUS established a COVID-19 interagency task force.

U.S. Department of State issued authorized departure for all China posts. (*D)

31.01 US public health emergency

The Trump administration declared the coronavirus outbreak to be a public health emergency in the United States, setting quarantines of Americans who had recently been to certain parts of China. CDC officials said it was the first quarantine order issued by the federal government in over 50 years.

Azar also announced a temporary suspension of entry into the United States of foreign nationals

who had been in China in the previous 14 days. The ban was effective Feb. 2.

Meanwhile, officials began funneling all flights from China to the U.S. to one of seven airports that were designated ports of entry: New York, San Francisco, Seattle, Honolulu, Los Angeles, Chicago and Atlanta. (*U)

02.02– 08.02 (2 / N/A)
Public Health Policies

02.02 U.S. Department of State issued a Level 4 travel advisory for China. (*D)

06.02 First death in US

Autopsies on the bodies of two people who died at home on Feb. 6 and Feb. 17 showed they were positive for the virus, a California county announced April 21.

Previously, the first U.S. death had been thought to occur Feb. 29 outside Seattle. The autopsy findings revealed that the virus may have been spreading in U.S. communites earlier than previously known. The two people died during a time when very limited testing was available only through the CDC, and the agency's testing criteria restricted testing to only individuals with a known travel history and who sought medical care for specific symptoms. (*U)

08.02 The first U.S. citizen died from COVID-19 in Wuhan. (*N)

09.02– 15.02 (2 / N/A)
Public Health Policies

11.02 COVID-19

The WHO announced a formal name for the coronavirus – COVID-19. Meanwhile, China reported its highest daily coronavirus death toll, the 103 additional fatalities pushing the total past 1,100. "With 99% of cases in China, this remains very much an emergency for that country, but one that holds a very grave threat for the rest of the world," WHO's Dr. Tedros Adhanom Ghebreyesus said.

The CDC confirmed the 13th U.S. coronavirus case, and about 800 Americans evacuated from Wuhan remained under quarantine. At a rally in New Hampshire, Trump said that, "in theory" once the weather warmed up, "the virus" would "miraculously" go away. (*U)

16.02– 22.02 (2 / N/A)
Public Health Policies

21.02 Pandemic 'likely'

Dr. Nancy Messonnier, director of the CDC's National Center for Immunization and Respiratory Diseases, told reporters that U.S. health officials were preparing for the

coronavirus to become a pandemic. "We're not seeing community spread here in the United States, yet, but it's very possible, even likely, that it may eventually happen," she said. (*U)

23.02– 29.02 (18 / 5)
Socio-Economic Policy Packages

24.02 The U.S. stock market plummeted over coronavirus fears, after the Dow Jones Industrial Average experienced the worst day in two years. (*N)

Public Health Policies

25.02 NIH clinical trial of remdesivir to treat COVID-19 began[1]

26.02 CDC reported community spread; Pence to lead task force

The CDC confirmed an infection in California that would represent the first U.S. person to contract the virus despite not visiting a foreign country recently or coming in contact with an infected patient. This brought the number of coronavirus cases detected in the U.S. to 15, with 12 of them related to travel and the other two to direct contact with a patient.

Meanwhile, Trump announced that Vice President Mike Pence would lead the administration's coronavirus response.

---

1   www.nih.gov/news-events/news-releases/nih-clinical-trial-remdesivir-treat-covid-19-begins

"We're very, very ready for this," Trump said at a press conference. "The risk to the American people remains very low." (*U)

28.02 Flawed test kits

Messonnier told reporters that the CDC had taken steps to address problems with flawed test kits mailed to state and local labs. The agency had also expanded criteria for coronavirus testing. (*U)

VPOTUS announced Ambassador Debbie Birx as White House COVID-19 Response Coordinator. (*D)

29.02 President Donald Trump announced additional travel restrictions involving Iran and increased warnings about travel to Italy and South Korea. (*N)

FDA began to open up testing

In an effort to increase testing, the Food and Drug Administration announced it would be opening up its emergency authorization process to allow new testing technologies at hospitals and health care facilities nationwide.

U.S. Surgeon General Jerome Adams echoed CDC guidance encouraging Americans not to buy face masks needed by medical professionals. "They are NOT effective in preventing general public from catching Coronavirus, but if healthcare providers can't get them to care for sick patients, it puts them

and our communities at risk," he said on Twitter.

A man in Washington state died after contracting the coronavirus – what was initially thought to be the first death from the new disease in the U.S. Gov. Jay Inslee declared a state of emergency in Washington hours later, saying that the outbreak "could likely be a worldwide pandemic." (*U)

01.03– 07.03 (1,271 /27)

Socio-Economic Policy Packages

03.03 U.S. surpassed 100 cases (*U)

CDC lifted restrictions for virus testing

The CDC issued new guidance that allowed anyone to be tested for the virus without restriction. Previously, only those who had traveled to an outbreak area, who had close contact with people diagnosed with COVID-19, or those with severe symptoms, could get tested. (*A)

06.03 Austin, Texas, cancels the SXSW conference and festivals amid the coronavirus concerns, following the cancellation of other high-profile events across the country.

Vice President Mike Pence announced that 21 people aboard the Grand Princess, a cruise ship being held off the coast of California, tested positive

for the coronavirus. (*N)

'Anybody' can get a test

While touring the CDC headquarters in Atlanta, Trump told reporters: "Anybody that wants a test can get a test. That's what the bottom line is." (*U)

Socio-Economic Policy Packages

06.03 Trump signed an $8.3 billion emergency spending package (CORONAVIRUS PREPAREDNESS AND RESPONSE SUPPLEMENTAL APPROPRIATIONS ACT) to combat the coronavirus outbreak, as the number of global cases hit 100,000. (*N)

08.03– 14.03 (5,495 /64)

Public Health Policies

11.03 Travel ban on Europe; WHO declared pandemic

Trump addressed the nation on the coronavirus outbreak and outlined strict travel restrictions on passengers arriving in the United States from hard-hit portions of Europe. Three days later, he added the United Kingdom and Ireland to the ban.

The WHO declared that the spread of COVID-19 had become a pandemic, which the organization had defined as "the worldwide spread of a new disease." Infections outside China had increased 13-fold in two weeks, WHO's direc-

tor general said. In that same time, the number of countries hit by the outbreak had tripled. (*U)

Trump announced a new restriction on many foreign travelers from 26 countries in Europe, except for Ireland and the United Kingdom, for the next 30 days.

The NBA suspended all basketball games after a player for the Utah Jazz preliminarily tested positive for COVID-19, the disease caused by the new coronavirus.

Trump announced a new restriction on many foreign travelers from 26 countries in Europe, except for Ireland and the United Kingdom, for the next 30 days.(*N)

12.03 US testing rollout 'a failing'

Dr. Anthony Fauci, director of the National Institute of Allergy and Infectious Diseases, said the testing logjam constituted a "failing" of the nation's health care system. "The idea of anybody getting (a coronavirus test) easily, the way people in other countries are doing it – we're not set up for that," Fauci told Congress. "That is a failing." (*U)

MLB announced that it would suspend spring training and delay the start of the regular baseball season by at least two weeks.

The NHL announced that it would pause its hockey season. The league's commissioner did not set an end date for the suspension.

The NCAA canceled both the men's and women's college basketball tournaments, known as March Madness, after most conferences suspended their postseason tournaments. (*N)

Socio-Economic Policy Packages

12.03 Fed said it would pump more than $1 trillion into financial system[2]

Public Health Policies

13.03 States across the U.S., including Michigan, Pennsylvania and Maryland, announced plans to close schools over the coronavirus concerns.

Trump tweeted that some cruise lines, including Princess Cruises, Norwegian and Royal Caribbean, would suspend outbound trips, at his request, for 30 days. (*N)

President Trump announced Friday that the government was partnering with private companies to set up drive-through coronavirus testing sites[3]

Socio-Economic Policy Packages

13.03 Trump declared national emergency

Trump declared the coronavirus pandemic to be a national emergency. Trump said the move would free up nearly $50 billion in additional disaster funding and would allow HHS to waive regulations and laws to deliver coronavirus testing quicker. (*U)

Potential costs of COVID-19 treatment for people with employer coverage

To address concerns over costs associated with COVID-19, Vice President Pence met with a group of large private insurers, who agreed to waive copayments and deductibles for COVID-19 tests. However, America's Health Insurance Plans (AHIP) clarified that the out-of-pocket costs for treatment – such as hospitalizations for more serious cases – would not be waived, meaning people with private insurance who faced deductibles could be on the hook for large costs[4].

Trump gave people with student loans a break[5]

International Tension

13.03 Class action filed against China over COVID-19 outbreak[6]

15.03– 21.03 (32,910 / 328)

Public Health Policies

15.03 The White House announced that the European travel ban would be extended to include the U.K. and Ireland.

The number of confirmed cases in the U.S. surpassed 3,000, with New York, California and Washington recording the most confirmed cases. The national death toll rose to 61.

Twenty-nine additional states, including New York, Massachusetts, South Carolina and Hawaii, announced school closures.

The Centers for Disease Control and Prevention released guidelines recommending "that for the next 8 weeks, organizers (whether groups or individuals) cancel or postpone in-person events that consist of 50 people or more throughout the United States." (*N)

U.S. State Department issued Global Level 3 Health Advisory: Do Not Travel. (*D)

Socio-Economic Policy Packages

15.03 Fed cut rates to zero, launches $700 billion quantitative easing program[7]

Public Health Policies

16.03 15 days to slow the spread

Trump issued guidelines that called for Americans to avoid social gatherings of more than 10 people for the next 15 days and to limit discretionary travel, among other guidelines. Trump said the country may be dealing with a number of restrictions through July or August as a result of the virus. He acknowledged the economy may be heading into a recession. (*U)

Canada announced plans to close the border to noncitizens, as the country's number of confirmed cases rose to 339 with one death. The border restrictions included some exceptions, including for

---

2   www.cnbc.com/2020/03/12/fed-to-pump-more-than-500-billion-into-short-term-bank-funding-expand-types-of-security-purchases.html

3   www.washingtonpost.com/health/under-heavy-fire-trump-administration-takes-steps-to-expand-coronavirus-testing/2020/03/13/f86b481e-6525-11ea-acca-80c22bbee96f_story.html

4   www.healthsystemtracker.org/brief/potential-costs-of-coronavirus-treatment-for-people-with-employer-coverage/

5   www.cnbc.com/2020/03/13/mnuchin-may-suspend-student-loan-repayments-amid-coronavirus-outbreak.html

6   www.law.com/dailybusinessreview/2020/03/13/class-action-filed-against-china-over-covid-19-outbreak/?slretu rn=20200405115550#

7   www.cnbc.com/2020/03/15/federal-reserve-cuts-rates-to-zero-and-launches-massive-700-billion-quantitative-easing-program.html

U.S. citizens.

San Francisco imposed strict prohibitions on residents leaving their homes "except for essential needs," becoming the first city in the U.S. to introduce such extreme measures in response to the pandemic.

MLB announced that the start of the season would be pushed back eight weeks, per guidance from the CDC.

President Trump advised all Americans to avoid gatherings of 10 or more people, to avoid going to bars and restaurants and to halt discretionary travel. The guidelines, from the administration's coronavirus task force, would remain in effect for 15 days.

U.S. researchers administered the first shot to the first person in a test of an experimental coronavirus vaccine. Even if the trials went well, health officials warned that a vaccine would not be widely available for at least 12 to 18 months.

NASCAR announced it would postpone all races until at least the beginning of May. (*N)

Department of State approved worldwide depar-

ture of American Citizens from overseas. (*D)

NIH clinical trial of investigational vaccine for COVID-19 began[8]

Socio-Economic Policy Packages

16.03 Wall Street plunged again, as the Dow Jones Industrial Average sank by 3,000 points and the S&P 500 and Nasdaq were down by around 12 percent by the closing bell. (*N)

Public Health Policies

17.03 The Kentucky Derby was postponed until September, along with several other major sporting events, including soccer's 2020 European Championships.

Maryland's governor postponed the state's primary election, a day after Ohio's primary was called also off. Florida and Illinois and Arizona proceeded with their primaries.

West Virginia, the last state in the U.S. without a confirmed coronavirus case, recorded its first. Confirmed cases across the country rose to more than 5,800 and the death toll surpassed 100. (*N)

Coronavirus now present in all 50 states.

Centers for Disease Control and Prevention

recommended that travelers defer all cruise travel worldwide and avoid all nonessential travel to China. (*D)

Socio-Economic Policy Packages

17.03 Trump invoked the Defense Production Act, a wartime authority that allowed him to direct industry to produce critical equipment. (*U)

Northern Californians ordered to 'shelter in place'. (*A)

Fed took new steps to keep money flowing.

The central bank took big steps to keep money flowing in the U.S. economy: it established a Primary Dealer Credit Facility, which provided short-term funding to big financial firms, and a Commercial Paper Funding Facility to purchase corporate paper from issuers.[9]

Public Health Policies

18.03 Canada and the U.S. agreed to close its borders to all "non-essential traffic."

The WHO announced an international trial to gather data about which treatments were most effective for the coronavirus. Participants in the so-called solidarity trial included Argentina, Cana-

da, France, Norway, South Africa, Spain, Switzerland and Thailand. (*N)

CDC report showed that all ages were at risk

A CDC report found that among the roughly 12% of COVID-19 cases in the U.S. known to need hospitalizations, about 1 in 5 were among people ages 20 to 44. (*U)

Socio-Economic Policy Packages

18.03 Trading halted on Wall Street for the fourth time in two weeks. The Dow Jones Industrial Average closed with a loss of just over 1,300 points and the S&P fell by 5 percent. (*N)

The Trump administration suspended refugee admissions until April 6 due to the coronavirus pandemic. (*N)

President Trump signed a coronavirus aid bill into law. The Families First Coronavirus Response Act would provide free coronavirus testing and ensure paid emergency leave for those infected or caring for a family member with the illness, while also providing additional Medicaid funding, food assistance and unemployment benefits. (*N)

The U.S. Treasury and Internal Revenue Service (IRS) announced non-cor-

8   www.nih.gov/news-events/news-releases/nih-clinical-trial-investigational-vaccine-covid-19-begins

9   www.cnbc.com/2020/03/17/the-federal-reserve-is-adding-another-program-to-aid-lending-to-businesses-and-households.html
     www.cnbc.com/2020/03/17/fed-announces-move-to-help-businesses-get-short-term-funding-in-commercial-paper-market.html

porate tax filers can defer any owed income up to $1 million until July 15, 2020, without penalties or interest.[10]

The U.S. Department of Housing and Urban Development issued a 60-day moratorium on foreclosures and evictions for single family homeowners with FHA-insured mortgages and had CARES Act flexibilities for Community Development Block Grant recipients.[11]

U.S. Department of Labor announced availability of up to $100 million in national health emergency dislocated worker grants in response to Covid-19 outbreat.[12]

Public Health Policies

19.03 The U.S. State Department raised the global travel advisory to Level 4: Do Not Travel, warning Americans against traveling internationally and for those abroad to consider returning immediately. (*N)

U.S. surpassed 10,000 cases (*U)

Socio-Economic Policy Packages

19.03 Connecticut delayed its presidential primary election to June. (*N)

California issued a statewide stay-at-home order asking residents to only leave the house if necessary. (*N)

Governors in 27 states activated the National Guard. Across those 27 states, more than 2,050 National Guard members were assisting with state response. (*D)

Public Health Policies

20.03 Cases in California exceeded 1,000, more than doubling from only three days ago. The new figures came one day after Gov. Gavin Newsom issued a statewide "stay-at-home" order for the state's 40 million residents. (*N)

New York Mayor Bill de Blasio said the nation's largest city was "now the epicenter of this crisis" in the U.S., with 5,151 coronavirus cases and 29 deaths. (*N)

Illinois and New York announced stay-at-home orders (*N)

Socio-Economic Policy Packages

20.03 Indiana postponed its presidential primary to June 2. (*N)

The Dow Jones Industrial Average sank by 916 points and the S&P 500

closed the day down 4.3 percent, marking its worst weekly performance since the 2008 financial crisis. (*N)

Tax day moved from April 15 to July 15.[13]

Delivering on President Trump's promise, Secretary DeVos suspended federal student loan payments, waived interest during national emergency.[14]

International Tension

20.03 White House announced an agreement with Mexico to restrict non-essential travel across shared border. (*D)

Public Health Policies

21.03 Coronavirus cases in New York State, the hardest-hit in the U.S., surpassed 10,000. (*N)

Socio-Economic Policy Packages

21.03 Gov. Phil Murphy of New Jersey issued a stay-at-home order for nearly all of the state's 9 million residents. (*N)

22.03– 28.03 (133,540 / 2,262)

Public Health Policies

22.03 Sen. Rand Paul, R-Ky., became the first known senator to test positive for coronavirus. (N)

Socio-Economic Policy Packages

22.03 Ohio Gov. Mike DeWine issued a new stay-at-home order for all non-essential workers.

Louisiana Gov. John Bel Edwards announced that the state would be under a stay-at-home order.

President Trump announced that he would activate the federal National Guard to assist Washington, California and New York, three of the states hit hardest by the pandemic.

A vote to advance a massive coronavirus stimulus bill failed in the Senate. Democrats said they were dissatisfied with worker protections in the Republican-written bill. (*N)

POTUS announced federal support to governors for use of the National Guard with 100% cost share for California, Washington, and New York. (*N)

Public Health Policies

23.03 New York Gov. Andrew Cuomo announced the state will begin three studies of potential coronavirus treatments in the coming week, as the state's number of confirmed cases grew to more than 20,000. (*N)

---

10   https://home.treasury.gov/news/press-releases/sm948

11   www.hud.gov/press/press_releases_media_advisories/HUD_No_20_042

12   www.dol.gov/newsroom/releases/eta/eta20200318

13   https://home.treasury.gov/news/press-releases/sm953

14   www.ed.gov/news/press-releases/delivering-president-trumps-promise-secretary-devos-suspends-federal-student-loan-payments-waives-interest-during-national-emergency

Socio-Economic Policy Packages

23.03 Massachusetts Gov. Charlie Baker issued a stay-at-home advisory and ordered all non-essential businesses to close.

Michigan Gov. Gretchen Whitmer signed a "stay home, stay safe" executive order to bar non-essential businesses from requiring employees to leave their homes.

Virginia Gov. Ralph Northam announced that schools would remain closed for the rest of the school year.

Rhode Island postponed its presidential primary until June 2.

Washington Gov. Jay Inslee issued a statewide "stay home" order, telling residents they must stay home unless they were "pursuing an essential activity."

West Virginia Gov. Jim Justice issued a statewide stay-at-home order, telling residents the disease caused by the coronavirus was "really serious stuff."

Hawaii and Alaska ordered businesses shuttered and told residents to stay home, becoming the latest states to implement sweeping measures to limit the movements of residents in order to halt the virus' spread.

Stocks plunged again, after an emergency fiscal stimulus package was twice rejected by the Senate and a new round of cash injection from the Federal Reserve failed to stem market declines. (*N)

Fed pledged asset purchases with no limit[15]

International Tension

23.03 Team USA's Olympic and Paralympic Committee surveyed more than 1,700 athletes and issued a statement urging the International Olympic Committee to postpone the 2020 Olympic Summer Games in Tokyo. (*N)

Public Health Policies

24.03 The White House warned people who had been in New York recently to quarantine themselves for 14 days if they left the state. With more than 25,000 cases, New York was the center of the coronavirus pandemic in the U.S. (*N)

Scramble for medical equipment descended into chaos as U.S. states and hospitals competed for rare supplies.[16]

Socio-Economic Policy Packages

24.03 Wall Street rebounded with the Dow Jones Industrial Average surging by more than 2,000 points for its biggest daily points gain ever. The increases came after news that a $2 trillion stimulus bill was close to approval. (*N)

Miami Mayor Francis Suarez, who tested positive for coronavirus and remained in quarantine, announced a shelter-in-place order for the city's residents.

Vermont Gov. Phil Scott issued a stay-at-home order for the state that included the closure of all non-essential businesses. The state had 95 confirmed coronavirus cases and 7 deaths.

President Trump approved disaster declarations for the states of Iowa and Louisiana. Iowa had 124 confirmed cases and reported its first death that day, while Louisiana had more than 1,300 cases and 46 deaths. (*N)

International Tension

24.03 Bipartisan resolution condemned China's handling of coronavirus outbreak.[17]

Public Health Policies

25.03 The WHO warned that the U.S. could become the global epicenter of the coronavirus pandemic. The country recorded 54,810 coronavirus cases, including 781 deaths. (*N)

Socio-Economic Policy Packages

25.03 President Trump approved disaster declarations for Florida, Texas and North Carolina.

Minnesota Gov. Tim Walz issued a stay-at-home order for the state's 5.6 million residents, other than those performing essential services.

Idaho Gov. Brad Little announced a stay-at-home order for at least 21 days.

The Senate passed a massive $2 trillion stimulus package designed to ease the economic blow from the coronavirus pandemic. The bill was subsequently sent to the House. (*N)

Public Health Policies

26.03 Deaths in the U.S. passed 1,000, as confirmed cases nationwide rose to more than 68,100.

The number of cases in California climbed past 3,000, while the number of deaths statewide stood at 65.

U.S. coronavirus cases surpassed China. The U.S. reported at least 82,474, with more than 1,100 deaths, while China reported 81,961 cases and more

15 www.cnbc.com/2020/03/23/fed-announces-a-slew-of-new-programs-to-help-markets-including-open-ended-asset-purchases.html

16 www.washingtonpost.com/business/2020/03/24/scramble-medical-equipment-descends-into-chaos-us-states-hospitals-compete-rare-supplies/

17 https://thehill.com/homenews/house/489253-bipartisan-resolution-condemns-chinas-handling-of-coronavirus-outbreak

than 3,000 deaths. (*N)

26.03 The U.S. surged past China and Italy to become the planet's most infected nation. More than 1,296 people had died in the U.S. (*U)

Socio-Economic Policy Packages

26.03 President Trump approved a major disaster declaration for New Jersey, as confirmed cases in the state soared to 4,402.

The Indianapolis 500, the world's oldest automobile race, had been postponed until Aug. 23.

Wall Street rallied for the third straight day, despite record-breaking unemployment claims in the U.S.

Montana Gov. Steve Bullock announced a stay-at-home directive, ordering residents to remain in their homes as much as possible and for nonessential businesses to temporarily close. The state also announced its first coronavirus death, in addition to a total of 90 confirmed cases. (*N)

Socio-Economic Policy Packages

27.03 Trump signed $2T stimulus package

President Donald Trump signed the largest stimulus package in U.S. history (The CARES Act).

The stimulus package was expected to provide $1,200 checks to many Americans – and more for families – while making available hundreds of billions of dollars for companies to maintain payroll through the crisis.

Trump also ordered his administration to use its authority under the Defense Production Act to force General Motors to expedite government contracts to build ventilators. (*U)

North Carolina Gov. Roy Cooper announced plans for a stay-at-home order for the state's 10 million-plus residents.

Utah Gov. Gary Herbert issued a statewide stay-at-home order for at least two weeks.

Alaska issued a mandate barring in-state travel between communities except in support of critical infrastructure or personal needs. (*N)

POTUS signed executive order to order the selected reserve and certain members of the individual ready reserve of the armed forces to active duty. (*D)

Public Health Policies

28.03 CDC issued travel advisory to New York area

The CDC issued a request asking residents of New York, New Jersey and Connecticut to curtail nonessential travel for 14 days.

Meanwhile, an infant younger than one year – who tested positive for the virus in Chicago – died. (*U)

The U.S. Food and Drug Administration authorized the emergency use of a new, rapid coronavirus test that could give patients results in less than 15 minutes. (*N)

Socio-Economic Policy Packages

28.03 New York Gov. Andrew Cuomo announced that the state's primary election would be postponed from April 28 to June 23. (*N)

POTUS invoked the Defense Production Act, requiring GM to make ventilators. (*D)

29.03– 04.04 (318,748 / 9,052)

Public Health Policies

29.03 Two navy ships steamed to New York and Los Angeles to help with pandemic[18]

USNS Mercy began treating patients in Los Angeles. (*D)

Socio-Economic Policy Packages

29.03 White House extended social distancing guidelines

Trump announced that the White House would be extending its social distancing guidelines through April 30. "The peak in death rate is likely to hit in two weeks," Trump said. "Nothing would be worse than declaring victory before the victory is won." Trump said that he expected that, by June 1, "we will be well on our way to recovery."(*U)

'Project Airbridge' to expedite arrival of needed supplies, White House said[19]

Public Health Policies

30.03 A U.S. Navy hospital ship arrived at New York Harbor on Monday to help relieve local hospitals being overwhelmed by coronavirus patients.[20]

USNS Comfort arrived in New York five days ahead of schedule, providing 1,000 patient beds. (*D)

Socio-Economic Policy Packages

30.03 Virginia Gov. Ralph Northam issued a stay-at-home order for the state's 8.5 million residents as coronavirus cases in the state topped 1,000.

Arizona Gov. Doug Ducey ordered a stay-at-home directive for the nearly 7.3 million residents of his state. The state had 1,157

---

18   www.wsj.com/articles/two-navy-ships-steam-to-new-york-and-los-angeles-to-help-with-pandemic-11585488166

19   www.npr.org/sections/coronavirus-live-updates/2020/03/29/823543513/project-airbridge-to-expedite-arrival-of-needed-supplies-white-house-says

20   https://thehill.com/policy/defense/490136-navy-hospital-ship-arrives-in-new-york

confirmed coronavirus cases and 20 deaths.

President Trump approved a disaster declaration for Rhode Island and Pennsylvania. The number of confirmed cases in Rhode Island rose to more than 400, while more than 4,000 cases and 49 deaths were confirmed in Pennsylvania. (*N)

Public Health Policies

31.03 The 531st and 9th Army Field Hospitals began receiving patients at the Javits Center in New York.

The 627th Army Field Hospital and 47th Combat Support Hospital deployed to Seattle. (*D)

Socio-Economic Policy Packages

31.03 Wall Street ended one of the worst quarters in stock market history, an indication of the devastating economic impact of the pandemic.

South Carolina Gov. Henry McMaster ordered all non-essential businesses in the state to close.

The Federal Bureau of Prisons ordered a lockdown of its facilities in an effort to curb the spread of the coronavirus.

Maine Gov. Janet Mills issued a "stay healthy at home mandate" requiring people to stay at their residence except for essential work.

President Trump approved disaster declarations for Montana and Ohio. (*N)

17,250 National Guardsmen were supporting COVID-19 at the direction of their governors in 10 states, two territories, and the District of Columbia. (*D)

Public Health Policies

01.04 USNS Comfort began seeing patients in New York. (*D)

Socio-Economic Policy Packages

01.04 Pennsylvania Gov. Tom Wolf placed the entire state under a stay-at-home order, as the number of confirmed cases hit 5,805 with at least 74 deaths.

Florida Gov. Ron DeSantis issued a stay-at-home order for the entire state after weeks of resistance. Florida reported nearly 7,000 confirmed cases and 87 deaths.

West Virginia Gov. Jim Justice announced that the state's primary will be delayed until June 9.

The governors of Mississippi and Georgia announced new shelter-in-place orders for their states. (*N)

The federal government took a big step toward protecting renters by issuing a 120-day moratorium

on evictions from federally subsidized housing or from a property with a federally backed mortgage loan (under CARES ACT). And a USA TODAY analysis showed that at least 34 states had issued broader moratoriums on evictions[21]

Public Health Policies

02.04 DOD expanded-medical support at the Javits Federal Medical Station in New York, Kay Bailey Hutchinson Federal Medical Station in Dallas, and the Morial Federal Medical Station in New Orleans to treat COVID-19 patients. (*D)

Socio-Economic Policy Packages

02.04 The U.S. Department of Labor released new figures that showed a record 6.6 million Americans filed for unemployment benefits the previous week, a sign of the pandemic's mounting toll on the U.S economy.

The Democratic National Committee postponed its summer convention in Milwaukee from July to the week of August 17.

Tennessee Gov. Bill Lee announced a statewide stay-at-home order. (*N)

In the U.S., a record 6.65 million Americans filed first-time jobless claims the previous week, the Labor Department said.

That number would later be revised up by 219,000 to an all-time high of 6.86 million. (*U)

Public Health Policies

03.04 CDC recommended use of face masks

The Trump administration advised people to start wearing face masks in public to stop the spread of the coronavirus, a reversal on previous guidance that urged people not to wear masks. (*U)

Socio-Economic Policy Packages

03.04 The U.S. Supreme Court announced that it would scrap the oral argument schedule, which included nine cases, for the rest of the term.

Alabama Gov. Kay Ivey ordered residents who weren't essential workers to stay at home unless getting takeout food, groceries or gas.

Montana Gov. Steve Bullock issued a directive allowing the state's June 2 primary to be conducted by mail in an effort to limit the spread of the coronavirus. (*N)

19,700 National Guardsmen were supporting COVID-19 at the direction of their governors. In just one day, 420 West Virginia guardsmen delivered PPE to 55 counties, delivered 5,500 meals, assisted at two drive-through test-

---

21 www.usatoday.com/story/news/nation/2020/03/31/paying-rent-during-coronavirus-many-states-offer-relief-renters/5086542002/

ing sites and conducted 20 training missions; Maryland guardsmen distributed 1M+ pieces of PPE; Tennessee guardsmen were supporting 35 testing sites. (*D)

Public Health Policies

04.04 The Coral Princess cruise ship, which had been stranded at sea with at least 12 people with coronavirus aboard, arrived at Port Miami in Florida. The ship was carrying a total of 1,020 passengers and 878 crew.

New Jersey reported 200 deaths in the past 24 hours, bringing the state's total number of fatalities to 846. The state, the second worst-hit in the U.S., also recorded 34,124 confirmed cases.

More than 150 crew members of a U.S. Navy aircraft carrier whose captain was relieved of command after raising concerns about the coronavirus tested positive. More than 1,500 sailors on the USS Theodore Roosevelt were moved ashore after a letter written by Capt. Brett Crozier was leaked. (*N)

POTUS announced over 1,000 military medical personnel would be deployed to New York City to augment those currently in place. (*D)

05.04– 11.04 (533,837 / 21,500)

Public Health Policies

05.04 DOD had constructed eight military field hospital sites around the country with 22 additional sites expected to be online in the next two weeks.

Secretary of Defense states Javits would be the largest hospital in the United States with 2,500 bed capacity. (*D)

Public Health Policies

06.04 POTUS announced 3M had agreed to provide 166M+ masks for frontline health care workers. (*D)

Socio-Economic Policy Packages

06.04 Wisconsin Gov. Tony Evers signed an executive order suspending all in-person voting for the state's April 7 primary and moved the date of the election to June 9. Hours later, the Wisconsin Supreme Court overturned the governor, siding with the Republican-controlled legislature that had appealed his order.

Indiana Gov. Eric Holcomb issued a new executive order extending the state's stay-at-home measures for another 14 days.

South Carolina Gov. Henry McMaster ordered the

state's 5 million residents to stay home, becoming the last state east of the Mississippi River to issue such a coronavirus-related mandate. South Carolina had 2,232 confirmed cases and 48 deaths. (*N)

Public Health Policies

07.04 New York saw its "largest single-day increase" in deaths, with the state's fatalities rising by 731 in the past 24 hours. The state had 138,836 confirmed cases and 5,489 total deaths.

New York City suffered its deadliest 24 hours of the coronavirus pandemic, after a spike of 806 new fatalities brought the city's total death toll to more than 4,000. (*N)

Navy expeditionary medical facility at Ernest M. Morial Convention Center in New Orleans, LA, began taking patients.

Seattle field hospital opened with 250 beds and New Orleans field hospital opened with 150 beds. (*D)

Socio-Economic Policy Packages

07.04 Wisconsin's primary election went on as planned despite the state being under stay-at-home orders. (*N)

Public Health Policies

08.04 New York suffered its highest single day of deaths with 779 new

fatalities in the past 24 hours. Despite the grim milestone, Gov. Andrew Cuomo said there were signs that the state appears to be slowing down the virus' spread. Cuomo also announced that all voters in the state will be able to cast absentee ballots in the June 23 Democratic primary election. (*N)

Socio-Economic Policy Packages

08.04 New Jersey Gov. Phil Murphy announced plans to delay the state's primary elections from June 2 to July 7 due to the coronavirus pandemic. (*N)

FEMA COVID-19 supply chain task force: supply chain stabilization[22]

Public Health Policies

09.04 The number of confirmed coronavirus cases in New York reached 151,598, more than any country except the United States.

Second coronavirus vaccine trial began in the U.S.

New York reported 799 deaths from coronavirus in one day, its highest daily toll yet in the pandemic, bringing the state's total number of fatalities to 7,067.

Pennsylvania emerged as a coronavirus hotspot after a surge in new cases. The state reported a total of 18,228 cases statewide

---

22   www.fema.gov/news-release/2020/04/08/fema-covid-19-supply-chain-task-force-supply-chain-stabilization

and 338 deaths.

The U.S. Centers for Disease Control and Prevention extended indefinitely the government's March 14 no-sail order for cruise ships. (*N)

Evidence that first COVID-19 cases in NYC came from Europe

A new study found evidence that the first COVID-19 cases in New York City originated in Europe and occurred as early as February. (*A)

NIH clinical trial of hydroxychloroquine, a potential therapy for COVID-19, began.[23]

Socio-Economic Policy Packages

09.04 Another 6.6 million American workers filed first-time unemployment claims for the week ending April 4, bringing the cumulative total to 16 million over the past three weeks. (*N)

Federal Reserve announced actions to provide up to $2.3T in loans to support the economy. (*D)

Public Health Policies

10.04 US marked deadliest day

More than 2,000 people in the U.S. died of coronavirus on Good Friday, a new daily high in the nation's fight against COVID-19. Dr. Deborah Birx, coordinator of the White House coronavirus task force, said that the U.S. had not "reached the peak" of the pandemic but that there were "encouraging" signs that the curves were flattening or lowering. (*U)

Apple and Google announced a rare partnership to try to use smartphone technology to trace the spread of the coronavirus pandemic. (*N)

In New York City, the USNS Comfort was treating 64 patients and the Javits Center was treating 255.

366 military medical personnel were augmenting New York City hospitals.

The USNS Mercy wa currently treating 15 patients in Los Angeles.

The Navy Expeditionary Medical Facility detachment at the Hutchinson Center, Dallas, was 90% complete with setup and was positioned to treat patients. (*D)

Socio-Economic Policy Packages

10.04 DOD received approval from the White House Task Force to execute the first Defense Production Act Title 3 project responding to COVID-19. The $133M project will increase domestic production capacity of N95 masks to over 39M in the next 90 days. (*D)

Public Health Policies

11.04 The United States surpassed Italy in the number of coronavirus deaths, becoming the worst-hit country in the world. Deaths in the U.S. totaled 18,860 people, compared to 18,849 in Italy, according to a tally from Johns Hopkins University. (*U)

Coronavirus deaths in the United States passed the 20,000 mark, with over a half million confirmed cases nationwide. More than half of the deaths were concentrated in three states: New York, with 8,627; New Jersey with 2,183; and Michigan, with 1,392.

Coronavirus cases spiked aboard the USS Theodore Roosevelt more than a week after its captain, Brett Crozier, was relieved of duty for sounding the alarm about an outbreak on the ship. A U.S. Navy sailor assigned to the USS Theodore Roosevelt would later die of coronavirus complications on April 13. (*N)

Socio-Economic Policy Packages

11.04 Wyoming became the final state to receive a major disaster declaration, meaning such declarations were in effect for every state in the country. (*N)

With POTUS approving Wyoming's disaster declaration, a major disaster declaration had been issued in all 50 states for the first time in American history. (*D)

12.04– 18.04 (733,593 / 35,530)

Public Health Policies

12.04 New York City, the hardest-hit city in the U.S., saw its death toll surge past 6,000. The city's health officials reported at least 6,182 fatalities. (*N)

Public Health Policies

13.04 Wyoming reported its first coronavirus-related death, meaning all 50 states had at least one fatality in the pandemic. Nationwide, there were more than 22,000 deaths and more than half a million confirmed cases.

The U.S. Food and Drug Administration cleared the first saliva test to diagnose COVID-19. The test initially would be available through hospitals and clinics affiliated with Rutgers University in New Jersey. (*N)

Socio-Economic Policy Packages

11.04 The Supreme Court announced it would hear half of the remaining cases of the term by telephone conference call — a first in the court's history — with the justices and the lawyers calling in remotely.

---

23   www.nih.gov/news-events/news-releases/nih-clinical-trial-hydroxychloroquine-potential-therapy-covid-19-begins

The governors of several northeastern states, including New York, New Jersey, Connecticut and Pennsylvania, outlined the first steps each state will take towards easing lockdown restrictions. The Democratic officials said each state would form a panel of experts to monitor the outbreak in the region and help devise a plan to slowly reopen parts of each state.

The governors of three West Coast states, Washington, Oregon and California, announced that they would work on a shared approach to reopening their economies.

The U.S. Department of the Treasury announced that about 80 million Americans would begin to receive their coronavirus payments. (*N)

Trump claimed total authority over the states, saying: "The president of the United States calls the shots." He was challenged by governors, who said he did not have the constitutional right to reopen the country without their involvement.[24]

A month after emergency declaration, Trump's promises largely unfulfilled.[25]

Public Health Policies

14.04 All 50 states

reported deaths

All 50 states reported at least one death, and more than 23,000 Americans died. President Donald Trump said his administration would "halt" funding to the WHO as it conducted a review of the global organization's handling of the pandemic. (*U)

Socio-Economic Policy Packages

14.04 Senate majority leader Mitch McConnell announced that the Senate would not reconvene until May 4. (*N)

International Tension

14.04 President Trump announced plans to halt funding for the World Health Organization, accusing the agency of "severely mismanaging and covering up" the coronavirus crisis. Trump previously threatened to cut off funding after the WHO criticized his response to the epidemic. (*N)

Socio-Economic Policy Packages

15.04 Protests erupted over stay-at-home orders

Demonstrators drove thousands of vehicles to Michigan's state Capitol, protesting the state's stay-at-home order. Protests also erupted in

Kentucky, Oklahoma and North Carolina. (*U)

Demonstrators in Michigan clogged the streets around the state Capitol, protesting Gov. Gretchen Whitmer's stay-at-home orders. A similar demonstration against coronavirus lockdown measures was previously held in Ohio on April 13. (*N)

Public Health Policies

16.04 Officials across the U.S. were racing to provide coronavirus tests to diagnose infections and to identify recovered patients with antibodies that may help others battle the disease.

An anonymous tip led to the discovery of 17 bodies crowded into a four-person morgue at one of New Jersey's largest nursing homes. (*N)

Socio-Economic Policy Packages

16.04 White House issued guidance to reopen

The White House issued guidelines to states aimed at easing social distancing restrictions and reopening parts of the country. About 14% of the U.S. workforce had filed for unemployment in the past month. (*U)

President Donald Trump announced new federal guidelines for reopening the U.S. that put the onus

on governors for making decisions about their own state economies. (Guidelines for Opening Up America Again, a three-phased approach based on the advice of public health experts. These steps will help state and local officials when reopening their economies, getting people back to work, and continuing to protect American lives.).[26]

Aircraft manufacturer Boeing said it would resume plane production starting the week of April 20th at its Washington state facilities in a "phased approach," after operations had been suspended due to the coronavirus epidemic.

Ohio Gov. Mike DeWine announced his intention to "start opening Ohio back up," saying the first phase of the planned reopening would begin on May 1.

Seven midwestern governors announced they are forming a regional pact to plan for the reopening of their respective economies.

The small business loan program was officially out of cash: the Small Business Administration said in a statement that it had run out of money for the Paycheck Protection Program.

---

24   www.theguardian.com/us-news/2020/apr/25/us-coronavirus-timeline-trump-cases-deaths

25   www.npr.org/2020/04/13/832797592/a-month-after-emergency-declaration-trumps-promises-largely-unfulfilled

26   www.whitehouse.gov/openingamerica/

The latest jobless claim numbers were announced: around 5 million more people filed for first-time unemployment claims in the week ending April 11, as the job market in every sector of the economy continued to be devastated by the coronavirus pandemic. (*N)

International Tension

16.04 At least four class-action suits filed against China, seeking trillions over Coronavirus outbreak in U.S.[27]

Public Health Policies

17.04 Health officials in New York City estimated that the city's coronavirus death toll surpassed 12,000. The city's death toll jumped in recent days as a result of the inclusion of "probable" fatalities in daily tallies.

A federal judge Friday night ruled that Tennessee had to continue allowing abortions amid a temporary ban on nonessential medical procedures that's aimed at slowing the spread of COVID-19. (*N)

NIH to launch public-private partnership to speed COVID-19 vaccine and

treatment options[28]

Socio-Economic Policy Packages

17.04 NBA Commissioner Adam Silver announced the league would withhold 25 percent of player pay starting with their May 15 checks. Silver added that games that were not played due to the pandemic would not be rescheduled and said it remained impossible to make any decisions about whether to resume the remainder of the season.

President Trump encouraged anti-lockdown groups in a series of tweets calling to "liberate" Minnesota, Michigan and Virginia.

Hawaii Gov. David Ige ordered the state's beaches to close. The state reported 553 confirmed cases and 9 deaths.

Florida reopened certain beaches, South Carolina reopened certain boat ramps as states began to loosen restrictions.

Two days after thousands of protesters in Michigan gathered to decry their state's stay-at-home order, Trump tweeted to "LIBERATE MINNESOTA", "LIBERATE MICHIGAN" and "LIBERATE VIRGINIA".

Protesters in other states followed suit.[29]

USDA announced Coronavirus Food Assistance Program[30]

International Tension

17.04 President Trump said his administration would "end that grant (to Wuhan lab) very quickly."[31]

Public Health Policies

18.04 Deaths mounted in certain places: Los Angeles County health officials said Saturday they recorded the largest daily tally of coronavirus deaths, 81.

More than 700,000 people in the United States had tested positive for coronavirus. The U.S. led all countries in reported deaths with 36,734. (*N)

19.04– 25.04 (944,041 / 48,865)

Public Health Policies

19.04 The federal agency that oversaw nursing homes announced new transparency measures requiring the disclosure of coronavirus cases to patients' families and public health officials. (*N)

POTUS announced he will use the Defense Pro-

duction Act to increase COVID-19 testing swab production in one U.S. facility by over 20 million additional swabs per month. (*D)

Socio-Economic Policy Packages

19.04 Shake Shack, one of several large restaurant chains that secured federal loans through the coronavirus stimulus law meant to help small businesses, said that it was giving all $10 million back. (*N)

Public Health Policies

20.04 The Navajo Nation, which sprawled across three states, reported 1,197 positive coronavirus cases, a per capita infection rate 10 times higher than Arizona and the third-highest infection rate in the country behind New York and New Jersey.

The Department of Homeland Security announced that it would continue its travel restrictions with Canada and Mexico for another 30 days.

New York's daily death toll dropped below 500 for the first time since April 2.

Robert Redfield, director of the Centers for Disease Control and Prevention,

27 www.newsweek.com/china-class-action-lawsuits-covid-19-1498400

28 www.nih.gov/news-events/news-releases/nih-launch-public-private-partnership-speed-covid-19-vaccine-treatment-options

29 www.theguardian.com/us-news/2020/apr/25/us-coronavirus-timeline-trump-cases-deaths

30 www.usda.gov/media/press-releases/2020/04/17/usda-announces-coronavirus-food-assistance-program

31 www.whitehouse.gov/briefings-statements/remarks-president-trump-vice-president-pence-members-coronavirus-task-force-press-briefing-april-17-2020/

warned that a second wave of the coronavirus was bound to be much worse next winter. The comments came during an interview with The Washington Post. (*N)

Socio-Economic Policy Packages

20.04 States announced plans to reopen

The governors of Tennessee, South Carolina and Georgia announced various measures aimed at easing restrictions on some businesses in their states. (*U)

The NYC Pride March was canceled for the first time in a half-century, along with all in-person events leading up to the annual June event. (*N)

Tennessee Gov. Bill Lee announced he would not extend the state's stay-at-home order and plans on reopening businesses next week. The state reported 7,238 confirmed cases and 152 deaths.

Georgia Gov. Brian Kemp announced that the first phase of reopening businesses in the state would begin on April 24. There were 18,947 confirmed cases and 733 deaths due to coronavirus in the state of Georgia.

South Carolina Gov. Henry McMaster announced plans to reopen many

non-essential businesses effective immediately, and said beaches in the state would reopen the next day. South Carolina reported 4,439 confirmed cases and 124 deaths due to coronavirus.

Oil prices plunged into negative territory as global demand plummeted

President Trump said that he was temporarily suspending immigration to the United States in response to the coronavirus pandemic and the "need to protect jobs." (*N)

Protests erupted again over coronavirus shelter-in-place orders...Colorado, Michigan, Ohio, Kentucky, Minnesota, North Carolina, Utah, western New York state and Washington state had all seen protests in recent days.[32]

Protests against lockdown in Texas, California and seven other states as calls to end stay-at-home orders grow...California, Florida, Texas, Arizona, Colorado, Montana, Washington, Tennessee, and Illinois all saw protesters gather in large numbers.[33]

POTUS released memorandum on providing continued federal support for governors' use of the National Guard to respond to COVID-19

and facilitate economic recovery. (*D)

International Tension

20.04 Chinese officials spoke out against President Trump's remarks about suspicions that the coronavirus outbreak originated from a laboratory in the city of Wuhan. China's Foreign Ministry spokesman Geng Shuang called the remarks irresponsible, and said they spread conspiracy theories and politicized the crisis. (*N)

McSally & Blackburn to Introduced the Stop COVID Act to hold China accountable for the spread of the Coronavirus[34]

Public Health Policies

21.04 FDA approved home-testing kit

LabCorp, a global life sciences company based in North Carolina, received FDA authorization for kits that enable people to collect nasal swab samples at home and mail them to a laboratory for testing. (*U)

Milwaukee's health commissioner said officials identified seven people who appeared to have contracted the coronavirus through activities related to the April 7 election in Wisconsin.

Officials in Silicon Valley reported two virus-related

deaths that predated a Washington state fatality previously believed to be the first victim of COVID-19 in the United States. (*N)

Autopsy reveled 1st US COVID-19 death was earlier than previously thought. The CDC confirmed that tissue from an individual in Santa County, California, who died Feb. 6 tested positive for COVID-19 . That death occurred weeks earlier than the COVID-19 deaths in the Seattle area Feb. 26 that were previously believed to be the nation's first. (*A)

Socio-Economic Policy Packages

21.04 Hundreds of protesters gathered at state capitols in North Carolina and Missouri to protest stay-at-home orders.

The Senate passed a nearly $500 billion interim coronavirus bill that included additional money for the small business loan program as well as for hospitals and testing.

Washington Gov. Jay Inslee said that the state won't be able to lift many of the stay-at-home restrictions implemented to fight the coronavirus by May 4, when the current directive was set to expire. (*N)

---

32   www.cnn.com/2020/04/20/us/protests-coronavirus-stay-at-home-orders/index.html

33   www.newsweek.com/protest-lockdown-stay-home-orders-coronavirus-covid-19-texas-california-1498897

34   www.mcsally.senate.gov/news/press-releases/mcsally-and-blackburn-to-introduce-the-stop-covid-act-to-hold-china-accountable-for-the-spread-of-the-coronavirus

DOD announced details for $133M Defense Production Act Title 3 COVID-19 project. Three companies awarded contracts to increase U.S. domestic N95 mask production by over 39M in the next 90 days: 3M ($76M), O&M Halyward ($29M), and Honeywell ($27.4M). (*D)

International Tension

21.04 Missouri became first state to sue China over coronavirus response.[35]

Public Health Policies

22.04 Texas' ban on abortions prompted by the coronavirus pandemic ended, and clinics said they were resuming services.

A top official at Health and Human Services said he was ousted from his job this week for pushing back on demands that he signed off on a coronavirus treatment that was advocated by the president.

Illinois reported a new daily high in coronavirus cases, 2,000, as experts projected the state would peak in mid-May. Illinois had more than 35,000 cases reported in the state, the sixth-most in the country.

Tyson Foods suspended operations at an Iowa plant that was critical to the nation's pork supply but had been devastated by a growing coronavirus outbreak. (*N)

Socio-Economic Policy Packages

22.04 President Trump issued temporary suspension in new immigrant visas for the next 60 days. (*D)

Las Vegas Mayor Carolyn Goodman offered up her 650,000 constituents as a "control group" against shutdown orders while bitterly complaining that her tourism-reliant city was being economically ravaged.

Gov. Kevin Stitt announced plans to reopen businesses across Oklahoma beginning on April 24, using the three-phase plan issued by the White House as its guide.

State and local governments facing dire financial straits due the pandemic would have to wait until at least May before Congress considered further relief, Senate Majority Leader Mitch McConnell indicated. (*N)

International Tension

22.04 Mississippi to sue China over response to coronavirus outbreak[36]

Public Health Policies

23.04 President Donald Trump suggested exploring disinfectants as a possible treatment for COVID-19 infections — an extremely dangerous proposition that could kill people, medical experts warned.

More than 15,000 New York City residents had likely died from complications brought on by coronavirus, in another grim milestone.

New York City Mayor Bill de Blasio said the number of people with the coronavirus admitted to hospitals and the total number in intensive care had both declined. (*N).[37]

Socio-Economic Policy Packages

23.04 The House passed a nearly $500 billion interim coronavirus bill that included additional money for the small-business loan program, as well as for hospitals and testing, making way for the legislation to become law by the end of the week.

Ruth's Chris Steak House would return the $20 million coronavirus small business loan it procured from the government's

$350 billion Paycheck Protection Program, the company announced.

Colleges and universities across the U.S. were still waiting for most of the $6.3 billion set aside by Congress to help students struggling to pay for food, housing and child care during the coronavirus pandemic.

New jobless claims numbers showed another 4.4 million Americans filed claims in the week ending April 18th. Since the start of the coronavirus pandemic, more than 26 million people had requested unemployment benefits. (*N)

The House of Representatives approved another relief bill to help small businesses and hospitals, after previous funds for small businesses fell into the hands of large companies such as Shake Shack and Potbelly.[38]

Kushner-backed program (Project Airbridge) chartering flights to address hospital shortages raised questions in Congress[39]

Public Health Policies

24.04 Trump claimed he was being sarcastic about the disinfectant. The US surpassed 50,000 Covid-related deaths.[40]

35 https://thehill.com/homenews/state-watch/493929-missouri-becomes-first-state-to-sue-china-over-coronavirus-response
36 https://thehill.com/homenews/state-watch/494143-mississippi-to-sue-china-over-response-to-coronavirus-outbreak
37 www.theguardian.com/us-news/2020/apr/25/us-coronavirus-timeline-trump-cases-deaths
38 www.theguardian.com/us-news/2020/apr/25/us-coronavirus-timeline-trump-cases-deaths
39 https://abcnews.go.com/Politics/kushner-backed-program-charters-flights-medical-supplies-behalf/story?id=70291872
40 www.theguardian.com/us-news/2020/apr/25/us-coronavirus-timeline-trump-cases-deaths

Socio-Economic Policy Packages

24.04 POTUS signed into law the Paycheck Protection Program and Health Care Enhancement Act, providing additional funding to support Americans impacted by the coronavirus.(*D)

(On April 3, PPP started to accept applications. On April 16, the program ran out of initial funding. It resumed application on April 27, some estimated it would run out money again in 2-14 days.)[41] [42]

The law authorized an additional $310 billion to the Paycheck Protection Program, $50 billion to the Economic Injury Disaster Loan (EIDL) program and $10 billion for EIDL grants.[43]

International Tension

24.04 President Donald Trump's administration abruptly cut funding to a non-profit conducting research on virus transmission between bats and humans, over unfounded rumors linking it to a research institute in Wuhan.[44]

26.04– 02.05 (1,137,695 / 61,435)

Socio-Economic Policy Packages

26.04 Hundreds gathered in Pacific Beach for anti-lockdown protest.[45]

Public Health Policies

27.04 President Donald J. Trump unveiled the Opening Up America Again Testing Overview and Testing Blueprint designed to facilitate state development and implementation of the robust testing plans and rapid response programs described in the President's Opening Up America Again Guidelines.[46]

White House canceled another Trump coronavirus briefing

Monday's coronavirus briefing had been canceled by the White House, leaving the future of the near-daily televised addresses in doubt after they became increasingly contentious.[47]

Public Health Policies

28.04 The United States surpassed 1M confirmed coronavirus cases, a third of all cases around the globe. So far, over 56,000 have died and 112,000 have recovered in the United States. (*D)

Public Health Policies

29.04 NIH clinical trial showed Remdesivir accelerated recovery from advanced COVID-19[48]

Socio-Economic Policy Packages

24.04 US GDP turned negative, worst since 2008

America's first-quarter GDP, fell at a 4.8% annualized rate. It was the first contraction of the US economy since the first quarter of 2014, and the worst drop since the fourth quarter of 2008, the height of the financial crisis.[49]

American workers filed 26.5 million initial claims since March 14, according to the seasonally adjusted numbers.[50]

Public Health Policies

30.04 More than 80 percent of hospitalized covid patients in Georgia were African American, study found[51]

International Tension

30.04 Trump claimed to have evidence coronavirus started in Chinese lab but offered no details[52]

Public Health Policies

01.05 US allowed use of 1st drug (Remdesivir), shown to help virus recovery[53]

Socio-Economic Policy Packages

01.05 Which states were reopening, which remained on lockdown, and why there's not a national plan to restart US businesses. That led to inconsistencies among governors' orders, and some confusion among residents.[54]

---

41   www.sba.gov/funding-programs/loans/coronavirus-relief-options/paycheck-protection-program

42   www.claconnect.com/resources/articles/2020/trump-to-sign-ppp-hce-act-310-billion-in-additional-funding-to-restart-ppp

43   www.whitehouse.gov/briefings-statements/remarks-president-trump-signing-ceremony-h-r-266-paycheck-protection-program-health-care-enhancement-act/

44   www.businessinsider.com/trump-cut-research-funds-bat-virus-conspiracy-theories-politico-2020-4

45   www.sandiegouniontribune.com/news/politics/story/2020-04-26/hundreds-gather-in-pacific-beach-for-anti-lockdown-protest-100-new-covid-19-cases-reported-in-region

46   www.whitehouse.gov/briefings-statements/statement-press-secretary-126/

47   https://nypost.com/2020/04/27/white-house-cancels-another-trump-coronavirus-briefing/

48   www.nih.gov/news-events/news-releases/nih-clinical-trial-shows-remdesivir-accelerates-recovery-advanced-covid-19

49   www.cnn.com/2020/04/29/economy/us-economy-downturn-coronavirus/index.html

50   www.cnn.com/2020/04/23/economy/unemployment-benefits-coronavirus/index.html

51   www.washingtonpost.com/health/more-than-80-percent-of-hospitalized-covid-patients-in-georgia-were-african-american-study-finds/2020/04/29/a71496ea-8993-11ea-8ac1-bfb250876b7a_story.html

52   www.theguardian.com/us-news/2020/apr/30/donald-trump-coronavirus-chinese-lab-claim

53   https://apnews.com/9abbfec50de663093cadb0d6cd39c0d2

54   www.wired.com/story/which-states-reopening-lockdown/

International Tension

02.05 A US researcher who worked with a Wuhan virology lab gave 4 reasons why a coronavirus leak would be extremely unlikely.[55]

03.05– 09.05 (1,313,395 / 73,981)

Socio-Economic Policy Packages

05.05 Meat prices went up. USDA officials pointed to supply chain disruption[56]

Administration to phase out Coronavirus Task Force[57]

Public Health Policies

06.05 Pfizer, NYU working on innovative coronavirus vaccine that could be ready by end of summer[58]

International Tension

06.05 China Ambassador to U.S. urged end to 'blame game' over pandemic[59]

Public Health Policies

08.05 The U.S. Food and Drug Administration authorized the first test that used saliva, rather than an uncomfortable nasal swab, to diagnose COVID-19.

The National Institute of Allergy and Infectious Disease began a trial looking at the effects of remdesivir combined with a second drug, called baricitinib, on treating COVID-19. (*N)

Socio-Economic Policy Packages

08.05 A monthly employment report released by the Department of Labor showed that the U.S. economy lost an unprecedented 20.5 million jobs in April, and the unemployment rate soared to 14.7 percent. (*N)

Public Health Policies

09.05 The F.D.A. approved the first antigen test for detecting the virus

Three children had died of a mysterious syndrome linked to the virus.[60]

10.05– 16.05 (1,473,107 / 83,417)

Public Health Policies

10.05 Johnson & Johnson aimed to produce 1 billion coronavirus vaccines for next year[61]

Public Health Policies

12.05 The Trump administration signed a $138 million deal with the makers of an innovative syringe designed to be used in developing countries in an effort to ramp up the nation's capacity to administer a possible COVID-19 vaccine. The goal of the public-private initiative, called Project Jumpstart, was to facilitate the production of 100 million prefilled syringes by the end of 2020 and more than 500 million in 2021 in the event a vaccine became available. (*N)

Socio-Economic Policy Packages

13.05 Fauci told US Congress that states faced serious consequences if they reopened too quickly[62]

International Tension

13.05 The FBI and the U.S. Department of Homeland Security's cybersecurity agency issued a stark and unusual warning asserting that China's efforts to hack health care and pharmaceutical companies posed a "significant threat" to the nation's response to the coronavirus pandemic. (*N)

Public Health Policies

14.05 The CDC issued a health alert to physicians about what had emerged as a rare but potentially deadly condition linked to COVID-19 in children. The illness, known as "multisystem inflammatory syndrome in children" or MIS-C, had been reported in at least 19 states and Washington, D.C. (*N)

Socio-Economic Policy Packages

14.05 CDC released six one-page checklists providing guidance to schools, businesses, restaurants and more on when and how to safely reopen. (*U)

Socio-Economic Policy Packages

15.05 New White House coronavirus task force members announced.[63]

Unveiling vaccine effort, Trump said country would be back with or without one[64]

55 www.businessinsider.com/why-coronavirus-did-not-leak-from-wuhan-lab-researcher-2020-4

56 www.newsweek.com/will-price-meat-go-usda-officials-say-yes-point-supply-chain-disruption-coronavirus-1501842

57 www.nytimes.com/2020/05/05/us/politics/coronavirus-task-force-trump.html

58 www.nbcnews.com/news/us-news/pfizer-nyu-working-innovative-coronavirus-vaccine-could-be-ready-end-n1200776

59 www.bloomberg.com/news/articles/2020-05-06/china-ambassador-to-u-s-urges-end-to-blame-game-over-pandemic

60 www.nytimes.com/2020/05/09/us/coronavirus-news-updates.html

61 www.cnn.com/world/live-news/coronavirus-pandemic-05-10-20-intl/index.html

62 www.cnn.com/world/live-news/coronavirus-pandemic-05-13-20-intl/index.html

63 www.cnn.com/us/live-news/us-coronavirus-update-05-15-20/index.html

64 www.cnn.com/2020/05/15/politics/trump-vaccine-effort-coronavirus/index.html

17.05– 23.05 (1,629,100 / 91,607)

Public Health Policies

18.05 A COVID-19 vaccine candidate developed by Moderna showed it can prompt an immune response in the human body, and was also found to be safe and well-tolerated in a small group of patients. (*N)

Socio-Economic Policy Packages

18.05 The majority of states were moving forward with phased-in approaches that often varied by county and city. (*U)

International Tension

18.05 President Donald Trump threatened to make the freeze on U.S. funding for the World Health Organization permanent. (*N)

Socio-Economic Policy Packages

19.05 CDC released longer guidance to reopen (*U)

24.05– 30.05 (1,923,547)

Public Health Policies

24.05 The White House announced a travel ban with Brazil that would bar anyone from entering the United States who had been in that country for the prior two weeks. (*N)

Public Health Policies

25.05 WHO said it was temporarily dropping hydroxychloroquine from its study of experimental COVID-19 treatments. (*U)

Public Health Policies

27.05 A large federal trial of remdesivir entered its next phase to test the effects of combining the antiviral drug with a pill to bring down inflammation. (*N)

Socio-Economic Policy Packages

27.05 More than 100,000 deaths in the US (*U)

Public Health Policies

29.05 The CDC reported that the coronavirus began quietly spreading in the U.S. as early as late January — before President Trump blocked air travel from China and a full month before community spread was first detected in the country. (*N)

31.05– 06.06 (1,923,547 / 103,834)

Socio-Economic Policy Packages

31.05 As thousands of Americans gathered in cities across the country to protest the in-custody death of George Floyd in Minneapolis, infectious disease experts worried that the large crowds and lack of social distancing could cause catastrophic setbacks for controlling the spread of the coronavirus. (*N)

Public Health Policies

01.06 Eli Lilly started the first COVID-19 antibody treatment trials in humans. The treatment used what were known as monoclonal antibodies made from people who were sick with the coronavirus. They were meant to work as natural antibodies did in the body by blocking the virus.

Public Health Policies

02.06 As mass protests continued across the U.S., a meta-analysis published in The Lancet found that social distancing was the most effective way to slow the spread of the coronavirus — more so than face coverings and eye protection. (*N)

Public Health Policies

03.06 New research from the University of Minnesota Medical School found that hydroxychloroquine was no better than a placebo at preventing symptoms of COVID-19 among people exposed to the virus.

An autopsy found that George Floyd, who died during an arrest in Minneapolis on May 25, had coronavirus. (*N)

International Tension

03.06 The Department of Transportation said in a statement that it planned to ban Chinese carriers from flying passengers to the U.S, after Beijing declined to increase the number of flights it allowed to the United States. (*N)

Public Health Policies

04.06 The medical journal The Lancet on Thursday retracted a large study on the use of hydroxychloroquine to treat COVID-19 because of potential flaws in the research data. The study, published two weeks ago, found no benefit to the drug — and suggested its use may even increase the risk of death. (*N)

Socio-Economic Policy Packages

04.06 Several U.S. states across the South appeared to be grappling with upticks in infections, as Alabama, South Carolina and Virginia saw new cases climb 35 percent or more in the week that ended May 31 compared with the previous week.

The United States Department of Agriculture Farm Service Agency (FSA) issued $545 million in its first payments to farmers through the Coronavirus Food Assistance Program. (*N)

Socio-Economic Policy Packages

05.06 The Bureau of Labor Statistics released new figures showing that the U.S. economy gained 2.5 million jobs in May and the unemployment rate dropped to 13.3 percent, down from 14.7 percent in April. Black unemployment rose to 16.8 percent, up slightly from 16.7 last month, white unemployment came in at 12.4 percent, down from 14.9 percent. (*N)

07.06– 13.06
(2,068,210 / 109,084)

Socio-Economic Policy Packages

10.06 Texas experienced a spike in COVID-19 hospitalizations, setting a new record for three consecutive days. (*N)

Public Health Policies

11.06 The Defense Department's largest biomedical lab, the Walter Reed Army Institute of Research in Maryland, selected a lead COVID-19 vaccine candidate for additional research as well as two backup vaccine candidates. (*N)

Socio-Economic Policy Packages

11.06 Reports showed that coronavirus cases were rising in nearly half the states, as many places rolled back lockdowns. Gov. Brian Kemp signed an executive order that removed many restrictions in Georgia starting June 16, including allowing restaurants and movie theaters to no longer enforce maximums on the number of people who can sit together. (*N)

14.06– 20.06
(2,245,968 / 113,302)

Public Health Policies

16.06 Scientists at the University of Oxford said that they had identified what they called the first drug proven to reduce coronavirus-related deaths. A 6,000-patient trial of dexamethasone, a low-cost steroid, showed that it could reduce deaths of some hospitalized patients. Dexamethasone reduced deaths by a third in patients receiving ventilation, and by a fifth in patients receiving only oxygen treatment, the scientists said. (*NYT)

Public Health Policies

17.06 The World Health Organization halted research on whether hydroxychloroquine could be an effective treatment for COVID-19. Multiple studies had shown that the drug, an anti-malarial medicine also used to treat lupus and rheumatoid arthritis, had no impact on the coronavirus. (*N)

Public Health Policies

20.06 The NIH announced that it had halted a clinical trial evaluating the safety and effectiveness of drug hydroxychloroquine as a treatment for the coronavirus. (*C)

Socio-Economic Policy Packages

20.06 Southern U.S. states saw sharp rise in cases. Florida and South Carolina broke their single-day records for new cases. The news came as infection levels for Missouri and Nevada also reached new highs. (*NYT)

21.06– 27.06
(2,499,250 / 118,955)

Socio-Economic Policy Packages

25.06 Texas Gov. Greg Abbott paused reopening the state after Texas recorded the most daily deaths since May 20 and hospitals were inundated with "an explosion" of COVID-19 cases. (*N)

Socio-Economic Policy Packages

26.06 The governors of Florida and Texas closed down bars to slow down the spread of the coronavirus that was rampaging at record levels through their states. (*N)

28.06– 04.07
(2,838,558 / 122,453)

Socio-Economic Policy Packages

28.06 California Gov. Gavin Newsom ordered seven counties, including Los Angeles, to shutter bars as coronavirus cases surged in the state. (*N)

Public Health Policies

29.06 Gilead Sciences, the maker of a drug shown to shorten recovery time for severely ill COVID-19 patients said it would charge $2,340 for a typical treatment course for people covered by government health programs in the United States and other developed countries.The price for remdesivir would be $3,120 for patients with private insurance. (*N)

Socio-Economic Policy Packages

30.06 The E.U. to reopen borders on July 1 and bar travelers from the U.S. (*NYT)

Socio-Economic Policy Packages

01.07 19 states and cities slowed or backtracked their reopenings[65]

05.07– 11.07
(3,230,991 / 127,201)

Socio-Economic Policy Packages

05.07 Florida surpassed 200,000 confirmed coronavirus cases as the state reported more than 10,000 new positives for four straight days. (*N)

Socio-Economic Policy Packages

06.07 U.S. deaths surpassed 130,000 as Dr. Anthony S. Fauci urged citizens to avoid crowds. (*NYT)

SEVP modified temporary exemptions for nonimmigrant students taking online courses during fall 2020 semester[66]

---

65   www.businessinsider.com/states-and-cities-slowing-pausing-coronavirus-reopening-plans-2020-6
66   www.ice.gov/news/releases/sevp-modifies-temporary-exemptions-nonimmigrant-students-taking-online-courses-during

Public Health Policies

07.07 The number of coronavirus cases in the U.S. surpassed three million.

The WHO acknowledged "emerging evidence" of the airborne spread of the coronavirus, after a group of scientists wrote a letter urging the global body to update its guidance on how the respiratory disease was spread. (*N)

Socio-Economic Policy Packages

07.07 Trump insisted schools 'must open' in fall, said he would 'put pressure' on governors to do so[67]

International Tension

07.07 The United States officially notified the United Nations of its withdrawal from the World Health Organization. The withdrawal was expected to take effect July 6, 2021. (*N)

International Tension

08.07 Harvard, MIT sued Trump administration over international student visas[68]

12.07– 18.07 (3,692,061 / 132,273)

Socio-Economic Policy Packages

13.07 Most of California was closing down again[69]

Public Health Policies

14.07 Trump, in full reversal, urged Americans to wear masks[70]

Socio-Economic Policy Packages

14.07 Trump administration dropped plan to deport international students in online-only classes[71]

Public Health Policies

15.07 White House striped CDC of data collection role for COVID-19 hospitalizations[72]

19.07– 25.07 (4,158,341 / 138,625)

Public Health Policies

24.07 FDA authorized the first coronavirus test for asymptomatic cases and for those who didn't think they were infected at all.[73]

25.07 More people died in Houston in July than in the past four months combined.[74]

26.07– 01.08 (4,596,299 / 146,614)

Public Health Policies

27.07 A vaccine being developed by the Vaccine Research Center at the National Institutes of Health's National Institute of Allergy and Infectious Diseases, in partnership with the biotechnology company Moderna, entered Phase 3 testing. (*C)

Socio-Economic Policy Packages

31.07 A Covid-19 outbreak at a Georgia sleep away camp this June could have implications for school reopening, CDC said.[75]

Public Health Policies

01.08 Infections swamped the US, which recorded 42% of all its coronavirus cases in July.

02.08– 08.08 (4,967,754 / 153,905)

Public Health Policies

02.08 Dr. Deborah L. Birx, the Trump administration's coronavirus coordinator, said the nation was in a "new phase" of the coronavirus epidemic that was much more sprawling across the country than last spring's outbreaks in major cities like New York and Seattle.

Admiral Brett Giroir said 85 or 90 percent of individuals wearing a mask and avoiding crowds, "essentially — gives you the same outcome as a complete shutdown".[76]

05.08 A coronavirus vaccine could be ready for frontline responders by December, health expert said.[77]

07.08 People in many parts of the US were moving around as much as they did before the pandemic started.[78]

67 https://abcnews.go.com/Politics/trump-insists-schools-open-fall-local-authorities-hold/story?id=71648610

68 https://abcnews.go.com/Politics/harvard-mit-sue-trump-administration-international-student-visas/story?id=71637154

69 www.latimes.com/science/newsletter/2020-07-13/california-closing-down-again-coronavirus-today

70 www.politico.com/news/2020/07/14/trump-urges-americans-to-wear-masks-361836

71 www.politico.com/news/2020/07/14/trump-administration-drops-plan-to-deport-international-students-in-online-only-classes-361053

72 www.npr.org/sections/health-shots/2020/07/15/891351706/white-house-strips-cdc-of-data-collection-role-for-covid-19-hospitalizations

73 www.cnn.com/world/live-news/coronavirus-pandemic-07-24-20-intl/index.html

74 www.cnn.com/world/live-news/coronavirus-pandemic-07-25-20-intl/index.html

75 https://us.cnn.com/2020/07/31/health/georgia-camp-coronavirus-outbreak-cdc-trnd/index.html

76 www.msn.com/en-us/news/us/birx-says-u-s-coronavirus-epidemic-is-in-a-new-phase/ar-BB17tW3K

77 www.cnn.com/world/live-news/coronavirus-pandemic-08-05-20-intl/index.html

78 www.cnn.com/world/live-news/coronavirus-pandemic-08-07-20-intl/index.html

Socio-Economic Policy Packages

07.08 Johns Hopkins University and Princeton University became the latest academic institutions to rescind plans for in-person classes this fall, announcing that they would instead conduct undergraduate instruction entirely online.

New York Governor Andrew Cuomo said New York schools can reopen in-person but left it up to districts to determine if, when and how.[79]

08.08 Texas reported its highest 7-day Covid-19 positivity rate since pandemic began.[80]

09.08– 15.08 (5,336,362 / 161,373)

Public Health Policies

09.08 US surpassed 5 million coronavirus cases.[81]

Socio-Economic Policy Packages

09.08 Trump signed executive measures for pandemic relief, billed as a federal eviction ban, a payroll tax suspension, relief for student borrowers and $400 a week for the unemployed. [82]

Public Health Policies

10.08 Expert said children may be able to spread coronavirus like they spread the common cold.[83]

International Tension

10.08 Top US health official met with Taiwan President Tsai Ing-wen in highest-level summit for decades.[84]

Public Health Policies

11.08 US government stroke $1.525 billion deal with Moderna for 100 million doses of its Covid-19 vaccine.[85]

12.08 New White House recommendations encouraged mask use in schools, but didn't require it.

Colleges and universities in Los Angeles must remain mostly closed, officials said.

Arizona school district reopened for in-person classes.[86]

13.08 The pandemic had a "broad impact" on mental health issues, according to CDC survey.

Every New York City public school would have a certified nurse when they reopen, mayor said.[87]

Socio-Economic Policy Packages

13.08 California's Covid-19 death rate remained high as overall cases and hospitalizations dropped.

Former Vice President and 2020 president candidate Biden called for national mask mandate.

Biden and his Vice President candidate Harris received first joint health briefing from experts on Covid-19.

First-time jobless claims fell below 1 million for the first time since March.[88]

14.08 More than 96% of schools in California to begin the academic year online.[89]

Public Health Policies

15.08 In Covid-19 hotspots across the US, Latino and Black people were hit particularly hard.[90]

16.08– 22.08 (5,641,585 / 168,245)

23.08– 29.08 (5,929,256 / 174,772)

Public Health Policies

29.08 Public health experts raised a new concern over coronavirus testing in US: the standard tests were diagnosing huge numbers of people who may be carrying relatively insignificant amounts of the virus, and underscored the need for more widespread use of rapid tests, even if there were less sensitive.[91]

Trump program to cover uninsured Covid-19 patients fell short of promise.[92]

30.08– 05.09 (6,214,166 / 180,655)

Public Health Policies

30.08 US would revive global virus-hunting effort ended last year.[93]

79 www.nytimes.com/2020/08/07/world/covid-19-news.html
80 www.cnn.com/world/live-news/coronavirus-pandemic-08-08-20-intl/index.html
81 www.cnn.com/world/live-news/coronavirus-pandemic-08-09-20-intl/index.html
82 www.nytimes.com/2020/08/09/world/coronavirus-covid-19.html
83 www.cnn.com/world/live-news/coronavirus-pandemic-08-10-20-intl/index.html
84 www.cnn.com/world/live-news/coronavirus-pandemic-08-10-20-intl/index.html
85 www.cnn.com/2020/08/11/health/moderna-vaccine-government-deal/index.html
86 www.cnn.com/world/live-news/coronavirus-pandemic-08-12-20-intl/index.html
87 www.cnn.com/world/live-news/coronavirus-pandemic-08-13-20-intl/index.html
88 www.cnn.com/world/live-news/coronavirus-pandemic-08-13-20-intl/index.html
89 www.cnn.com/world/live-news/coronavirus-pandemic-08-14-20-intl/index.html
90 www.cnn.com/world/live-news/coronavirus-pandemic-08-15-20-intl/index.html
91 www.nytimes.com/2020/08/29/health/coronavirus-testing.html?referringSource=articleShare
92 www.nytimes.com/2020/08/29/health/Covid-obamacare-uninsured.html?referringSource=articleShare
93 www.nytimes.com/2020/08/30/health/predict-pandemic-usaid.html?referringSource=articleShare

01.09 Patients treated with antibody therapy saw 80% reduction in relative risk of death, study found.[94]

The Trump administration said it would not join a global effort to develop, manufacture and equitably distribute a coronavirus vaccine.[95]

02.09 Coronavirus symptoms can last much longer than initially thought, experts said.[96]

06.09– 12.09
(6,446,653 / 185,771)

Public Health Policies

08.09 Nine vaccine makers signed safety pledge in race for Covid-19 vaccine.[97]

09.09 US greatly undercounted coronavirus cases at the beginning of the pandemic, missing 90% of them – mostly because of a lack of testing, a new study found.

US to end limit on international arrivals from certain countries to 15 airports.[98]

10.09 Technology around developing Covid-19 vaccine may improve flu vaccine effectiveness, health expert said.

AstraZeneca denied news reports that suggested its coronavirus vaccine trial was stopped because of a case of transverse myelitis – a rare inflammatory condition of the spinal cord.[99]

11.09 Moderna increased minority numbers among volunteers in Covid-19 vaccine trial.[100]

12.09 Even children with no symptoms can spread Covid-19, CDC report showed.[101]

13.09– 19.09
(6,726,486 / 191,300)

Public Health Policies

14.09 Nearly 550,000 children in the US had been diagnosed with Covid-19 since the onset of the pandemic.[102]

15.09 Study found some evidence convalescent plasma helped coronavirus patients.[103]

16.09 CDC director said Covid-19 vaccine for general public likely to be available in 2021.

CDC study found coronavirus rarely killed children, but minorities at higher risk.[104]

20.09– 26.09
(7,037,157 / 196,561)

Public Health Policies

22.09 National Institutes of Health to expand Covid-19 convalescent plasma trials.[105]

23.09 More than 587,000 children in US had tested positive for Covid-19 since the beginning of the coronavirus pandemic earlier this year.[106]

24.09 Johnson & Johnson's coronavirus vaccine was fourth to begin Phase 3 trials in the US.[107]

26.09 Johnson and Johnson vaccine produced strong immune response, early results said.[108]

29.09– 03.10
(7,336,775 / 201,352)

Public Health Policies

29.09 Moderna coronavirus vaccine showed "acceptable safety" and immune response in older adults.[109]

Biotechnology company Regeneron released some early results of tests using its antibody cocktail in coronavirus patients, and said it seemed to reduce levels of the virus and improve symptoms in patients.[110]

30.09 The Bill & Melinda Gates Foundation signed a new joint agreement, along with 16 pharmaceutical companies, to commit to scaling up manufacturing of

94 www.cnn.com/world/live-news/coronavirus-pandemic-09-01-20-intl/index.html

95 www.washingtonpost.com/world/coronavirus-vaccine-trump/2020/09/01/b44b42be-e965-11ea-bf44-0d31c85838a5_story.html

96 www.cnn.com/world/live-news/coronavirus-pandemic-09-02-20-intl/h_0eb19f7f7298250b70d61760f550307d

97 www.cnn.com/world/live-news/coronavirus-pandemic-09-08-20-intl/index.html

98 www.cnn.com/world/live-news/coronavirus-pandemic-09-09-20-intl/index.html

99 www.cnn.com/world/live-news/coronavirus-pandemic-09-10-20-intl/index.html

100 www.cnn.com/world/live-news/coronavirus-pandemic-09-11-20-intl/index.html

101 www.cnn.com/world/live-news/coronavirus-pandemic-09-12-20-intl/index.html

102 www.cnn.com/world/live-news/coronavirus-pandemic-09-14-20-intl/index.html

103 www.cnn.com/world/live-news/coronavirus-pandemic-09-15-20-intl/index.html

104 www.cnn.com/world/live-news/coronavirus-pandemic-09-16-20-intl/index.html

105 www.cnn.com/world/live-news/coronavirus-pandemic-09-22-20-intl/index.html

106 www.cnn.com/world/live-news/coronavirus-pandemic-09-23-20-intl/index.html

107 www.cnn.com/world/live-news/coronavirus-pandemic-09-24-20-intl/index.html

108 www.cnn.com/world/live-news/coronavirus-pandemic-09-26-20-intl/index.html

109 www.cnn.com/world/live-news/coronavirus-pandemic-09-29-20-intl/index.html

110 www.cnn.com/2020/09/29/health/regeneron-covid-19-early-antibody-treatment-results/index.html

Covid-19 vaccines at "an unprecedented speed" and making sure that approved vaccines reach broad global distribution as early as possible.[111]

01.10 Hope Hicks, one of President Trump's top aides, tested positive for coronavirus.

The US Food and Drug Administration won't allow political pressure to interfere with the agency's decision-making on a potential Covid-19 vaccine, FDA Commissioner Dr. Stephen Hahn said.

Loss of smell and taste were a strong sign that someone was infected with Covid-19, according to new research published Thursday.[112]

02.10 Trump announced that he and his wife both tested positive for the coronavirus.[113]

Trump received a dose of an experimental antibody cocktail being developed by the drug maker Regeneron, in addition to several other drugs, including zinc, vitamin D and the generic version of the heartburn treatment Pepcid.[114]

Trump received cutting-edge combination treatment: remdesivir, an antiviral medication; dexamethasone, a steroid only recently shown to reduce death rates in severe cases; and an experimental cocktail of monoclonal antibodies, designed to turn back the virus shortly after infection.

About 80% of deaths in the U.S. from COVID-19 occurred in those 65 or older, according to CDC.[115]

03.10 A Rose Garden supreme court announcement packed with Covid-19 red flags.[116]

Little evidence that White House offered contact tracing, guidance to hundreds potentially exposed.[117]

04.10– 10.10 (7,672,220 / 206,135)

Public Health Policies

04.10 Trump's oxygen levels dropped and he was given dexamethasone, potentially signaling a 'severe' case of Covid-19.[118]

National Security Council required masks for staff members after the virus spread in the West Wing of the White House.[119]

06.10 FDA issued guidance on emergency use authorization for COVID-19 vaccines and development and licensure of vaccines to prevent COVID-19.[120]

07.10 34 White House staffers and other contacts had been infected with the coronavirus in recent days.[121]

08.10 A coronavirus outbreak centered at the White House exploded in the week since Trump said he tested positive on October 2. At least three dozen people so far were known to have contracted the virus, but the true number was unknown absent a running update from the White House.[122]

10.10 Trump held event at White House a week after coronavirus diagnosis.[123]

US saw highest number of daily coronavirus cases since August.[124]

Trump offered a lavish endorsement for a treatment he had received while hospitalized. Trump's insistence on getting an E.U.A. (emergency-use authorization) for the Regeneron antibodies was an extraordinary intervention into a process that was usually left to career scientists at the FDA.[125]

111 www.cnn.com/world/live-news/coronavirus-pandemic-09-30-20-intl/h_024eb86aee8f0af1fbf17228a4cb0c8b

112 www.cnn.com/world/live-news/coronavirus-pandemic-10-01-20-intl/index.html

113 www.cnn.com/2020/10/01/politics/hope-hicks-positive-coronavirus/index.html

114 www.nytimes.com/live/2020/10/02/world/covid-19-coronavirus#leaders-who-have-caught-the-virus-boris-johnson-jair-bolsonaro-and-now-trump

115 https://time.com/5895439/trump-covid-19-coronavirus-age/

116 www.statnews.com/2020/10/03/hugs-handshakes-and-few-masks-rose-garden-supreme-court-announcement-packed-with-covid19-red-flags/

117 www.washingtonpost.com/health/white-house-covid-contact-tracing/2020/10/03/2a6b8e2a-05a1-11eb-897d-3a6201d6643f_story.html

118 www.nytimes.com/live/2020/10/04/world/trump-covid-live-updates#trumps-oxygen-levels-dropped-and-he-was-given-dexamethasone-potentially-signaling-a-severe-case-of-covid-19

119 www.nytimes.com/live/2020/10/04/world/trump-covid-live-updates#the-national-security-council-now-requires-masks-for-staff-members

120 www.fda.gov/news-events/fda-brief/fda-brief-fda-issues-guidance-emergency-use-authorization-covid-19-vaccines

121 www.businessinsider.com/leaked-fema-report-34-people-trump-orbit-coronavirus-2020-10

122 https://nymag.com/intelligencer/article/trump-white-house-orbit-tested-positive-covid.html

123 www.nytimes.com/video/us/elections/100000007388931/trump-white-house-event-coronavirus.html

124 www.cnn.com/2020/10/10/health/us-coronavirus-saturday/index.html

125 www.nytimes.com/2020/10/10/health/covid-vaccine-treatment-fda-emergency.html?referringSource=articleShare

11.10– 17.10 *(8,056,170 / 210,997)*

Public Health Policies

12.10 Johnson & Johnson paused coronavirus vaccine trial due to "unexplained illness" in volunteer.

US experienced high coronavirus death rates during the pandemic, even when compared to other countries with high Covid-19 mortality, according to a study published Monday in the medical journal JAMA.

More than half of US states saw an increase in new Covid-19 cases, with five states -- Montana, New Mexico, North Carolina, Tennessee and Vermont -- reporting a jump of more than 50% in one week.[126]

13.10 Pfizer to start testing its vaccine in kids as young as 12. It would be the first coronavirus vaccine trial to include children in the US.

Eli Lilly paused trial of its monoclonal antibody to treat Covid-19 for safety reasons.

US saw 20% more deaths than expected this year, most due to Covid-19, research found.[127]

17.10 US recorded over 70,000 cases in one day for the first time since July.[128]

18.10– 24.10 *(8,522,418 / 216,652)*

Public Health Policies

20.10 FDA commissioner Stephen Hahn and a band of agency scientists stood up to the president's pressure to speed up emergency authorization of vaccines and treatments, after months of caving to pressures from the White House.[129]

Covid-19 patients were almost 19 times more likely to experience acute respiratory distress syndrome, twice as likely to need intensive care and five times more likely to die than flu patients, according to national Veterans Health Administration data from more than 9,000 patients with either Covid-19 or influenza.

Blood from the most severely ill Covid-19 patients may be the best for use in convalescent plasma therapy, according to a new study from Johns Hopkins University.[130]

21.10 CDC redefined close contact with someone with Covid-19 to include cumulative exposure. The new definition included exposures adding up to a total of 15 minutes spent six feet or closer to an infected person. Previously, the CDC defined a close contact as 15 minutes of continuous exposure to an infected individual.[131]

A third coronavirus surge took root in the U.S.[132]

22.10 FDA approved the antiviral drug Veklury (remdesivir) for use in adult and pediatric patients 12 years of age and older and weighing at least 40 kilograms (about 88 pounds) for the treatment of COVID-19 requiring hospitalization. Veklury was the first treatment for COVID-19 to receive FDA approval.[133]

23.10 US set a daily record of over 85,000 new cases on Friday, breaking a single-day record set on July 16 by more than 9,000 cases. Hospitalizations were up 40 percent and deaths were creeping up in several states.[134]

24.10 4 Pence aides tested positive for the Coronavirus.[135]

25.10–31.10 *(9,077,689 / 222,316)*

Public Health Policies

26.10 Eli Lilly said its antibody treatment did not work on hospitalized virus patients.[136]

27.10 Washington, Oregon and Nevada joined California's vaccine-review plan.[137]

30.10 US broke daily record with over 99,000 new cases as surge quickened.[138]

US surpassed 9 million coronavirus cases.

About 20% of grocery store workers had Covid-19, and most didn't have symptoms, study found.[139]

126 www.cnn.com/world/live-news/coronavirus-pandemic-10-12-20-intl/index.html

127 www.cnn.com/world/live-news/coronavirus-pandemic-10-13-20-intl/index.html

128 www.nytimes.com/live/2020/10/17/world/covid-coronavirus

129 www.nytimes.com/2020/10/20/health/covid-vaccines-fda-trump.html?referringSource=articleShare

130 www.cnn.com/world/live-news/coronavirus-pandemic-10-20-20-intl/index.html

131 www.cnn.com/world/live-news/coronavirus-pandemic-10-21-20-intl/index.html

132 www.nytimes.com/live/2020/10/20/world/covid-19-coronavirus-updates

133 www.fda.gov/news-events/press-announcements/fda-approves-first-treatment-covid-19

134 www.nytimes.com/live/2020/10/23/world/covid-19-coronavirus-updates

135 www.nytimes.com/live/2020/10/24/world/covid-19-coronavirus-updates

136 www.nytimes.com/live/2020/10/26/world/covid-19-coronavirus-updates

137 www.nytimes.com/live/2020/10/27/world/covid-19-coronavirus-updates

138 www.nytimes.com/live/2020/10/30/world/covid-19-coronavirus-updates

139 www.cnn.com/world/live-news/coronavirus-pandemic-10-30-20-intl/index.html